METHODS IN MOLECULAR BIOLOGY

Series Editor
John M. Walker
School of Life and Medical Sciences
University of Hertfordshire
Hatfield, Hertfordshire, UK

For further volumes:
http://www.springer.com/series/7651

For over 35 years, biological scientists have come to rely on the research protocols and methodologies in the critically acclaimed *Methods in Molecular Biology series.* The series was the first to introduce the step-by-step protocols approach that has become the standard in all biomedical protocol publishing. Each protocol is provided in readily-reproducible step-by-step fashion, opening with an introductory overview, a list of the materials and reagents needed to complete the experiment, and followed by a detailed procedure that is supported with a helpful notes section offering tips and tricks of the trade as well as troubleshooting advice. These hallmark features were introduced by series editor Dr. John Walker and constitute the key ingredient in each and every volume of the *Methods in Molecular Biology* series. Tested and trusted, comprehensive and reliable, all protocols from the series are indexed in PubMed.

Mitochondrial Gene Expression

Methods and Protocols

Edited by

Michal Minczuk

Medical Research Council Mitochondrial Biology Unit, University of Cambridge, Cambridge, UK

Joanna Rorbach

Division of Molecular Metabolism, Department of Medical Biochemistry and Biophysics, Karolinska Institutet, Solna, Sweden; Max Planck Institute Biology of Ageing - Karolinska Institutet Laboratory, Karolinska Institutet, Stockholm, Sweden

Humana Press

Editors
Michal Minczuk
Medical Research Council
Mitochondrial Biology Unit
University of Cambridge
Cambridge, UK

Joanna Rorbach
Division of Molecular Metabolism
Department of Medical Biochemistry and Biophysics
Karolinska Institutet
Solna, Sweden

Max Planck Institute Biology of Ageing - Karolinska
Institutet Laboratory
Karolinska Institutet
Stockholm, Sweden

ISSN 1064-3745 ISSN 1940-6029 (electronic)
Methods in Molecular Biology
ISBN 978-1-0716-0833-3 ISBN 978-1-0716-0834-0 (eBook)
https://doi.org/10.1007/978-1-0716-0834-0

This Humana imprint is published by the registered company Springer Science+Business Media, LLC, part of Springer Nature.
The registered company address is: 1 New York Plaza, New York, NY 10004, U.S.A.

Preface

From the discovery of the mitochondrial genome (mtDNA) in 1963 to the most recent cryo-EM model of the human mitochondrial ribosome, the scientific community has been gaining better understanding of how the expression of mtDNA is regulated. In mammals, this pathway is necessary for the synthesis of 13 proteins that are encoded by mtDNA and translated by a specialized, membrane-attached mitoribosome to form the catalytic core of the oxidative phosphorylation complexes. The significantly compacted mitochondrial genome, the limited set of uniquely structured transcripts, and the need for the proteins to be co-translationally inserted into the membrane and co-assembled with nuclear-encoded subunits have substantial consequences for the mitochondrial gene expression machinery. In fact, all stages of mitochondrial gene expression differ significantly from the analogous stages for bacterial pathways and eukaryotic pathways for nuclear-encoded genes.

Mitochondrial dysfunction has been implicated in many metabolic and degenerative diseases, cancer, and aging; therefore, a deeper understanding of the processes of mitochondrial gene expression has a great importance not only for uncovering fundamental aspects of organelle and cell function, but also for human disease.

This volume presents the recent advancements in the field of mitochondrial gene expression: from mtDNA replication and transcription, through translation to membrane insertion of the final protein products. Each chapter provides an overview of the particular process and a detailed protocol that can be applied to study this process by a variety of research laboratories. Investigators who are new to the field are offered an opportunity to access a focused collection of protocols for an entire range of methods, whereas investigators with previous experience in the field will find the volume useful for the perspective on complementary approaches and for the plethora of practical guidelines, often invaluable for a successful examination.

We are most grateful to the authors for their efforts in contributing to this volume and generous sharing of their protocols and technical expertise. We would like to also acknowledge the help of Delia-Denisa Dunka during the final stages of preparation of this volume.

Cambridge, UK
Solna, Sweden
Stockholm, Sweden

Michal Minczuk
Joanna Rorbach

Contents

Contributors

ALEXEY AMUNTS • *Science for Life Laboratory, Department of Biochemistry and Biophysics, Stockholm University, Solna, Sweden; Department of Medical Biochemistry and Biophysics, Karolinska Institutet, Stockholm, Sweden*

ILIAN ATANASSOV • *Proteomics Core Facility, Max Planck Institute for Biology of Ageing, Cologne, Germany*

ANTONI BARRIENTOS • *Department of Neurology, University of Miami Miller School of Medicine, Miami, FL, USA; Department of Biochemistry and Molecular Biology, University of Miami Miller School of Medicine, Miami, FL, USA*

ROLANDO BERLINGUER-PALMINI • *Newcastle University Bioimaging Unit, Newcastle University, Medical School, Newcastle Upon Tyne, UK*

LUKASZ S. BOROWSKI • *Institute of Biochemistry and Biophysics, Polish Academy of Sciences, Warsaw, Poland; Institute of Genetics and Biotechnology, Faculty of Biology, University of Warsaw, Warsaw, Poland*

IAN BRIERLEY • *Department of Pathology, University of Cambridge, Cambridge, UK*

ANDREAS CARLSTRÖM • *Department of Biochemistry and Biophysics, Stockholm University, Stockholm, Sweden*

AUSTIN CHOI • *Department of Neurology, University of Miami Miller School of Medicine, Miami, FL, USA*

ZOFIA M. CHRZANOWSKA-LIGHTOWLERS • *Wellcome Centre for Mitochondrial Research, Newcastle University Biosciences Institute, Newcastle University, Medical School, Newcastle Upon Tyne, UK*

BETTY CHUNG • *Department of Pathology, University of Cambridge, Cambridge, UK*

MIRIAM CIPULLO • *Division of Molecular Metabolism, Department of Medical Biochemistry and Biophysics, Karolinska Institutet, Solna, Sweden; Max Planck Institute Biology of Ageing—Karolinska Institutet Laboratory, Karolinska Institutet, Stockholm, Sweden*

ROBERT ENGLMEIER • *Cryo-Electron Microscopy, Bijvoet Center for Biomolecular Research, Utrecht University, Utrecht, The Netherlands*

MARIA FALKENBERG • *Department of Medical Biochemistry and Cell Biology, University of Gothenburg, Gothenburg, Sweden*

ERIKA FERNANDEZ-VIZARRA • *MRC Mitochondrial Biology Unit, University of Cambridge, Cambridge, UK*

ALEKSANDRA FILIPOVSKA • *Harry Perkins Institute of Medical Research, Nedlands, WA, Australia; ARC Centre of Excellence in Synthetic Biology, QEII Medical Centre, Nedlands, WA, Australia; Centre for Medical Research, The University of Western Australia, QEII Medical Centre, Nedlands, WA, Australia; Telethon Kids Institute, Northern Entrance, Perth Children's Hospital, Nedlands, WA, Australia; School of Molecular Sciences, The University of Western Australia, Crawley, WA, Australia*

FRIEDRICH FÖRSTER • *Cryo-Electron Microscopy, Bijvoet Center for Biomolecular Research, Utrecht University, Utrecht, The Netherlands*

CHRISTOPH FREYER • *Max Planck Institute Biology of Ageing—Karolinska Institutet Laboratory, Division of Molecular Metabolism, Department of Laboratory Medicine, Karolinska Institutet, Stockholm, Sweden; Department of Medical Biochemistry and*

Biophysics, Karolinska Institutet, Stockholm, Sweden; Centre for Inherited Metabolic Diseases, Karolinska University Hospital, Stockholm, Sweden

HEIKO GIESE • *Molecular Bioinformatics, Institute of Computer Science, Goethe-University, Frankfurt am Main, Germany*

ANDREW HAMILTON • *School of Medicine, Dentistry and Nursing, Glasgow University, Glasgow, UK*

JULIANA HEIDLER • *Functional Proteomics, ZBC, Goethe-University, Frankfurt am Main, Germany*

EDUARD HOFSETZ • *Cologne Excellence Cluster on Cellular Stress Responses in Aging-Associated Diseases (CECAD), University of Cologne, Cologne, Germany; Institute for Mitochondrial Diseases and Aging, Medical Faculty, University of Cologne, Cologne, Germany*

PITTER F. HUESGEN • *Central Institute for Engineering, Electronics and Analytics, ZEA-3, Forschungszentrum Jülich, Jülich, Germany*

YUMA ISHIGAMI • *Department of Chemistry and Biotechnology, Graduate School of Engineering, University of Tokyo, Tokyo, Japan*

MARITA ANNIKA ISOKALLIO • *Max Planck Institute for Biology of Ageing, Cologne, Germany*

ANNA V. KOTRYS • *Institute of Biochemistry and Biophysics, Polish Academy of Sciences, Warsaw, Poland*

IRINA KUZNETSOVA • *Harry Perkins Institute of Medical Research, Nedlands, WA, Australia; ARC Centre of Excellence in Synthetic Biology, QEII Medical Centre, Nedlands, WA, Australia; Centre for Medical Research, The University of Western Australia, QEII Medical Centre, Nedlands, WA, Australia*

ROBERT N. LIGHTOWLERS • *Wellcome Centre for Mitochondrial Research, Newcastle University Biosciences Institute, Newcastle University, Medical School, Newcastle Upon Tyne, UK*

JEAN-CLAUDE MARTINOU • *Department of Cell Biology, University of Geneva, Genève, Switzerland*

JANA MEISTERKNECHT • *Functional Proteomics, ZBC, Goethe-University, Frankfurt am Main, Germany*

MICHAL MINCZUK • *Medical Research Council Mitochondrial Biology Unit, University of Cambridge, Cambridge, UK*

RONIT NIR • *Department of Molecular Genetics, Weizmann Institute of Science, Rehovot, Israel*

MARTIN OTT • *Department of Biochemistry and Biophysics, Stockholm University, Stockholm, Sweden*

SARAH F. PEARCE • *Division of Molecular Metabolism, Department of Medical Biochemistry and Biophysics, Karolinska Institutet, Solna, Sweden; Max Planck Institute Biology of Ageing—Karolinska Institutet Laboratory, Karolinska Institutet, Stockholm, Sweden*

AARON FRASER PHILLIPS • *Department of Developmental Genetics, Skirball Institute of Biomolecular Medicine, New York University School of Medicine, New York, NY, USA*

YASMIN PROCTOR-KENT • *Wellcome Centre for Mitochondrial Research, Newcastle University Biosciences Institute, Newcastle University, Medical School, Newcastle Upon Tyne, UK*

OLIVER RACKHAM • *Harry Perkins Institute of Medical Research, Nedlands, WA, Australia; ARC Centre of Excellence in Synthetic Biology, QEII Medical Centre, Nedlands, WA, Australia; School of Pharmacy and Biomedical Sciences, Curtin University, Bentley, WA, Australia; Curtin Health Innovation Research Institute, Curtin University, Bentley, WA, Australia; Telethon Kids Institute, Northern Entrance, Perth Children's Hospital, Nedlands, WA, Australia*

JOANNA RORBACH • *Division of Molecular Metabolism, Department of Medical Biochemistry and Biophysics, Karolinska Institutet, Solna, Sweden; Max Planck Institute Biology of Ageing—Karolinska Institutet Laboratory, Karolinska Institutet, Stockholm, Sweden*

MAGDALENA RZEPKA • *Department of Biochemistry and Biophysics, Stockholm University, Stockholm, Sweden*

AZADEH SARFALLAH • *Department of Biochemistry & Molecular Biology, Sidney Kimmel Cancer Center, Thomas Jefferson University, Philadelphia, PA, USA*

ALDEMA SAS-CHEN • *Department of Molecular Genetics, Weizmann Institute of Science, Rehovot, Israel*

FLORIAN A. SCHOBER • *Department of Molecular Medicine and Surgery, Karolinska Institutet, Stockholm, Sweden; Max Planck Institute Biology of Ageing—Karolinska Institutet Laboratory, Division of Molecular Metabolism, Department of Laboratory Medicine, Karolinska Institutet, Stockholm, Sweden*

SCHRAGA SCHWARTZ • *Department of Molecular Genetics, Weizmann Institute of Science, Rehovot, Israel*

AGNEL SFEIR • *Department of Developmental Genetics, Skirball Institute of Biomolecular Medicine, New York University School of Medicine, New York, NY, USA*

VIVEK SINGH • *Science for Life Laboratory, Department of Biochemistry and Biophysics, Stockholm University, Solna, Sweden; Department of Medical Biochemistry and Biophysics, Karolinska Institutet, Stockholm, Sweden*

JOHANNES N. SPELBRINK • *Radboud Center for Mitochondrial Medicine, Department of Paediatrics, Radboudumc, Nijmegen, The Netherlands*

JAMES BRUCE STEWART • *Max Planck Institute for Biology of Ageing, Cologne, Germany*

TAKEO SUZUKI • *Department of Chemistry and Biotechnology, Graduate School of Engineering, University of Tokyo, Tokyo, Japan*

TSUTOMU SUZUKI • *Department of Chemistry and Biotechnology, Graduate School of Engineering, University of Tokyo, Tokyo, Japan*

ROMAN J. SZCZESNY • *Institute of Biochemistry and Biophysics, Polish Academy of Sciences, Warsaw, Poland*

DMITRY TEMIAKOV • *Department of Biochemistry & Molecular Biology, Sidney Kimmel Cancer Center, Thomas Jefferson University, Philadelphia, PA, USA*

MARCO TIGANO • *Department of Developmental Genetics, Skirball Institute of Biomolecular Medicine, New York University School of Medicine, New York, NY, USA*

ALEKSANDRA TRIFUNOVIC • *Cologne Excellence Cluster on Cellular Stress Responses in Aging-Associated Diseases (CECAD), University of Cologne, Cologne, Germany; Institute for Mitochondrial Diseases and Aging, Medical Faculty, University of Cologne, Cologne, Germany*

JAY P. UHLER • *Department of Medical Biochemistry and Cell Biology, University of Gothenburg, Gothenburg, Sweden*

SELMA L. VAN ESVELD • *Radboud Center for Mitochondrial Medicine & Center for Molecular and Biomolecular Informatics, Radboud Institute for Molecular Life Sciences, Radboudumc, Nijmegen, The Netherlands*

LINDSEY VAN HAUTE • *Medical Research Council Mitochondrial Biology Unit, University of Cambridge, Cambridge, UK*

ILKA WITTIG • *Functional Proteomics, ZBC, Goethe-University, Frankfurt am Main, Germany*

ANNA WREDENBERG • *Max Planck Institute Biology of Ageing—Karolinska Institutet Laboratory, Division of Molecular Metabolism, Department of Laboratory Medicine, Karolinska Institutet, Stockholm, Sweden; Department of Medical Biochemistry and Biophysics, Karolinska Institutet, Stockholm, Sweden; Centre for Inherited Metabolic Diseases, Karolinska University Hospital, Stockholm, Sweden*

VANESSA JOANNE XAVIER • *Department of Cell Biology, University of Geneva, Genève, Switzerland*

MASSIMO ZEVIANI • *MRC Mitochondrial Biology Unit, University of Cambridge, Cambridge, UK*

MATTHEW ZORKAU • *Wellcome Centre for Mitochondrial Research, Newcastle University Biosciences Institute, Newcastle University, Medical School, Newcastle Upon Tyne, UK*

Chapter 1

In Vitro Analysis of mtDNA Replication

Jay P. Uhler and Maria Falkenberg

Abstract

Human mitochondrial DNA is a small circular double-stranded molecule that is essential for cellular energy production. A specialized protein machinery replicates the mitochondrial genome, with DNA polymerase γ carrying out synthesis of both strands. According to the prevailing mitochondrial DNA replication model, the two strands are replicated asynchronously, with the leading heavy-strand initiating first, followed by the lagging light-strand. By using purified recombinant forms of the replication proteins and synthetic DNA templates, it is possible to reconstitute mitochondrial DNA replication in vitro. Here we provide details on how to differentially reconstitute replication of the leading- and lagging-strands.

Key words mtDNA, Replication, In vitro, Mitochondria, DNA polymerase

1 Introduction

Mitochondrial DNA (mtDNA) in humans is a 16.6 kb circular double-stranded molecule encoding several essential subunits of the oxidative phosphorylation system [1, 2]. The DNA is replicated by a dedicated mitochondrial replisome, many proteins of which share homology to phage or bacterial proteins. The core proteins of the mitochondrial replisome are DNA polymerase POLγ (one catalytic POLγA subunit and a dimer of the POLγB accessory subunit) [3], TWINKLE helicase [4], and the mitochondrial single-stranded DNA (ssDNA) binding protein, mtSSB [5].

MtDNA replication is initiated from two strand-specific origins, one for each strand—the origin of heavy (H)-strand DNA replication (OriH), and the origin of light (L)-strand DNA replication (OriL). According to the strand-displacement model of mtDNA replication, both strands are replicated asynchronously in a continuous and unidirectional manner [6]. Replication starts with synthesis of the leading H-strand from OriH. As the nascent H-strand is elongated, it displaces the parental H-strand into single-stranded form. After approximately 11 kb, the replisome passes OriL which adopts an activated stem-loop structure [6]. Lagging L-strand synthesis

Michal Minczuk and Joanna Rorbach (eds.), *Mitochondrial Gene Expression: Methods and Protocols*,
Methods in Molecular Biology, vol. 2192, https://doi.org/10.1007/978-1-0716-0834-0_1,

initiates and proceeds in the opposite direction using the displaced single-stranded H-strand as template. H- and L-strand DNA syntheses then progress continuously until two completed daughter molecules are formed.

In 2004, our lab was the first to reconstitute a functional minimal mitochondrial replisome in vitro, using purified human recombinant proteins and artificial DNA templates [7]. In the absence of any other proteins, POLγ can synthesize DNA products from a primed single-stranded template but it has difficulty bypassing secondary structures. For efficient DNA replication, the other core factors are required. For lagging-strand (mimicking mtDNA L-strand synthesis) replication on ssDNA, mtSSB is added to stimulate POLγ polymerase activity by removing secondary structures in the template strand. For leading-strand replication (mimicking mtDNA H-strand synthesis) on dsDNA, TWINKLE is required in the reaction to separate the DNA duplex.

With additional proteins and specifically designed templates, it is possible to reconstitute a system that approaches the complexity of the in vivo process. For example, the entire lagging-strand replication cycle, from initiation to termination, has been recently reconstituted in vitro [8]. Here we focus on reconstituting the elongation phase of mtDNA replication using circular templates. The main steps of the method are template preparation, followed by the replication reaction itself, gel electrophoresis, and visualization. We provide details on all these steps for both the lagging- and the leading-strand.

2 Materials

Prepare all solutions with ultrapure water and molecular grade reagents. Unless indicated otherwise, store reagents as instructed by the manufacturer.

2.1 DNA Template Preparation

1. pBluescript SK+ (pBS-SK+) (Stratagene) (*see* **Note 1**).
2. XL1-blue MRF′ supercompetent cells (Stratagene).
3. XL1-blue MRF′ supercompetent cells freshly transformed with pBS-SK+, on 2 × YT agar plates.
4. DNA oligonucleotide primers:
   (a) Lagging-strand primer: 5′-ATCTCAGCGATCTGTCTATTTCGTTCAT-3′ (*see* **Note 2**).
   (b) Leading-strand primer: 5′-42[T]ATCTCAGCGATCTGTCTATTTCTTCAT-3′ (*see* **Note 3**).
5. 2× YT medium: Add 16 g bacto tryptone, 10 g bacto yeast extract, and 5 g NaCl to 900 mL of water and dissolve. Adjust pH to 7.0 with 5N NaOH. Adjust volume to 1 L with water. Sterilize by autoclaving.

6. VCSM13 Interference-Resistant Helper Phage (Stratagene).
7. Ampicillin (100 mg/mL).
8. Kanamycin (50 mg/mL).
9. QIAprep® spin M13 kit (Qiagen).
10. PEG/NaCl solution (20%/2.5 M): Dissolve 100 g PEG-8000 (20% w/v) and 75 g NaCl (2.5 M) in 400 mL water by stirring. Bring to a final volume of 500 mL.
11. Annealing buffer (10×): 1 M NaCl, 0.2 M Tris–HCl, pH 7.5.
12. Illustra Microspin G-25 column (GE Healthcare).
13. T4 polynucleotide kinase (T4 PNK) (NEB).
14. 10× T4 PNK buffer (NEB).
15. EasyTides® adenosine 5′-triphosphate [γ-^{32}P] ([γ-^{32}P] ATP) (3000 Ci/mmol) (PerkinElmer).
16. T100 thermal cycler (BIO-RAD).
17. KOD Hot Start DNA Polymerase (NOVAGEN).
18. QIAquick PCR Purification Kit (QIAGEN).

2.2 DNA Replication Assays

1. Protein dilution buffer: 20 mM Tris–HCl, pH 7.5, 10% glycerol, 0.5 mM EDTA, 0.2 M NaCl, 1 mM DTT, 0.1 mg/mL BSA. Store at −20 °C in 1 mL aliquots.
2. Lagging-strand replication buffer: 25 mM Tris–HCl, pH 7.5, 10 mM $MgCl_2$, 0.1 mg/mL BSA, 1 mM DTT, 10 μM dATP, 10 μM dTTP, 10 μM dGTP, 10 μM dCTP (*see* **Notes 4** and **5**).
3. 6× Stop solution: 90 mM EDTA, 6% SDS, 30% glycerol, 0.25% (w/v) bromophenol blue. Store aliquots at 4 °C and keep a working aliquot at room temperature. Preheat to 37 °C just before use to be sure that the SDS is not precipitated.
4. Leading-strand replication buffer: 25 mM Tris–HCl, pH 7.5, 10 mM $MgCl_2$, 1 mM DTT, 100 μg/mL bovine serum albumin (BSA), 4 mM ATP, 10 μM dATP, 10 μM dGTP, 10 μM dTTP, 10 μM dCTP, and 2 μCi α-^{32}P dCTP (3000 Ci/mmol) (*see* **Notes 4** and **5**).
5. Leading-strand stop solution: 10 mM Tris–HCl, pH 7.5, 0.2 M NaCl, 1 mM EDTA and 0.1 mg/mL glycogen. Per 200 μL, add 1.6 μL of 20 mg/mL proteinase K (final 100 μg/mL) and 1.6 μL of 10% SDS (final 0.5%) right before use.
6. dATP, dTTP, dCTP, and dGTP (individual 100 mM solutions) (Invitrogen).
7. α-^{32}P dCTP (3000 Ci/mmol) (PerkinElmer).

8. Alkaline loading buffer: 18% (w/v) ficoll® 400, 300 mM NaOH, 60 mM EDTA, pH 8.0, 0.15% (w/v) bromocresol green, and 0.25% (w/v) xylene cyanol.
9. 95% Ethanol (EtOH).
10. 70% EtOH.
11. Purified recombinant POLγA [9].
12. Purified recombinant POLγB [9].
13. Purified recombinant mtSSB [9].
14. Purified recombinant TWINKLE (only needed for leading-strand reactions; [9]).

2.3 Gel Electrophoresis and Visualization

1. Agarose.
2. 10× Tris boric acid EDTA (TBE) buffer (Invitrogen).
3. 1× TBE running buffer—prepare fresh.
4. Alkaline running buffer: 50 mM NaOH, 1 mM EDTA—prepare fresh.
5. OWL A1 gel electrophoresis system (Thermo Scientific).
6. 1 kb DNA ladder (NEB), 5′-labeled with [γ-^{32}P] ATP using T4 PNK (NEB) according to the manufacturer's protocol.
7. GD 2000 slab gel dryer (Hoefer).
8. Razor blade.
9. Whatman® 3MM filter paper.
10. Multi-fold paper towels.
11. Cling film.
12. Super RX-N Medicine X-ray film (Fuji).
13. Film cassette with intensifying screen (Kodak).
14. X-ray film processor (Kodak X-OMAT 1000).
15. FLA-7000 Phosphorimaging system (Fujifilm) (*see* **Note 6**).

3 Methods

3.1 Template Preparation

The construction of the two strand-specific templates is illustrated in Fig. 1. In both cases, the circular template strand is obtained by isolating ssDNA from the pBS-SK+ vector. pBS-SK+ ssDNA is then combined with one of two primers, depending on which strand-specific template is needed. It is possible to construct other types of templates if desired (*see* **Note 7**).

3.1.1 ssDNA pBS-SK+ Isolation

1. Supplement 25 mL of 2× YT medium with 25 μL of 100 mg/mL ampicillin and 45 μL of VCSM13 helper phage. Distribute the medium into five culture flasks, 5 mL in each.

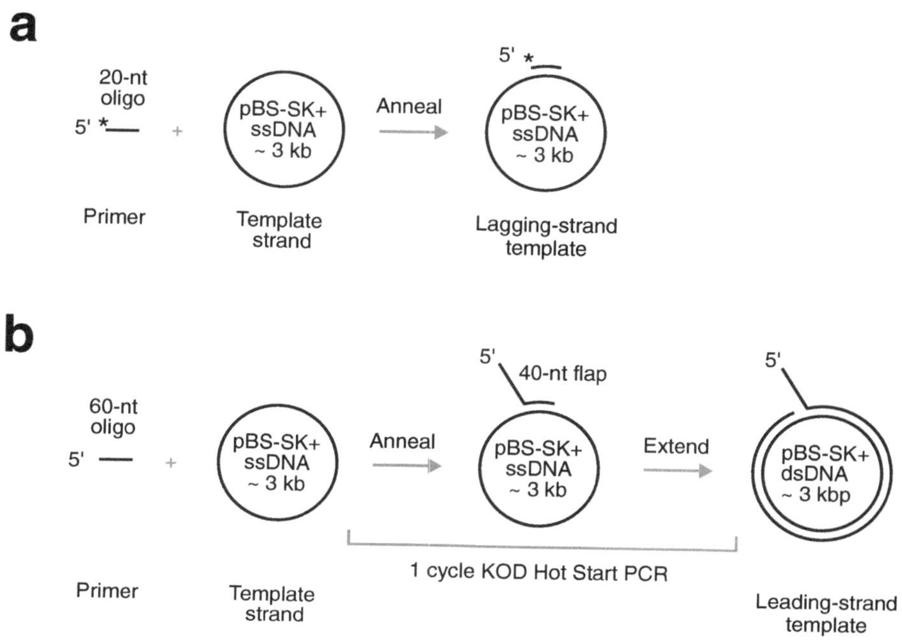

Fig. 1 Schematic of template construction. The same ssDNA isolated from pBS (pBS-SK+ ssDNA) is used as the template strand for both the leading- and lagging-strand templates. (**a**) For the lagging-strand template, pBS-SK+ ssDNA is annealed to a 20-nt primer oligonucleotide labeled on the 5′-end (asterisk). (**b**) For the leading-strand template, the pBS-SK+ ssDNA template strand is annealed to a 60-nt long flap-forming oligonucleotide (40-nt non-complementary, 20-nt complementary to pBS-SK+) for 1 cycle of PCR to produce a dsDNA template

2. Inoculate each with XL1-blue MRF′ cells freshly transformed with pBS-SK+ and grow at 37 °C in a shaking incubator. After 2 h, add 7 μL of 50 mg/mL kanamycin per 5 mL culture, and continue culturing overnight.
3. The next morning, pool the cultures together into a 50 mL conical centrifuge tube. Centrifuge at 25,000 × *g*, 10 min, 4 °C.
4. Transfer the upper 90% of supernatant into a new 50 mL Falcon tube, discard the rest.
5. Add 4.4 mL of PEG/NaCl solution to the recovered supernatant. Mix and incubate on ice, 2 h. Centrifuge 10,000 × *g*, 15 min, 4 °C. A white pellet should be visible.
6. Discard supernatant. Centrifuge 4000 × *g*, 3 min, 4 °C, and remove residual supernatant.
7. Resuspend pellet in 1 mL PBS. Add 10 μL MP buffer (QIAprep® spin M13 kit). Incubate samples 4 min, room temperature.
8. Follow the QIAprep® spin M13 kit handbook instructions from **steps 6** to **13**. In brief, transfer to two spin columns.

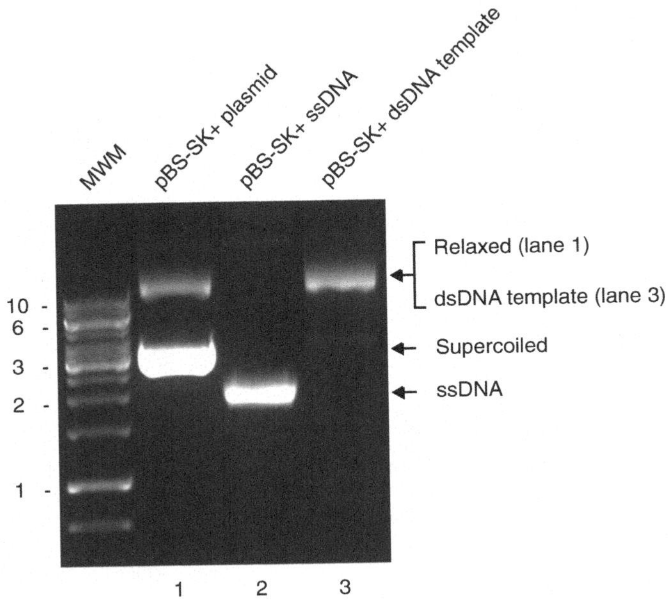

Fig. 2 Validation of template construction. Two steps of template preparation—(1) isolation of the pBS-SK+ ssDNA template strand (*see* Subheading 3.1.1), and (2) conversion to the leading-strand pBS-SK+ dsDNA template after PCR (*see* Subheading 3.1.4)—were verified by agarose gel electrophoresis (1% with 0.1 μg/mL ethidium bromide). The pBS-SK+ plasmid control (lane 1) shows both supercoiled and relaxed forms. pBS-SK+ ssDNA migrates slightly faster than the supercoiled pBS-SK+ plasmid (compare lanes 2 and 1). pBS-SK+ dsDNA template runs similarly to relaxed pBS-SK+ plasmid (compare lanes 3 and 1). MWM: molecular weight marker (GeneRuler™1 kb DNA ladder), sizes in kilobase, but will not give an accurate size reference (*see* **Note 12**)

Centrifuge at 8000 rpm (6,010 × *g*), 15 s. Discard flow-through. Add 0.7 mL PB buffer, centrifuge 8000 rpm (6,010 × *g*), 15 s. Discard flow-through. Add 0.7 mL PB buffer again, incubate 1 min, centrifuge 8000 rpm (6,010 × *g*), 15 s. Discard flow-through. Add 0.7 mL PE buffer, centrifuge 8000 rpm (6,010 × *g*). Discard flow-through and centrifuge 8000 rpm (6,010 × *g*), 15 s. Place column in a new 1.5 mL microcentrifuge tube. Add 100 μL EB buffer, incubate at room temperature, 10 min. Centrifuge 8000 rpm (6,010 × *g*), 30 s.

9. Store the eluted ssDNA at −20 °C (aliquot to avoid freeze thaw cycles).
10. Check purified ssDNA on a 1% agarose gel (TBE buffer). The pBS-SK+ plasmid can be run alongside as a comparison (Fig. 2, lanes 1 and 2).
11. Measure the concentration of the ssDNA and calculate the molarity (*see* **Note 8**).

3.1.2 Lagging-Strand Primer Labeling

1. Label the lagging-strand primer at the 5′-end by combining in the following order 1 μL (10 pmol) of the primer, 17.5 μL water, 2.5 μL of 1× T4 PNK buffer, 1 μL (10 U) of T4 PNK, and 3 μL (3000 Ci/mmol) of [γ-^{32}P] ATP in a 1.5 mL reaction tube.
2. Incubate at 37 °C for 60 min.
3. Transfer to 65 °C for 20 min to inactivate T4 PNK.
4. Remove unincorporated nucleotides using an illustra Microspin G-25 column according to the manufacturer's instructions.
5. Store the labeled oligonucleotide at −20 °C.

3.1.3 Lagging-Strand Template Preparation

1. The lagging-strand template consists of the pBS-SK+ ssDNA template strand annealed to the 5′-end labeled lagging-strand primer. To construct it, prepare an annealing reaction in a PCR tube using 1.5 pmol of labeled primer (Subheading 3.1.2) and 1 pmol of pBS-SK+ ssDNA (from Subheading 3.1.1) (*see* **Note 9**). Add water to a final volume of 45 μL.
2. Place the tube in a thermal cycler and heat the sample at 75 °C for 10 min, then add 5 μL of 10× annealing buffer.
3. Cool the sample from 75 °C to room temperature using a temperature drop of 0.5 °C/min.
4. Aliquot [please provide the volume] and keep at −20 °C.
5. Template yield will be 1 pmol per reaction, assuming 100% successful annealing (*see* **Note 10**). The template can be diluted to a suitable working concentration in water (10 nM is recommended) and stored at −20 °C.

3.1.4 Leading-Strand Template Preparation

1. The leading-strand template is pBS-SK+ dsDNA with a 5′-tail. To prepare it, pBS-SK+ ssDNA is converted to dsDNA in a second-strand synthesis reaction using KOD polymerase (required reagents supplied in KOD polymerase kit). Combine in a PCR tube 5 pmol of the leading-strand primer (unlabeled; labeling of the product occurs by α-^{32}P dCTP incorporation during the replication reaction), 2 pmol of the pBS-SK+ ssDNA (from Subheading 3.1.1), 5 μL 10× KOD buffer, 3 μL 25 mM $MgSO_4$, 5 μL 2 mM dNTPs, water up to 49 μL, and 1 μL KOD Hot Start polymerase.
2. Place reaction in a thermal cycler and perform 1 cycle of polymerization as follows: 95 °C 3 min, 50 °C 5 min, 70 °C 35 min.
3. Purify the DNA using the QIAquick PCR Purification Kit (this also removes the excess free primer oligonucleotide).

4. Check the yield of dsDNA by running 5 μL of the reaction on a 1% agarose gel (*see* **Note 11**) along with 5–10 μL ssDNA pBS-SK+ (*see* **Note 12**) for comparison (Fig. 2, lanes 1 and 3).
5. Measure the concentration and calculate the molarity of the template. The template can be diluted to a suitable working concentration in water (10 nM is recommended) and stored at −20 °C.

3.2 Lagging-Strand Replication Reaction

The lagging-strand reaction is carried out using the primed single-stranded circular template. POLγ will elongate the primer and progress around the template until reaching the 5′-end of the primer (Fig. 3). The reaction can be modified for increased

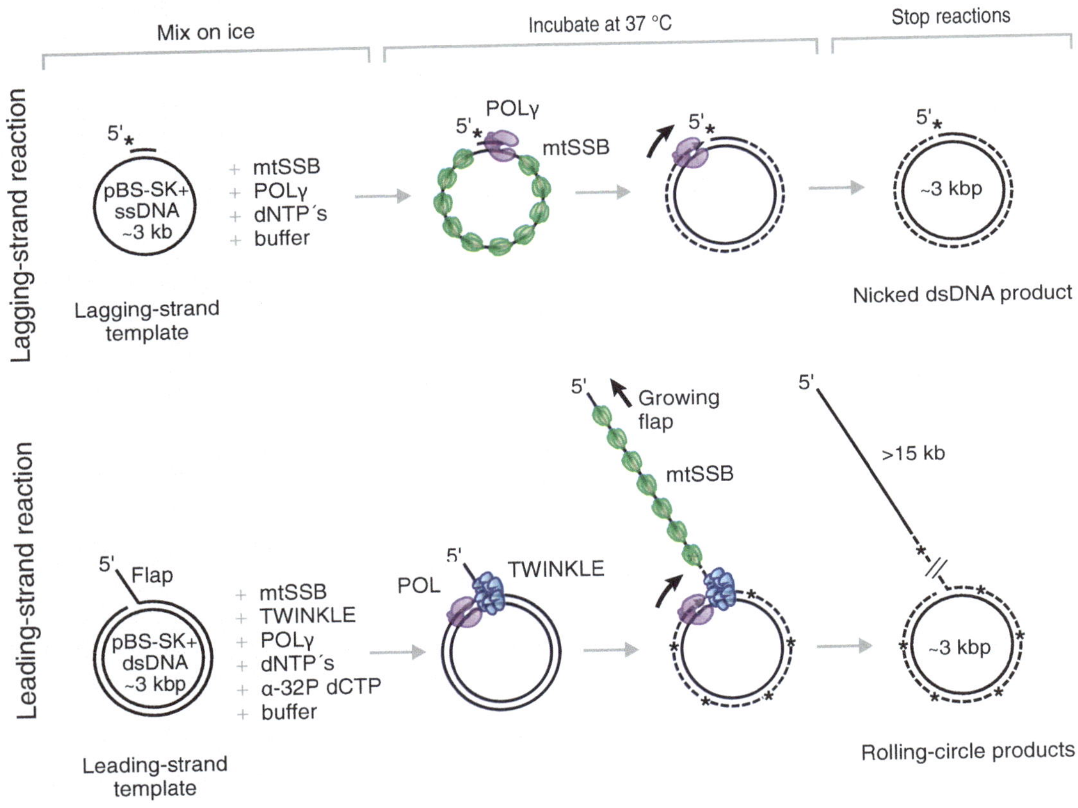

Fig. 3 Schematic of the DNA replication reactions. The key steps (mix, incubate, and stop) are indicated above the panels. For the lagging-strand replication reaction (top panel), the ssDNA template becomes coated with mtSSB and Polγ replicates the template from the primer to form a dsDNA product. For the leading-strand replication reaction (bottom panel), TWINKLE loads onto the 5′-flap, and Polγ initiates replication from the 3′-end of the nick. The replisome continues around the template in a rolling-circle mode of replication, first displacing the non-template strand, and then the newly synthesized DNA over many rounds. The newly synthetized ssDNA flap becomes coated with mtSSB. The products have extended 5′-tails of varying length (indicated with a double-slash), reaching over 15 kb in length. Asterisks—radiolabel; dashed line—nascent DNA; black curved arrows—direction of DNA synthesis

complexity if desired (*see* **Note 13**). Details on protein expression and purification are beyond the scope of this chapter and can be found elsewhere (see references in Subheading 2). His-tagged versions of mtSSB, POLγA and POLγB (all lacking the mitochondrial targeting sequence) can be expressed in insect cells using the baculovirus system and purified using affinity and ion exchange chromatography. Proteins are then diluted to the desired stock concentrations (please see below). The reaction is sensitive to salt, therefore note the salt concentration for each pooled protein stock (*see* **Note 14**). Proteins are usually aliquoted as 3–10 μL aliquots stored at −80 °C. The proteins are frozen in liquid nitrogen. Each aliquot is used only once. On average we keep the proteins with the following approximate concentrations: mtSSB, 10 μM, calculated as a tetramer; POLγA, 1 μM; POLγB, 1.5 μM, calculated as a dimer.

1. Perform everything on ice (a metal rack is recommended) unless stated otherwise. Add proteins last and thaw just before use.
2. Set up the desired number of reactions as per Table 1, depending on the type of experiment to be performed. In practice, several reactions are needed for an experiment and the reactions are carried out in several steps, as described in the following points. A master reaction mix without the proteins is prepared.
3. In the simplest case of a time course experiment, for example, the following five reactions are needed: 0, 5, 10, 15, and 30 min. Label five microcentrifuge tubes 1–5, add 4 μL of 6× stop buffer to each, and set aside at room temperature so that the SDS does not precipitate.
4. For mtSSB and template preincubation, in a separate tube, prepare a master reaction mixture for six reactions (five reactions plus one extra for pipetting errors) in the following order:
   (a) 87.6 μL water.
   (b) 3 μL Tris–HCl (pH 7.8) 1 M.
   (c) 1.2 μL $MgCl_2$ 1 M.
   (d) 1.2 μL DTT 100 mM.
   (e) 1.2 μL BSA 10 mg/mL.
   (f) 1.2 μL dGTP 10 mM.
   (g) 1.2 μL dATP 10 mM.
   (h) 1.2 μL dTTP 10 mM.
   (i) 1.2 μL dCTP 10 mM.
   (j) 6 μL of 10 nM lagging-strand template.
   (k) 3 μL of 10 μM mtSSB tetramer.
   (Total of 6 × 18 μL master reaction mixtures).

Table 1
Lagging-strand replication reaction

Component	Final concentration	Per 20 μL reaction
Water	–	14.6 μL
Tris–HCl pH 7.8 1 M	25 mM	0.5 μL
$MgCl_2$ 1 M	10 mM	0.2 μL
DTT 100 mM	1 mM	0.2 μL
BSA 10 mg/mL	100 μg/mL	0.2 μL
dGTP 10 mM	10 μM	0.2 μL
dATP 10 mM	10 μM	0.2 μL
dTTP 10 mM	10 μM	0.2 μL
dCTP 10 mM	10 μM	0.2 μL
Template 10 nM	0.5 nM	1 μL
mtSSB tetramer 10 μM	250 nM	0.5 μL
POLγA 150 nM	7.5 nM	1 μL
POLγB dimer 225 nM	11.25 nM	1 μL

The table shows a typical setup for a 20 μL reaction

Mix gently and leave on ice for 5–10 min so mtSSB can coat the ssDNA template.

5. For POLγA and POLγB preincubation, in a separate tube, combine POLγA and POLγB together as follows: 6 μL of 150 nM POLγA (diluted from 1 μM to 150 nM in protein dilution buffer) and 6 μL of 225 nM POLγB (diluted from 1.5 μM to 225 nM in protein dilution buffer). Mix gently and leave on ice for 5–10 min to allow the POLγ holoenzyme to form (*see* **Note 15**).
6. To start replication reactions, add the master mix reaction to the preincubated POLγ holoenzyme, mix gently. Immediately remove 20 μL and transfer to tube 1 (prepared with stop buffer in **step 2**), mix and set aside at room temperature. This is the "0" time point. Immediately place the remainder of the reaction in a heating block set at 37 °C and start the timer.
7. To stop reactions, at the 5 min time point, remove 20 μL from the reaction mixture and add to tube 2 containing stop solution. Mix and set aside at room temperature. Repeat this procedure at the 10 min, 20 min, and 30 min time points for tubes 3, 4, and 5 respectively. Samples can be stored at room temperature at this point (*see* **Note 16**).

3.3 Agarose Gel Electrophoresis

1. To prepare a 1% agarose gel, dissolve 2 g of agarose in 200 mL of 1× TBE buffer in a microwave. Allow agarose solution to cool to ~60 °C before pouring into a gel tray (dimensions 14 cm by 24 cm). Immediately insert a comb with medium well width (30 μL capacity per well) at one end of the gel. Allow gel to set.
2. Place the gel in a running tank and fill with 1× TBE buffer so that the gel is just covered. Fill wells with buffer if necessary.
3. Load half of each sample (12 μL of) per well (*see* **Note 17**). Optionally, a molecular weight marker can be included as a general guide, but note that it will not provide an accurate size reference (*see* **Note 18**).
4. Run the gel at room temperature at 130 V for 4 h, or until the bromophenol blue dye has run approximately 12 cm into the gel.

3.4 Visualization

1. Remove the gel from the tank, allow excess buffer to drain away. If desired, cut away the lower section of the gel (below the bromophenol blue) which contains the excess unannealed primer, and discard in the radioactivity waste.
2. Place the trimmed gel on top of two 3MM filter papers (precut to be slightly larger than the gel) by allowing the gel to slowly slide out of the tray directly onto the paper. Optionally, place five sheets of multi-paper towel on the gel dryer to decrease the radioactive background. On top of that, place the gel/3MM stack, gel side up. Cover the gel with cling film. Dry the gel at 60 °C for 2 h under vacuum (*see* **Note 19**).
3. Transfer the dried gel including the 3MM backing (throw the paper towels into the radioactive waste) to a cassette and expose to a phosphorimaging screen for 1 h, or up to overnight. Scan using a phosphorscanner and re-expose if necessary. Alternatively, expose to autoradiography film at −80 °C for 1 h to several days, depending on signal strength. Develop in an X-ray film processor, or by hand. A representative result of a lagging-strand time course is shown in Fig. 4a. Should reactions be suboptimal, it may be due to template quality, protein quality, NaCl, or sample storage issues (*see* **Note 20**).

3.5 Leading-Strand Replication Reaction

We use the rolling-circle (RC) mechanism to reconstitute leading-strand replication (Fig. 3). The template has a nick on the non-template strand that provides a 3′-end to serve as the primer for POLγ. The 5′-end of the nick forms a single-stranded flap on which TWINKLE can load. The non-template strand is displaced by TWINKLE, and grows in length as the replisome continues around the template. Once initiated, the replisome continues

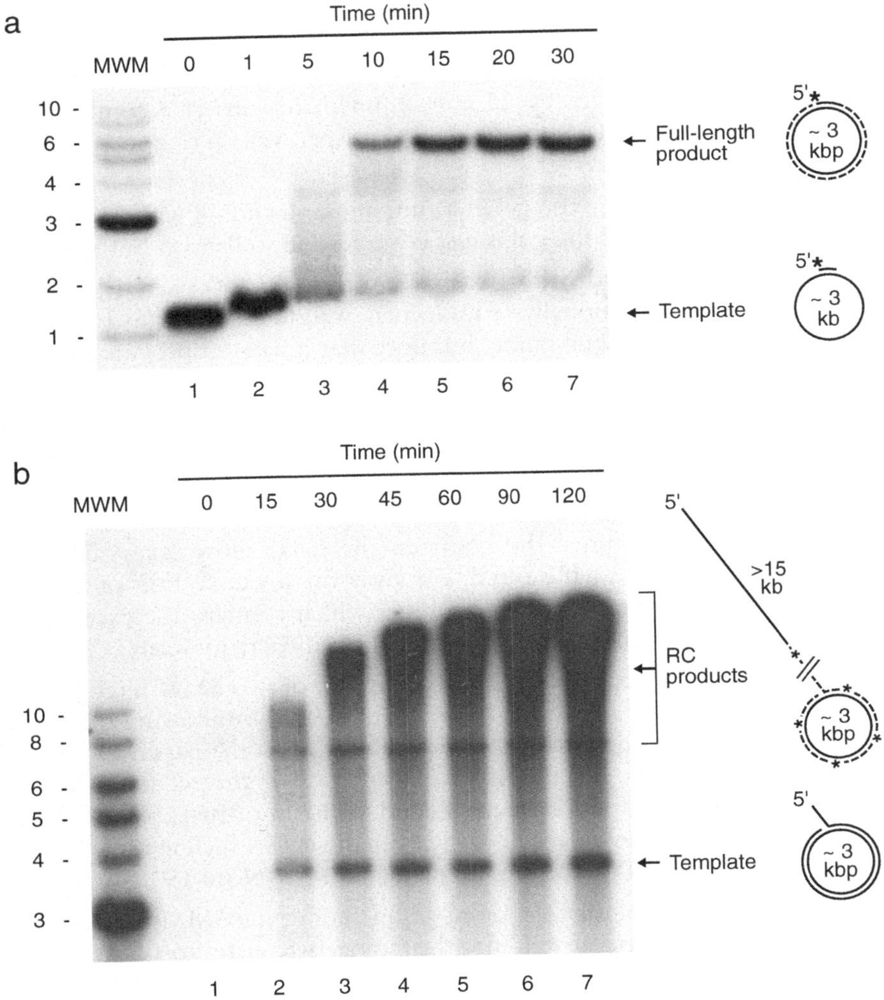

Fig. 4 Time course of DNA replication. (**a**) A time course of lagging-strand replication obtained from a dried gel. Schematics of the template and product are shown on the right (*see* Fig. 1a for details). DNA synthesis begins within the first minute (lane 2), and full-length products accumulate by 10 min (lane 4). Note that the molecular weight marker (MWM; sizes in kilobase) serves as a general reference and is not an accurate measure of sample size (*see* **Note 18**). (**b**) A time course of leading-strand replication. Molecular weight marker (MWM) sizes given in kilobase. Schematics of the template and rolling-circle (RC) products are shown on the right (*see* Fig. 1b for details). The RC products have extended 5′-tails of varying length, forming a smear. Note that some unutilized template also becomes labeled during the reaction because POLγ can idle at the nick: the 3′-end is degraded and resynthesized by POLγ, resulting in α-^{32}P dCTP incorporation

around the template like a rolling-circle mode of replication, displacing the newly synthesized strand in the process. The reaction can be modified for increased complexity (*see* **Note 21**).

Table 2
Leading-strand replication reaction

Component	Final concentration	Per 20 μL reaction
Water	–	12.5 μL
Tris–HCl pH 7.5, 1 M	25 mM	0.5 μL
$MgCl_2$ 1 M	10 mM	0.2 μL
DTT 100 mM	1 mM	0.2 μL
BSA 10 mg/mL	100 μg/mL	0.2 μL
ATP 100 mM	4 mM	0.8 μL
dGTP 10 mM	100 μM	0.2 μL
dATP 10 mM	100 μM	0.2 μL
dTTP 10 mM	100 μM	0.2 μL
dCTP 1 mM	10 μM	0.2 μL
α-^{32}P dCTP 3000 Ci/mmol	2 μCi	0.3 μL
Template 10 nM	0.5 nM	1 μL
POLγA 150 nM	7.5 nM	1 μL
POLγB dimer 225 nM	11.25 nM	1 μL
mtSSB tetramer 10 μM	250 nM	0.5 μL
Twinkle hexamer 100 nM	5 nM	1 μL

The table shows a typical setup for a 20 μL reaction

The leading-strand replication reaction uses the same proteins as for the lagging-strand, plus TWINKLE (*see* Subheading 3.2 for further information on proteins): mtSSB, 10 μM, calculated as a tetramer; POLγA, 1 μM; POLγB, 1.5 μM, calculated as a dimer; TWINKLE, 0.5 μM calculated as a hexamer (*see* **Notes 22** and **23**). As for the lagging-strand, the leading-strand replication reaction is sensitive to salt (*see* **Note 24**).

1. Perform everything on ice (a metal rack is recommended) unless stated otherwise. Add proteins last and thaw just before use.
2. Set up the desired number of reactions as per Table 2, depending on the type of experiment to be performed. In practice, several reactions are needed for an experiment and the reactions are carried out in several steps, as described in the following points. A master reaction mix without the proteins is prepared. Separately, the proteins are combined and then mixed with the master mix to start the reaction.

3. In the simplest case of a time course experiment for example, the following five reactions are needed: 0, 15, 30, 45, and 60 min. Label five microcentrifuge tubes 1–5 and place on ice. In each tube, add 200 μL of leading-strand stop solution, plus 1.6 μL of 20 mg/mL proteinase K (final 100 μg/mL), and 1.6 μL of 10% SDS (final 0.5%).
4. To prepare a master reaction mixture, in a separate tube, make a master mix for six reactions (five reactions plus one extra for pipetting errors) in the following order:
   (a) 75 μL water.
   (b) 3 μL of 1 M Tris–HCl pH 7.5.
   (c) 1.2 μL 1 M $MgCl_2$.
   (d) 1.2 μL of 100 mM DTT.
   (e) 1.2 μL 10 mg/mL BSA.
   (f) 4.8 μL 100 mM ATP.
   (g) 1.2 μL each of 10 mM dGTP, 10 mM dATP, 10 mM dTTP.
   (h) 1.2 μL of 1 mM dCTP.
   (i) 1.8 μL α-^{32}P dCTP.
   (j) 6 μL of 10 nM template.
   (Total of 6 × 16.5 μL master reaction mixtures)
   Mix and leave on ice.
5. For POLγA and POLγB preincubation, in a separate tube, combine POLγA and POLγB together to allow the POLγ holoenzyme to form: 6 μL of 150 nM POLγA (diluted from 1 μM to 150 nM in protein dilution buffer) and 6 μL of 225 nM POLγB dimer (diluted from 1.5 μM to 225 nM in protein dilution buffer). Leave on ice for 5–10 min (*see* **Note 15**).
6. Combine all the proteins together by adding 3 μL of 10 μM mtSSB and 6 μL of 0.1 μM TWINKLE (diluted from 0.5 to 0.1 μM in protein dilution buffer) to the tube containing POLγ.
7. To start reactions, transfer the entire master reaction mixture to the tube containing the proteins, mix gently. Immediately remove 20 μL and transfer to tube 1 (prepared with stop solution in **step 3**), mix and keep on ice. This is the "0" time point. Immediately place the remainder of the reaction in a 37 °C heating block and start the timer.
8. To stop reactions, at the 15 min time point, remove 20 μL from the reaction mixture and transfer to tube 2, mix gently, and keep on ice. Repeat this procedure at the 30 min, 45 min, and 60 min time points for samples 3, 4, and 5 respectively, until all time points are collected.

9. Incubate samples for 45 min at 42 °C. During this incubation, proteinase K degrades the proteins.
10. Precipitate the DNA by adding 0.6 mL of ice-cold 95% ethanol and incubating at −20 °C for 30 min to overnight. Centrifuge 20 min at maximum speed (~21,000 × *g*), 4 °C. Pour off the EtOH very carefully, because the pellet will not be visible. Add 400 μL of ice-cold 70% EtOH to wash the pellet. Centrifuge 5 min at maximum speed (~21,000 × *g*), 4 °C. Pour off the EtOH on a Kleenex tissue paper by turning the tube upside down and press it against the tissue. Vacuum dry at 45 °C for 5 min, or put in a heating block, 45 °C for 15 min. Resuspend the pellet in 20 μL water and 4 μL alkaline loading buffer (*see* **Notes 25** and **26**).

3.6 Alkaline Gel Electrophoresis

1. Prepare a 0.8% denaturing alkaline agarose gel (50 mM NaOH and 1 mM EDTA) by dissolving 1.6 g agarose in 200 mL water in a microwave. Allow to cool to ~60 °C. Add 2 mL of 5 M NaOH and 400 μL of 0.5 M EDTA to the agarose solution. Pour into a gel tray (dimensions 14 cm by 24 cm), immediately insert a comb (30 μL capacity per well) and allow to set. Submerge in alkaline running buffer within a gel tank.
2. Load half of each sample (12 μL) per well (*see* **Note 17**). In one well load 1 μL of labeled 1 kb DNA ladder (*see* **Note 27**). Run the gel at room temperature at 26 V for 16–24 h.

3.7 Visualization

1. Remove the gel from the tank, allow excess buffer to drain. With a razor blade cut away the lower section (about 6–8 cm counting from the bottom) of the gel, which contains any free α-^{32}P dCTP, and discard in the radioactivity waste.
2. For gel drying, *see* **step 2**, Subheading 3.4. The gel will turn yellow upon drying because of the NaOH.
3. Use phosphorimaging or autoradiography to visualize the dried gel as described in **step 3**, Subheading 3.4. The results of a typical leading-strand time course are shown in Fig. 4b. Should reactions be suboptimal, it may be due to template quality, protein quality, NaCl, or sample handling issues (*see* **Note 28**).

4 Notes

1. The + orientation allows recovery of sense strand ssDNA. If using pBS-SK-, antisense strand ssDNA is recovered and note that primers need to be designed accordingly. In principle, any desired sequences can be cloned into the pBS-SK vectors.

2. The primer anneals to position 2001–2028 in the pBS-SK+ vector. The optimal primer length for efficient replication initiation is 20–30 nt.
3. The 5′-42[T] sequence is non-complementary to the pBS-SK+ template strand, and forms a 5′ single-stranded flap needed for TWINKLE loading. The minimum flap length required for TWINKLE loading is 30 nt.
4. The end concentration of NaCl should be between 40 and 80 mM in the reaction for optimal activity. Normally, no extra salt is needed since it is added together with the proteins that are kept in high salt buffer.
5. The dNTP concentration can vary between 1 and 100 μM. High dNTP concentrations have a stimulatory effect on DNA synthesis.
6. Either X-ray film or phosphorimaging can be used for visualization. It is not necessary to have both systems available in the lab.
7. We have successfully used a range of templates, including oligo-based linear templates, oligo-based minicircles, as well as the larger pBS-SK-based templates described here. Take into account the template binding properties of the proteins when designing templates (*see* **Notes 2** and **3**). Also consider whether to label the template or the product. If products of varying size are expected (e.g., the leading-strand products), it is best to label the product so as not to dilute out the signal when separated on a gel. Products can be labeled by adding α-^{32}P dCTP in the replication reaction for example. If a product of defined size is expected (e.g., lagging-strand product), labeling the template is a good option. It is recommended to label the 5′-end of the primer. A 3′-end label is not recommended as it will be cleaved off by POLγ's 3′–5′ exonuclease activity.
8. Sometimes the ssDNA yield is low, in which case it is necessary to scale up by starting from 5 to 10 times more culture. Very weak bands high above the ssDNA band are sometimes visible in the gel, but these usually does not interfere with subsequent steps.
9. An excess of primer is added to promote 100% template formation. The presence of free primers in the template solution does not normally interfere with the replication reaction. However, the free primers can be removed after annealing using a Microspin S-200 HR column according to the manufacturer's instructions.
10. Annealing efficiency can be checked by 10% non-denaturing PAGE.

11. If second-strand synthesis was efficient, a clear dsDNA template band should be visible in the gel with few or no other bands. If other bands/smears are prominent, it is necessary to gel-purify the dsDNA band using a gel-purification kit.
12. As an additional control for dsDNA production, the pBS-SK+ plasmid nicked by a nicking enzyme (Nt.BspQI) can be run alongside as well. Note that a standard linear molecular weight marker can also be included, but it cannot be used for size determination of the circular sample DNA.
13. The lagging-strand reaction described here recapitulates the elongation phase of replication, but it can be easily adapted for increased functionality. For example, it is possible to couple it to replication initiation. For this the template is the same, except that it must contain the lagging-strand origin (OriL) sequence, and no pre-annealed primer oligonucleotide is required. Follow the standard reaction setup, and include POLRMT (100 fmol) and NTPs (250 μM) to enable de-novo priming. Another possibility is to couple the reaction to DNA ligation [9]. The standard lagging-strand template is suitable for this since the primer is 5′-end phosphorylated by the labeling reaction. Follow the standard reaction, and include 0.5 mM ATP and 15 nM mitochondrial DNA ligase 3. Note that it may be necessary to lengthen incubation times when increasing reaction complexity.
14. Salt in the replication reactions comes from the proteins or protein dilution buffer. The working salt range for the lagging-strand reaction is 40–80 mM NaCl. At 100 mM NaCl, the amount of full-length product decreases drastically. The reaction is completely inhibited at 160 mM NaCl. Also note that for some types of experiments it is necessary to correct for salt. In the case of a protein titration experiment, for example, make a serial dilution of the protein in dilution buffer and add the same total volume to each reaction so that the salt is kept constant.
15. POLγB is always added in excess to POLγA to be sure that the POLγ holoenzyme is formed.
16. Samples are best stored at room temperature, even for up to 1–2 weeks. We have found that freezing lagging-strand samples leads to dramatic loss of signal. Before gel loading, heat the samples at 37 °C for 5 min to ensure that the SDS is fully in solution.
17. Only half of each reaction is loaded, but if a stronger signal is needed, the whole reaction can be loaded. The advantage of loading half the reaction volume is that it is possible to rerun the gel if necessary.

18. The linear molecular weight marker cannot be used as a size reference for the circular sample DNA. If an exact size reference is desired, use nicked pBS-SK+ plasmid (*see* **Note 12**) labeled with [γ-^{32}P] ATP. Alternatively, run samples on a denaturing alkaline gel (*see* Subheading 3.6).
19. If gel drying is very slow, the temperature can be increased to 80 °C after 1 h. However, do not begin drying at 80 °C as this will cause the agarose to melt too fast and the lanes will be spread out.
20. There are several points to consider if lagging-strand reactions are suboptimal. The quality of the proteins used in the assays is critical. The purity of the protein should be more than 95% and free from contamination of nucleases and phosphatases. Poor template quality (*see* **Note 8**), too much NaCl in the reaction (*see* **Notes 4** and **14**), and improper storage/handling of samples (*see* **Note 16**) are also common sources of problems. Also see the relevant sections for further details.
21. With the RC reaction it is possible to couple leading-strand synthesis to lagging-strand synthesis [10]. This requires insertion of the OriL sequence into the template, and addition of POLRMT (100 fmol) and NTPs (250 μM) in the replication reaction. During the coupled RC reaction, the displaced non-template strand (containing OriL) emerges as the single-stranded lagging-strand template. Single-stranded OriL adopts the activated stem-loop structure which triggers POLRMT priming. To get specific initiation at OriL, optimal mtSSB concentrations need to be used. Start by performing an mtSSB concentration curve and use concentrations of mtSSB that can generate a lagging-strand product once per circle (please *see* [11] for details).
22. TWINKLE has a tendency to precipitate when freezing at higher concentrations.
23. TWINKLE can be a source of suboptimal assays. If necessary, perform a TWINKLE titration to determine the optimal concentration. This should be done routinely with every new batch of purified TWINKLE.
24. Salt in the replication reactions comes from the proteins or protein dilution buffer. The working salt range for the leading-strand reaction is 40–80 mM NaCl. At 100 mM NaCl, the amount of long leading-strand products decreases noticeably, and the reaction is completely inhibited at 120 mM NaCl. Also note that for some types of experiments, e.g., a protein titration, it is necessary to correct for salt (*see* **Note 14** for more details).
25. Samples can be stored at −20 °C at this point. Before loading, simply thaw them at room temperature.

26. DNA precipitation is time-consuming and there is the risk of losing pellets. This can be a cause for low signal. A rapid alternative is to stop each reaction by adding 1 μL of 0.5 M EDTA and 6 μL of alkaline loading buffer instead of stop solution. The samples are then ready for gel loading. It should be borne in mind that the free α-^{32}P dCTP will not be removed with the rapid method, and will cause higher background.
27. The 1 kb DNA ladder can be kept at −20 °C for several weeks. The half-time of the radioactivity is about 2 weeks, so simply load more if the ladder is older.
28. There are several possible sources of problems that could cause suboptimal leading-strand reactions. The main ones to consider are: poor template (*see* **Notes 8** and **11**) or protein quality (*see* **Note 20**), incorrect TWINKLE concentration (*see* **Note 23**), too much NaCl in the reaction (*see* **Notes 4** and **24**), and loss of pellet during ethanol precipitation (*see* **Note 26**). Also see the relevant sections for further details.

Acknowledgements

We thank lab members for their input, especially Majda Mehmedovic and Emily Hoberg for experimental demonstrations, and Örjan Persson, Yazh Muthukumar, and Hector Diaz for technical input. This work was supported by grants to MF from the Swedish Research Council; Swedish Cancer Foundation; European Research Council; the IngaBritt and Arne Lundberg Foundation; and the Knut and Alice Wallenberg Foundation.

References

1. Anderson S, Bankier AT, Barrell BG, de Bruijn MH, Coulson AR, Drouin J, Eperon IC, Nierlich DP, Roe BA, Sanger F, Schreier PH, Smith AJ, Staden R, Young IG (1981) Sequence and organization of the human mitochondrial genome. Nature 290(5806):457–465
2. Andrews RM, Kubacka I, Chinnery PF, Lightowlers RN, Turnbull DM, Howell N (1999) Reanalysis and revision of the Cambridge reference sequence for human mitochondrial DNA. Nat Genet 23(2):147. https://doi.org/10.1038/13779
3. Gray H, Wong TW (1992) Purification and identification of subunit structure of the human mitochondrial DNA polymerase. J Biol Chem 267(9):5835–5841
4. Spelbrink JN, Li FY, Tiranti V, Nikali K, Yuan QP, Tariq M, Wanrooij S, Garrido N, Comi G, Morandi L, Santoro L, Toscano A, Fabrizi GM, Somer H, Croxen R, Beeson D, Poulton J, Suomalainen A, Jacobs HT, Zeviani M, Larsson C (2001) Human mitochondrial DNA deletions associated with mutations in the gene encoding Twinkle, a phage T7 gene 4-like protein localized in mitochondria. Nat Genet 28(3):223–231. https://doi.org/10.1038/90058
5. Mignotte B, Barat M, Mounolou JC (1985) Characterization of a mitochondrial protein binding to single-stranded DNA. Nucleic Acids Res 13(5):1703–1716
6. Berk AJ, Clayton DA (1974) Mechanism of mitochondrial DNA replication in mouse L-cells: asynchronous replication of strands, segregation of circular daughter molecules, aspects of topology and turnover of an initiation sequence. J Mol Biol 86(4):801–824

7. Korhonen JA, Pham XH, Pellegrini M, Falkenberg M (2004) Reconstitution of a minimal mtDNA replisome in vitro. EMBO J 23 (12):2423–2429. https://doi.org/10.1038/sj.emboj.7600257
8. Al-Behadili A, Uhler JP, Berglund AK, Peter B, Doimo M, Reyes A, Wanrooij S, Zeviani M, Falkenberg M (2018) A two-nuclease pathway involving RNase H1 is required for primer removal at human mitochondrial OriL. Nucleic Acids Res 46:9471. https://doi.org/10.1093/nar/gky708
9. Macao B, Uhler JP, Siibak T, Zhu X, Shi Y, Sheng W, Olsson M, Stewart JB, Gustafsson CM, Falkenberg M (2015) The exonuclease activity of DNA polymerase gamma is required for ligation during mitochondrial DNA replication. Nat Commun 6:7303. https://doi.org/10.1038/ncomms8303
10. Wanrooij S, Fuste JM, Farge G, Shi Y, Gustafsson CM, Falkenberg M (2008) Human mitochondrial RNA polymerase primes lagging-strand DNA synthesis in vitro. Proc Natl Acad Sci U S A 105(32):11122–11127. https://doi.org/10.1073/pnas.0805399105
11. Miralles Fuste J, Shi Y, Wanrooij S, Zhu X, Jemt E, Persson O, Sabouri N, Gustafsson CM, Falkenberg M (2014) In vivo occupancy of mitochondrial single-stranded DNA binding protein supports the strand displacement mode of DNA replication. PLoS Genet 10(12): e1004832. https://doi.org/10.1371/journal.pgen.1004832

Chapter 2

In Vivo Analysis of mtDNA Replication at the Single Molecule Level and with High Resolution

Marco Tigano, Aaron Fraser Phillips, and Agnel Sfeir

Abstract

Single molecule analysis of replicating DNA (SMARD) is a powerful methodology that allows in vivo analysis of replicating DNA; identification of origins of replication, assessment of fork directionality, and measurement of replication fork speed. SMARD, which has been extensively used to study replication of nuclear DNA, involves incorporation of thymidine analogs to nascent DNA chains and their subsequent visualization through immune detection. Here, we adapt and fine-tune the SMARD technique to the specifics of human and mouse mitochondrial DNA. The mito-SMARD protocol allows researchers to gain in vivo insight into mitochondrial DNA (mtDNA) replication at the single molecule level and with high resolution.

Key words Mitochondrial DNA, mtDNA, mtDNA replication, DNA combing, DNA fibers, Thymidine analogs, mtDNA FISH

1 Introduction

Mitochondria are intracellular organelles that provide cellular energy in the form of ATP and impact a vast repertoire of cellular processes, including aging, apoptosis, and cancer. In humans, mitochondria maintain their own circular, 16.6 kb mitochondrial DNA (mtDNA). The small mitochondrial genome codes for proteins that are essential for respiration. All factors responsible for mtDNA replication and maintenance are encoded in the nuclear genome, translated within the cytosol, and imported into the mitochondria. The mechanism of mitochondrial DNA replication has been the subject of debate. In the early 1970s through the analysis of electron microscopy images, the lab of Jerome Vinograd and David Clayton proposed a unique mechanism of mtDNA replication, known as "the strand-displacement model" (SDM) [1, 2]. SDM hypothesizes an asynchronous mechanism that starts with the replication of the heavy mitochondrial DNA strand from

Michal Minczuk and Joanna Rorbach (eds.), *Mitochondrial Gene Expression: Methods and Protocols*, Methods in Molecular Biology, vol. 2192, https://doi.org/10.1007/978-1-0716-0834-0_2,

an origin termed O_H and proceeds unidirectionally. When ~two-thirds of the mtDNA molecule are replicated, a second origin, termed O_L, is exposed on the light strand and fires in the opposite direction to fully replicate the genome. In 2000, this model was challenged by Ian Holt's group with "the strand coupled model" (SCM), through the use of 2D gels to analyze mtDNA replication patterns [3]. The SCM hypothesize the synchronous replication of both mtDNA strands upon firing of O_H. This model was later amended with the RITOLs model, to include large RNA/DNA hybrids that cover the light strand before being replaced by DNA [4, 5].

The SDM is supported by microscopy techniques (such as electron microscopy and atomic force microscopy) which provides precise and detailed single molecule structural insights. On the other hand, the SCM/RITOLs is based on 2D-gel electrophoresis methods that examine bulk DNA molecules. In order to overcome the limitations of both approaches and provide a technique that enables in vivo and single molecule analysis of mtDNA replication, we successfully implemented the SMARD (Single Molecule Analysis of Replicated DNA) technique to the specifics of mitochondria. SMARD has been used in the past primarily to gain molecular insight into the mode of nuclear DNA replication [6–9]. The assay is based on the incorporation of thymidine analogs, 5-Chloro-2′-deoxyuridine (CldU) and 5-Iodo-2′-deoxyuridine (IdU) sequentially during DNA replication. Labeled DNA is then purified and stretched on the surface of glass coverslips coated with silane. Upon DNA combing, thymidine analogs are stained with specific antibodies that distinguish CldU from IdU. Using an epi-fluorescence microscope equipped with a 100× objective, or super resolution microscopy such as the DeltaVision OMX, it is possible to collect images of thousands of replicating mtDNA molecules. Analysis of the pattern of CldU and IdU incorporation provides insight into the directionality, speed, initiation, and termination of DNA replication.

We successfully applied SMARD to human and mouse mitochondria (to be termed mito-SMARD) [10]. Here, we present the full experimental methodology, divided in the following steps (Fig. 1a):

1. In vivo labeling of replicating mitochondrial DNA and crude mtDNA enrichment.
2. Preparation of aminosilane coated glass coverslips.
3. mtDNA linearization and purification from agarose plugs.
4. Molecular combing and fluorescent immunodetection.
5. mtDNA Fluorescent in situ Hybridization (FISH).

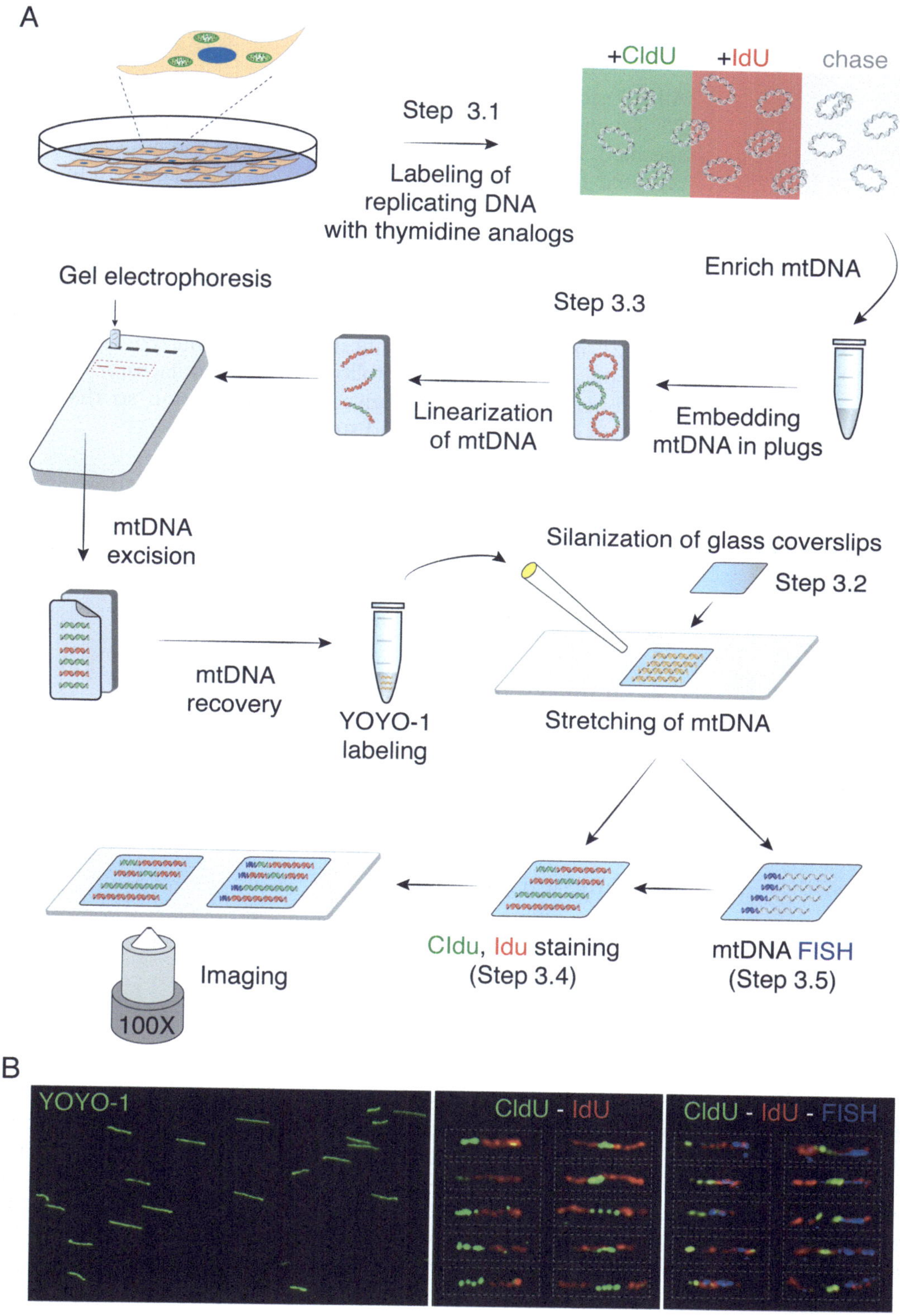

Fig. 1 Schematic of mito-SMARD procedure and expected results. (**a**) mito-SMARD graphical representation. All steps from labeling of replicating mtDNA with CldU and IdU (Subheading 3.1) to processing and

2 Materials

All solutions were prepared with ultrapure water (18 MΩ cm at 25 °C) and stored at the suggested temperatures unless otherwise specified. Frozen reagents should be aliquoted and not subjected to repeated freeze/thaw cycles. Unless a specific catalog number is provided, general providers can be used for purchasing reagents. The following list contains the reagents used throughout the entire experimental procedure. Thymidine analogs are light sensitive and stock solutions are prepared and stored in amber/brown microcentrifuge tubes. Antibodies are reconstituted and aliquoted following manufacturer specifications. Lyophilized fluorescent antibodies are reconstituted following the manufacturer specification, but with a final 50% glycerol concentration so that stock solutions can be aliquoted and stored at −20 °C.

2.1 In Vivo Labeling of Replicating Mitochondrial DNA and Crude mtDNA Enrichment

1. Culture Media appropriate for cellular line of interest.
2. 5-Iodo-2′-deoxyuridine (IdU; MP Biomedicals #2100357.2).
3. 5-Chloro-2′-deoxyuridine (CldU; MP Biomedicals #210547883).
4. Phosphate Buffered Saline 1× (PBS (1×)).
5. Trypsin.
6. QIAprep Spin Miniprep kit (Qiagen).

2.2 Preparation of Aminosilane Coated Glass Coverslips

1. (3-Aminopropyl) triethoxysilane (Sigma Aldrich).
2. High performance clover glasses (18 mm × 18 mm, $D = 0.17$, Zeiss).
3. Sodium dodecyl sulfate (SDS) 20%.
4. Nitric acid (HNO_3).
5. Hydrochloric acid (HCl) 37%.
6. Methanol.
7. Ethanol 95%.
8. 22 μm syringe filters.

Fig. 1 (continued) immunodetection (Subheadings 3.2 through 3.4 and 3.5) are indicated in the correct temporal order. mtDNA FISH (Subheading 3.5) is an additional, optional locus-specific detection step. (**b**) Examples of mtDNA molecules stained through mito-SMARD and imaged using a Nikon Eclipse Ti-V epifluorescence microscope equipped with 100×/1.45 NA objective. YOYO-1 staining, shown on the left, is used to assess the quality and concentration of the mtDNA sample before proceeding with immunodetection. Representative molecules replicating during the CldU (green) and IdU (red) pulses are shown on the right, with or without mtDNA FISH (blue)

2.3 mtDNA Linearization and Purification from Agarose Plugs

1. 2% agarose in PBS (1×).
2. Disposable plug molds (Biorad).
3. Restriction enzyme of choice and appropriate digestion buffer (1 mL for each sample).
4. Low melting point agarose (LMP, Thermo Fisher Scientific).
5. PBS (1×).
6. Ethidium bromide (EtBr).
7. TBE 0.5%: Tris–Borate–EDTA.
8. 1% Agarose in TBE 0.5%.
9. LMP Gel Digestion Buffer: TE pH 8, 100 mM NaCl, 0.1% 2-mercaptoethanol.

2.4 Molecular Combing and Fluorescent Immunodetection

1. Silanized coverslips.
2. Fisherbrand™ Superfrost™ Plus Microscope Slides (Fisher Scientific).
3. GELase (200 U, Epicentre Bio).
4. YOYO®-1 Iodide (491/509, Thermo Fisher Scientific).
5. 2-mercaptoethanol.
6. PBS (1×).
7. Post-Stretch Solution: Methanol 100%, 0.1% 2-mercaptoethanol.
8. Glutaraldehyde solution 25% (Sigma Aldrich).
9. Denaturation Buffer: 0.1N NaOH, 70% Ethanol, 0.1% 2-mercaptoethanol.
10. Fixation Buffer: 0.5% Glutaraldehyde in Denaturation Buffer.
11. Ethanol 70%, 95% and 100%.
12. IF Wash Buffer (0.03% Igepal CA-630 in PBS (1×)).
13. Staining Buffer: 3% BSA in PBS (1×).
14. Rat Anti BrdU (AbD Serotec).
15. Mouse Anti BrdU (BD Biosciences).
16. Alexa Fluor 488 Goat Anti-Rabbit IgG (H+L) (Thermo Fisher Scientific).
17. Alexa Fluor 568 Donkey Anti-Mouse IgG (Thermo Fisher Scientific).
18. Prolong gold antifade (Thermo Fisher Scientific).

2.5 mtDNA Fluorescent In Situ Hybridization (FISH)

Hybridization with FISH probes is a modification of the standard protocol for detection of CldU and IdU labels. The following components are required additionally:

1. 20× SSC buffer: 3 M NaCl, 0.3 M Sodium Citrate, pH 7.0.

2. High purity formamide.
3. 50% dextran sulfate solution.
4. DNA probes (*see* **Note 21**).
5. Probe Hybridization buffer (for 1 mL needed: 400 μL of high purity formamide, 100 μL of 20× SSC, 200 μL of 50% dextran sulfate solution, 100 ng of Probes, water to volume).
6. Biotinylated anti-streptavidin (Vector Labs).
7. Streptavidin-405 (Thermo Fisher Scientific).

3 Methods

All the procedures are carried out at room temperature unless otherwise stated. Steps involving thymidine analogs (CldU and IdU) or fluorophores should be carried out in a semi-dark environment.

3.1 In Vivo Labeling of Replicating Mitochondrial DNA and Crude mtDNA Enrichment

1. Human cells are split the day before pulsing with thymidine analogs, so that at collection they will not have exceed 80% confluency.
2. Cells are pulsed in standard media through sequential addition of 30 μM CldU or IdU followed by a chase phase of 2 h in standard media (*see* **Note 1**).
3. Wash cells with PBS (1×) and collect the sample through trypsinization.
4. Spin Cells for 5 min at 500 × *g* at RT and wash them once with PBS (1×) (*see* **Note 2**).
5. Purify an enriched fraction of mitochondrial DNA accordingly to Quispe-Tintaya et al. [11] using silica column and buffers from standard *E. coli* plasmid DNA preparation kit (QIAprep Spin Miniprep, *see* **Note 3**). Cells are resuspended in 300 μL of buffer P1, lysed with 300 μL of buffer P2 and the lysate is neutralized with 420 μL of buffer N3. Lysate is clarified by centrifugation for 10 min at maximum speed at RT and loaded on a silica column. The column is centrifuged for 1 min at maximum speed at RT. Bound DNA is washed once with 500 μL of buffer PB and twice with 750 μL of buffer PE. After the last wash spin for additional 2 min at maximum speed to dry ethanol residuals. During the process, warm an appropriate volume of elution buffer EB to 70 °C. Incubate the columns with 55 μL of warm EB for 5 min and finally elute with 1 min centrifugation at maximum speed. The eluate can be re-loaded on the column and spun again to increase the yield, or concentration can be increased by eluting in as little as 25 μL. DNA can be processed immediately or stored at −20 °C.

3.2 Preparation of Aminosilane Coated Glass Coverslips

1. A maximum of nine coverslips are placed in a glass petri dish.
2. Rinse with about 20 mL of pure water and add 2 mL of 20% SDS.
3. Shake at least 30 min at 70 rpm on an orbital shaker.
4. Pour off SDS and briefly rinse excess buffer with water. Add fresh water and shake coverslips for 30 min at 70 rpm. Repeat two additional washes with water.
5. Fill a glass petri dish with 20 mL of Nitric acid (HNO_3) and 10 mL of 37% HCl (*see* **Note 4**).
6. Holding a cover slip with plastic tweezers, drain excess water with a low flow of air and put the coverslip in the acid solution.
7. Gently seal each petri dish with parafilm. Incubate o/n in chemical hood.
8. Move coverslips using plastic tweezers to a new petri dish containing water. Wash for 5 min, shaking at 70 rpm. Repeat two additional washes. The acid solution can be discarded (*see* **Note 5**).
9. Wash coverslips with methanol for 5 min while shaking at 70 rpm.
10. Replace with 20 mL of fresh methanol. Add 400 μL of (3-aminopropyl) triethoxysilane dropwise while shaking at 70 rpm. Keep rotating for 1 h.
11. Wash coverslips with methanol for 5 min shaking at 70 rpm.
12. Wash coverslips with water for 5 min shaking at 70 rpm. Repeat washes 3 times.
13. Wash with 95% ethanol for 5 min shaking at 70 rpm shaking.
14. Dry coverslips with a low flow of air filtered through a 22 μm filter and store in a desiccator overnight before proceeding with DNA combing procedure (*see* **Note 6**).

3.3 mtDNA Linearization and Purification from Agarose Plugs

1. Prepare a 2% agarose solution in PBS (1×) and keep it at 55–60 °C.
2. Transfer 1 mL of 2% agarose in PBS (1×) to a microcentrifuge tube and place in a thermomixer set at 60 °C.
3. Incubate the 55 μL from **step 5** in Subheading 3.1 at 60 °C and mix at a 1:1 ratio with 2% agarose. Pipet few times up/down and cast 100 μL in a plug mold (*see* **Note 7**).
4. Incubate at RT for 5 min protected from light followed by 5 min at 4 °C.
5. Peel the bottom of the plug mold and using a tip slide the agarose plug into a brown microcentrifuge tube.
6. Wash the plug once with 1 mL of water for 30 min.

7. Wash the plug once with 500 μL of 1× restriction enzyme buffer of choice for 30 min.
8. Add 500 μL of fresh 1× restriction enzyme buffer. Add 10 μL of restriction enzyme of choice and resuspend it well by pipetting.
9. Incubate the plug o/n at 37 °C.
10. Cast a 1% low melting point agarose (LMP) gel in TBE 0.5% with regular amount of EtBr; use 1 mm combs matching the size of the plug mold. Let it solidify in the cold room protected from light.
11. Add some TBE 0.5% at the comb and carefully remove the comb from the gel.
12. Load each plug in the well along with a molecular marker of choice (*see* **Note 8**).
13. Seal the plugs with 1% regular agarose making sure that the plugs are totally sealed (*see* **Note 9**).
14. Run the gel for at least 2 h at 30–40 V in cold room.
15. Check for the mtDNA band running at 16.6 kb and cut the band as soon as it has run into the LMP gel (*see* **Note 10**).
16. Store the plug in an amber/brown microcentrifuge tube for few days at 4 °C, covered in LMP Gel Digestion Buffer and protected from light.
17. Cut 1 mm thick slices and put them in a new brown tube (*see* **Note 11**).
18. Cover the LMP agarose slices with 100 μL of LMP Gel Digestion Buffer.
19. Incubate the slices at 45 °C for 5 min protected from light.
20. Incubate the slices at 68 °C for 18 min protected from light.
21. Transfer one tube from 68 to 45 °C and equilibrate for 1 min. Add 3 μL of GELase 200 U in the tube to the top of the 100 μL. Avoid harsh mixing to preserve mtDNA integrity (*see* **Note 12**). Proceed in this way until all tubes have Gelase 200 U added.
22. Incubate for 2–3 h at 45 °C protected from light (*see* **Note 13**).
23. Add 10 μL of 2-mercaptoethanol on the top of the melted solutions without mixing.
24. Add 0.2 μL of YOYO®-1 Iodide on the top. Incubate o/n at RT protected from light.

3.4 Molecular Combing and Fluorescent Immunodetection

1. Prepare a superfrost slide by depositing two silanized coverslips along the long side of the slide (*see* **Note 14**).
2. Cut a 200 μL tip to make a wide mouth tip. Aspirate 8 μL of DNA from **step 24** in Subheading 3.3 and pipet it on the edge of the coverslip while avoiding touching the glass or the

coverslip. The DNA will be pulled by capillary action under the coverslip resulting into stretching of the mtDNA molecules (*see* **Note 15**).

3. Image the quality of the stretching by imaging YOYO®-1 with an epifluorescence microscope equipped with a 100× oil immersion objective (Fig. 1b and *see* **Note 16**).
4. Let the slide stand along a clean Kimwipe. Gently detach the coverslip to be processed with a razorblade letting the oil side to land on the wipe. Carefully wipe off imaging oil from the backside of the coverslip with a Kimwipe soaked in EtOH 70%.
5. Deposit the coverslip into a preassembled humid chamber and immediately cover with about 1 mL of Post-Stretch Solution until all combed coverslips have been removed and placed in the humidity chamber (*see* **Note 17**).
6. Remove the Post-Stretch solution and cover with Denaturation Buffer for exactly 9 min (*see* **Note 18**).
7. At the eighth minute of previous incubation prepare enough Fixation Buffer by adding glutaraldehyde 25% to Denaturation Buffer in order to achieve a final concentration of 0.5%.
8. Remove the Denaturation Buffer and cover with Fixation Buffer for 5 min.
9. Remove Fixation Buffer and rinse sequentially with EtOH 70%, EtOH 95%, and EtOH 100% for 2–3 min each (*see* **Note 19**).
10. Remove EtOH 100% and add Post-Stretch solution for at least 10 min.
11. Remove Post-Stretch solution and rinse with IF Wash Buffer until excess methanol is drained.
12. Block with Staining Buffer for 30 min.
13. Wash twice with IF Wash Buffer for 5 min each.
14. Incubate the coverslips for 1 h at room temperature with a mix of primary antibodies diluted in Staining Buffer as follow (80 μL per coverslip):
    (a) Rat Anti BrdU (reacts with CldU): 1:45.
    (b) Mouse Anti BrdU (reacts with IdU): 1:45.
15. Wash 3 times with IF Wash Buffer for 5 min each.
16. Incubate the coverslips for 1 h at room temperature with a mix of secondary antibodies diluted in Staining Buffer as follow (80 μL per coverslip):
    (a) Alexa Fluor 488 Goat Anti-Rabbit IgG: 1:250.
    (b) Alexa Fluor 568 Donkey Anti-Mouse IgG: 1:250.
17. Wash 3 times with IF Wash Buffer for 10 min each.

18. Wash once with PBS (1×).
19. Mount slides using Prolong gold antifade, allowing to dry overnight before sealing with nail polish (*see* **Note 20**).
20. Proceed with imaging (Fig. 1b) or store the mounted slides at −20 °C for up to several weeks.

3.5 mtDNA Fluorescent In Situ Hybridization (FISH)

mtDNA FISH allows visualization of specific sequences of mtDNA through biotynilated probes with co-staining of CldU and IdU (Fig. 1b and *see* **Note 21**). In order to perform mtDNA FISH, follow the experimental steps exactly as described in Subheading 3.4 until **step 12** (blocking). Substitute **steps 13** through **20** with the following steps:

13. Prepare Probe Hybridization solution.
14. Apply Enough Probe Hybridization solution to a clean glass slide (*see* **Note 22**).
15. Dry coverslips by allowing the excess methanol to run off the coverslip and wipe the non-DNA side with a Kimwipe.
16. Flip the coverslip on top of the Probe Hybridization solution so that the DNA side is in contact with the solution.
17. Allow to hybridize overnight in a humidity chamber at 37 °C.
18. Carefully remove the coverslips from the Probe Hybridization solution and place them in a humidity chamber with the DNA side up.
19. Wash the coverslips with 2× SSC for 3 min.
20. Wash with IF Wash Buffer for 3 min.
21. Wash with PBS (1×) for 3 min.
22. Block with Staining Buffer for 30 min.
23. Add Streptavidin-405 (1:250 dilution) in Staining Buffer for 30 min.
24. Wash twice with IF Wash Buffer for 5 min each.
25. Add biotinylated-anti-streptavidin (1:45 dilution) in Staining Buffer and incubate for 30 min.
26. Wash twice with IF Wash Buffer for 5 min each.
27. Add Streptavidin-405 (1:250 dilution) in Staining Buffer for 30 min.
28. Wash twice with IF Wash Buffer for 5 min each.
29. Incubate the coverslips for 1 h at room temperature with a mix of primary antibodies diluted in Staining Buffer as follow (80 μL per coverslip):
    (a) Biotinylated-anti-streptavidin: 1:45.
    (b) Rat Anti BrdU (reacts with CldU): 1:45.
    (c) Mouse Anti BrdU (reacts with IdU): 1:45.

30. Wash 3 times with IF Wash Buffer for 5 min each.
31. Incubate the coverslips for 1 h at room temperature with a mix of secondary antibodies diluted in Staining Buffer as follow (80 μL per coverslip):
    (a) Streptavidin-405: 1:250.
    (b) Alexa Fluor 488 Goat Anti-Rabbit IgG: 1:250.
    (c) Alexa Fluor 568 Donkey Anti-Mouse IgG: 1:250.
32. Wash 3 times with IF Wash Buffer for 10 min each.
33. Wash once with PBS (1×).
34. Mount slides using Prolong gold antifade, allowing to dry overnight before sealing with nail polish (*see* **Note 20**).
35. Proceed with imaging or store the mounted slides at −20 °C for up to several weeks.

4 Notes

1. The duration of CldU and IdU treatment should be tested and optimized for different cell lines and different types of analyses. For example, to discern the modes of mtDNA replication in human cells [10] optimal incubation times include 15 min of CldU followed by 90 min IdU and then, a 2-h chase period in which cells are incubated in standard medium lacking any thymidine analogs. Pulses of thymidine analogs are separated by two rapid washes with 1× PBS. Lastly, pulse-chase can be repeated an additional time to increase the number of labeled molecules.
2. Although fresh samples always guarantee better results, cellular pellets washed in PBS (1×) can be stored at −20 °C/−80 °C up to 1 month.
3. A crude mtDNA enriched fraction can be obtained by treating human/mouse cells as *E. coli* cultures carrying a plasmid of 16.6 kb. As recommended, we found that a total of 15 million cells can be easily processed at any given time, but cell line-specific optimization might be required. QIAprep Spin Miniprep kit was successfully used is suggested as first choice, but commercial kits based on alkaline precipitation lysis of bacterial cultures should also be compatible.
4. The HNO_3/HCl solution will turn orange. For all the measurements use a small glass beaker.
5. Prior to discarding the acid solution, it is necessary to neutralize pH with Sodium bicarbonate. Prepare a saturated solution of bicarbonate in water and pour it slowly in a glass tray where the HNO_3 dishes were previously placed. Keep adding bicarbonate solution and let it stand for at least 10 min.

6. Although pre-silanized coverslips are available commercially, the silanization procedure outlined above yields optimal results. The coverslips can be stored up to 4 days in a desiccator, protected from light.
7. While casting the plug, keep the tip at the edge of the mold to avoid formation of bubbles.
8. Loading the plugs into the wells of the gel might be challenging. Use a P200 pipette tip and a plastic inoculation loop to guide the plug when inserting it into the well.
9. Failure of sealing plugs will translate into a poor and slow running gel. Completely cover the well with agarose 1% and let it solidify before proceeding.
10. The mtDNA doesn't need to be resolved extensively. Once the DNA migrates out of the plug, the low melting point (LMP) gel can be processed. Excise a slice of the gel containing the mtDNA with a clean razor blade and move it on a piece of parafilm. The four external sides of the slice can be cut with a razor blade and set aside. Additional slices will be cut from the remaining portion of the processed slice.
11. Cutting very thin 1 mm slices of the gel is optimal to ensure complete solubilization of LMP agarose. According to the intensity of the 16.6 kb band in the gel, more than 1 mm slice can be processed at once. Alternatively, the original mtDNA enriched fraction can be eluted in smaller volumes from the miniprep column or more cells can be processed on one column. Determining the maximum number of cells per column is a critical step in order to ensure enough mtDNA in embedded in the agarose plug.
12. From this point it is imperative to avoid any mixing and/or pipetting to avoid mtDNA fragmentation. The incubation steps are long enough to allow diffusion of the reagents to the entire solution.
13. After the LMP agarose has been digested and the mtDNA released into solution, a small aliquot can be tested with a standard endpoint PCR to check for genomic DNA contamination.
14. Hold and move the coverslips with metal forceps and a razor-blade. Make sure the clean side of the coverslip (the upper one) will face the glass slide. Depositing the coverslips at the very border of the slide will help to recover them for IF processing.
15. As stated above, it is very important to avoid any kind of mixing of the sample to avoid shearing of mtDNA molecules. Aspirate the sample from the middle/bottom part of the tube.

16. If YOYO-1 imaging shows a good amount of stretched molecules (an intact full mtDNA molecule should be around 4–5 μm), the slides can be processed further. In the case that only few molecules are present, it's possible to follow suggestions from **Note 11** and process more slices/cells. For standard imagining a Nikon Eclipse Ti-V with 100×/1.45 NA objective was used. Alternatively, to image exact transitions between CldU/IdU, a super resolution DeltaVision OMX imaging station is more suitable.
17. Check frequently the level of the Post-Stretch solution because the methanol evaporates quickly. The coverslips can be incubated from 10 min to several hours, but drying should be avoided. Unless otherwise specified, the total volume of solutions is roughly estimated considering 1 mL per processed coverslip per solution.
18. Perform the denaturation and fixation steps with direct overhead lights turned off.
19. Overhead lights can be switched on during ethanol washes.
20. Although alternative mounting techniques can be used, we found these simple steps to perform very well and help minimize the number of bubbles in the mounting medium. Take a single coverslip with forceps holding the DNA side upward. Drain the liquid excess on a wipe and gently clean the remaining PBS (1×) from the non-DNA side with a Kimwipe. Placing the coverslip (DNA facing upward) at the edge of the bench, add 1–2 drops of Prolong Gold Antifade on the DNA side and gently deposit a clean superfrost microscope glass over it to mount it. Flip the slide on the bench and gently press the coverslip with a Kimwipe to drain excess mounting media.
21. Although other protocols can be used to obtain desired mtDNA biotinylated probes, optimization might be required. We used a MYtags protocol to generate a pool of 66 nt ssDNA biotinylated FISH probes covering 6.4 kb of mtDNA. ssDNA probes were generated following manufacturer instructions [12].
22. A hydrophobic marking pen is used to mark clean microscope slide with square boundaries slightly larger than the coverslip itself. The Probe Hybridization solution is applied to this region and the coverslips will be flipped on top of it.

Acknowledgement

Competing Interests: Agnel Sfeir is a cofounder and shareholder in Repare Therapeutics.

References

1. Clayton DA (1982) Replication of animal mitochondrial DNA. Cell 28(4):693–705
2. Kasamatsu H, Vinograd J (1973) Unidirectionality of replication in mouse mitochondrial DNA. Nat New Biol 241(108):103–105
3. Holt IJ, Lorimer HE, Jacobs HT (2000) Coupled leading- and lagging-strand synthesis of mammalian mitochondrial DNA. Cell 100 (5):515–524
4. Yang MY, Bowmaker M, Reyes A, Vergani L, Angeli P, Gringeri E, Jacobs HT, Holt IJ (2002) Biased incorporation of ribonucleotides on the mitochondrial L-strand accounts for apparent strand-asymmetric DNA replication. Cell 111(4):495–505
5. Yasukawa T, Reyes A, Cluett TJ, Yang MY, Bowmaker M, Jacobs HT, Holt IJ (2006) Replication of vertebrate mitochondrial DNA entails transient ribonucleotide incorporation throughout the lagging strand. EMBO J 25 (22):5358–5371. https://doi.org/10.1038/sj.emboj.7601392
6. Drosopoulos WC, Kosiyatrakul ST, Yan Z, Calderano SG, Schildkraut CL (2012) Human telomeres replicate using chromosome-specific, rather than universal, replication programs. J Cell Biol 197(2):253–266. https://doi.org/10.1083/jcb.201112083
7. Norio P, Kosiyatrakul S, Yang Q, Guan Z, Brown NM, Thomas S, Riblet R, Schildkraut CL (2005) Progressive activation of DNA replication initiation in large domains of the immunoglobulin heavy chain locus during B cell development. Mol Cell 20(4):575–587. https://doi.org/10.1016/j.molcel.2005.10.029
8. Norio P, Schildkraut CL (2001) Visualization of DNA replication on individual Epstein-Barr virus episomes. Science 294 (5550):2361–2364. https://doi.org/10.1126/science.1064603
9. Schultz SS, Desbordes SC, Du Z, Kosiyatrakul S, Lipchina I, Studer L, Schildkraut CL (2010) Single-molecule analysis reveals changes in the DNA replication program for the POU5F1 locus upon human embryonic stem cell differentiation. Mol Cell Biol 30(18):4521–4534. https://doi.org/10.1128/MCB.00380-10
10. Phillips AF, Millet AR, Tigano M, Dubois SM, Crimmins H, Babin L, Charpentier M, Piganeau M, Brunet E, Sfeir A (2017) Single-molecule analysis of mtDNA replication uncovers the basis of the common deletion. Mol Cell 65(3):527–538. e526. https://doi.org/10.1016/j.molcel.2016.12.014
11. Quispe-Tintaya W, White RR, Popov VN, Vijg J, Maslov AY (2013) Fast mitochondrial DNA isolation from mammalian cells for next-generation sequencing. BioTechniques 55 (3):133–136. https://doi.org/10.2144/000114077
12. Murgha YE, Rouillard JM, Gulari E (2014) Methods for the preparation of large quantities of complex single-stranded oligonucleotide libraries. PLoS One 9(4):e94752. https://doi.org/10.1371/journal.pone.0094752

Chapter 3

In Vitro Reconstitution of Human Mitochondrial Transcription

Azadeh Sarfallah and Dmitry Temiakov

Abstract

In vitro assay based on a reconstituted mitochondrial transcription system serves as a method of choice to probe the functional importance of proteins and their structural motifs. Here we describe protocols for transcription assays designed to probe activity of the human mitochondrial RNA polymerase and the transcription initiation complex using RNA–DNA scaffold and synthetic promoter templates.

Key words Mitochondrial transcription, RNAP, POLRTM, TFAM, TFB2M, Promoter

1 Introduction

Transcription of mitochondrial genes is driven by a single-subunit RNA polymerase (mtRNAP, or POLRMT), which makes near-genome size polycistronic transcripts [1]. To initiate transcription, mtRNAP is aided by two initiation factors—TFAM, which recruits polymerase to the promoter to form a pre-initiation complex, and TFB2M, which binds to mtRNAP-TFAM complex and assists in promoter melting and initiation of transcription [2]. Upon synthesis of ~15 nt-long transcript and TFB2M dissociation, mtRNAP clears the promoter, and recruits a transcription elongation factor, TEFM. Binding of TEFM renders mtRNAP processivity and prevents termination at the G-quadruplex terminator encoded in the CSB2 region of human mtDNA, downstream of the LSP promoter [3]. The first in vitro transcription assay based on purified protein components has been performed by Gustafsson's group and featured mtRNAP co-expressed with TFB2M using insect expression system [4]. The subsequent development of the assay involved reconstitution of the in vitro transcription system using highly purified recombinant forms of mtRNAP, TFAM, and TFB2M obtained by overexpression in *E. coli* cells, which allowed for mutagenesis of these proteins as well as for structural analysis of

Michal Minczuk and Joanna Rorbach (eds.), *Mitochondrial Gene Expression: Methods and Protocols*, Methods in Molecular Biology, vol. 2192, https://doi.org/10.1007/978-1-0716-0834-0_3,

transcription complex [5, 6]. Finally, the cross-linking and in vitro transcription experiments revealed the boundaries of the upstream promoter region in human mtDNA, completing development of an efficient initiation assay [2]. Here, we describe protocols that allowed us to probe the catalytic activity of human mtRNAP using primer extension assay and analyze the initiation stage of mitochondrial transcription at the conditions optimized for efficient RNA synthesis.

2 Materials

2.1 Reagents

All reagents were of a molecular biology grade. Ultrapure water was used to prepare all solutions, which were stored at −20 °C unless mentioned otherwise.

2.2 Proteins

The following variants of transcription proteins were used in the assay:

MtRNAP—His6-Δ119 mtRNAP (deletion of the first 119 residues to improve expression and solubility), purified using Ni-NTA chromatography, heparin-sepharose and size-exclusion chromatography as previously described [5].

TFAM—His6-Δ42 TFAM (a mature form of TFAM, deletion of the MTS, residues 1–42) purified using Ni-NTA chromatography, heparin-sepharose and size-exclusion chromatography as previously described [7].

TFB2M—His6-Δ20 TFB2M (a mature form of TFB2M, deletion of the predicted MTS, residues 1–20) purified using Ni-NTA chromatography, heparin-sepharose, and size-exclusion chromatography as previously described [5].

2.3 DNA and RNA Oligonucleotides

1. RNA primer for the RNA-DNA scaffold, mtRNA14 (5′–3′): AGUCUGCGGCGCGC
2. Template DNA strand for the RNA-DNA scaffold, mtTS2 (5′–3′): CGTCTGGCGTGCGCGCCGCTACCCCATG
3. Non-template DNA strand for the RNA-DNA scaffold, mtNT2 (5′–3′): CATGGGGTAATTATTTCGACGCCAG ACG
4. Light Strand Promoter (LSP) template DNA strand, TS-40LSP (5′–3′): GGCCCACAAATTTTATCTTTTGGC GGTATGCACTTTTAACAGTCACCCCCCAACTAACAC
5. LSP non-template DNA strand, NT-40LSP (5′–3′): GTGTTAGTTGGGGGGTGACTGTTAAAAGTGCA TACCGCCAAAAGATAAAATTTGTGGGCC

All oligonucleotides were dissolved in ultrapure water at 100 μM concentration and stored at −20 °C.

2.4 RNAP Catalytic Activity and Transcription Initiation Assays

1. T4 Polynucleotide Kinase (T4 PNK, 10,000 units/mL).
2. T4 PNK buffer (10×).
3. [γ-^{32}P] ATP (3000 Ci/mmol).
4. Duplex buffer (10×) [8]: 300 mM HEPES pH 7.5, 1 M Potassium Acetate. Store at room temperature.
5. Transcription buffer (10×): 200 mM Tris-HCl pH 7.9, 100 mM $MgCl_2$, 250 mM NaCl, 200 mM β-Mercaptoethanol, 1 mg/mL BSA (*see* **Notes 1** and **2**).
6. Ribonucleotide mix (10×): 3 mM ATP, 3 mM CTP, 3 mM GTP, and 0.5 mM UTP.
7. [α-^{32}P] UTP (800 Ci/mmol, 10 mCi/mL).
8. Transcription stop buffer (2×): 95% (v/v) formamide, 5 mM EDTA (pH 8.0), 0.025% SDS, 0.025% bromophenol blue, and 0.025% xylene blue.

2.5 Denaturing Polyacrylamide Gel Electrophoresis

1. Tris-Borate-EDTA (TBE) buffer (5×): 0.45 M Tris-base, 0.45 M Boric acid, and 0.01 M EDTA (*see* **Note 3**). Store at room temperature.
2. Acrylamide/Bis 19:1, 40% (w/v) solution: Store at 4 °C.
3. Ammonium persulfate (APS): 20% solution in water. Store at 4 °C.
4. *N*,*N*,*N*′,*N*′-tetramethylethane-1,2-diamine (TEMED). Store at 4 °C.
5. Urea.
6. Running Buffer: TBE (1×).
7. S2 sequencing gel electrophoresis system.

3 Methods

3.1 RNAP Catalytic Activity Assay

1. Label RNA primer by mixing 2.5 μL of mtRNA14 (100 μM), 0.5 μL of 10× T4 PNK buffer, 0.5 μL of T4 PNK (10,000 units/mL), 1 μL of [γ-^{32}P] ATP (3000 Ci/mmol), and 0.5 μL of water in 5 μL reaction and incubate the reaction for 30 min at 37 °C.
2. After the incubation, add to the reaction mix above 2.5 μL of the non-template DNA (mtNT2, 100 μM), 2.5 μL of the template DNA (mtTS2, 100 μM), and 15 μL of water in 25 μL reaction.
3. Anneal the RNA-DNA scaffold (10 μM) by heating the reaction mix for 7 min at 85 °C and cooling it down in a stepwise manner (1 °C/min) for 1 h using a thermocycler.

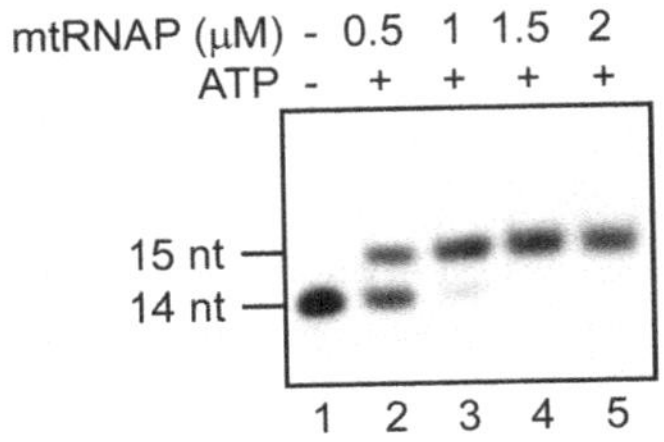

Fig. 1 RNAP catalytic activity assay. RNA-DNA scaffold (1 μM) (lane 1) was incubated with different concentrations of mtRNAP and extended with ATP (lanes 2–5) as described in the Methods. At the equimolar ratio of the RNA-DNA scaffold and mtRNAP, nearly 100% of the RNA is extended, indicating high catalytic activity of polymerase

4. For primer extension, mix 1 μL of the 10× transcription buffer, 1 μL of the labeled RNA-DNA scaffold (10 μM), 1 μL of Δ119-mtRNAP (10 μM), and 6 μL of water in 9 μL reaction (*see* **Note 4**).
5. Incubate the reaction mix for 5 min at room temperature.
6. To extend the RNA primer, add to the reaction 1 μL of ATP (1 mM) and incubate for 2 min at room temperature.
7. Stop the reaction by adding 10 μL of 2× transcription stop buffer and heat-inactivate the sample for 2 min at 95 °C.
8. Resolve the products of the reaction by electrophoresis using 20% polyacrylamide gel containing 7 M urea.
9. Expose the gel to the PhosphoImager screen and scan using Typhoon scanner (Fig. 1).

3.2 Transcription Initiation Assay

1. Prepare the double-stranded DNA template (5 μM) by mixing 2 μL of 10× duplex buffer, 1 μL of the NT-40LSP (100 μM), 1 μL of the TS-40LSP (100 μM), and 16 μL of water in 20 μL reaction in a PCR tube.
2. Anneal the templates by heating them for 7 min to 95 °C and cool down stepwise (1 °C/min) for 1 h to 25 °C using the thermocycler. Upon annealing, dilute the templates to 0.5 μM concentration using ultrapure water.
3. To perform the transcription initiation assay, combine 6.2 μL of water, 1 μL of transcription buffer (10×), 1 μL of the 10× ribonucleotide mix, 0.1 μL of [α-^{32}P]-UTP (800 Ci/mmol), 0.3 μL of Δ119-mtRNAP (5 μM), 0.3 μL of Δ20-TFB2M (5 μM), and 0.1 μL of Δ42-TFAM (5 μM) in 9 μL reaction mix (*see* **Note 5**).
4. Initiate transcription reaction by addition of 1 μL of the annealed DNA template (0.5 μM) to the reaction mix.
5. Incubate the reaction mix for 45 min at 36 °C (*see* **Note 6**).

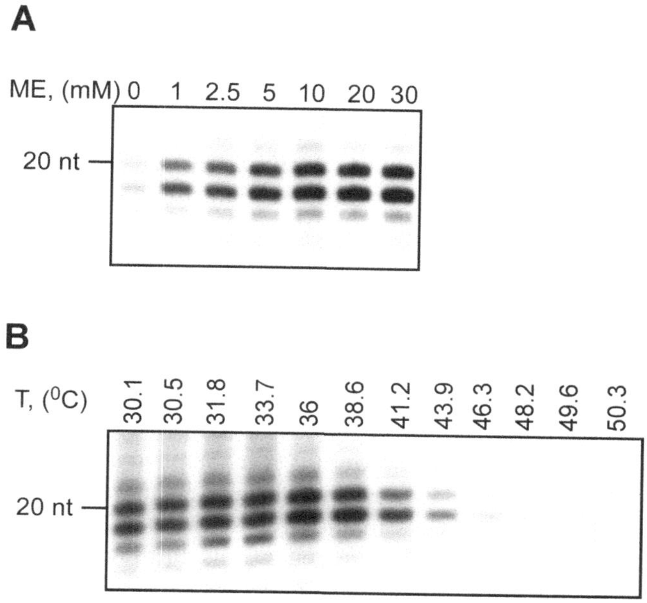

Fig. 2 Optimal conditions for in vitro transcription initiation assay. (**a**) The presence of a reducing agent is critical for efficient transcription initiation. Transcription reaction were performed in the presence of β-mercaptoethanol (ME) at the concentrations indicated. (**b**) Transcription initiation assay to determine the optimal temperature of the reaction. Transcription reactions were incubated at the temperatures indicated in a gradient thermocycler

6. Stop the reaction by adding 10 μL of the 2× transcription stop buffer and heating for 5 min at 95 °C.
7. Resolve the products of the reaction by electrophoresis using 20% polyacrylamide gel containing 7 M Urea (prepare the gel as described in Subheading 3.3).
8. Expose the gel to the PhosphoImager screen and scan using Typhoon scanner (Fig. 2).

3.3 Denaturing Polyacrylamide Gel Electrophoresis

1. To prepare 20% polyacrylamide gel, mix 21 g of urea (final concentration 7 M), 10 mL of TBE buffer (5×), and 25 mL of Acrylamide/Bis 19:1, 40% (w/v) solution. The final volume of the solution will be 50 mL.
2. Heat the mixture in a microwave for 30 s to dissolve urea.
3. Cool down the gel solution to prevent sudden polymerization.
4. Degas the gel solution using water bath sonicator for 5 min.
5. Assemble the glass plates.
6. Add 190 μL of 20% APS and 14 μL of TEMED.
7. Pour the gel in between the assembled glass plates and let it to polymerize at room temperature for at least 2 h.

4 Notes

1. The presence of a reducing agent is critical for efficient transcription initiation using human mitochondrial polymerase and transcription factors. The optimal β-mercaptoethanol concentration was determined to be 20 mM in transcription initiation assay (Fig. 2a).
2. As the backbone of the DNA has negatively charged phosphates, the two DNA strands repel each other, leading to locally single stranded regions. These open regions can facilitate TFAM-independent transcription initiation. However, in the presence of NaCl, the negatively charged phosphates are shielded, which prevents the DNA template breathing. Considering that the protein components of the transcription reaction will bring 15–25 mM NaCl into transcription reaction, we included 25 mM NaCl into transcription buffer to prevent unspecific transcription initiation [9]. It should be noted that the NaCl concentration should not exceed 100 mM to prevent dissociation of the initiation complex from promoter.
3. To dissolve boric acid, warm up deionized water before use.
4. To test the activity of the purified recombinant mtRNAP in a primer extension assay, we recommend titrating mtRNAP concentration (e.g., 0.5, 1, 1.5, and 2 μM). At the equimolar ratio of the RNA-DNA scaffold and mtRNAP (at 1 μM concentration in the reaction described above) nearly a 100% extension of RNA from 14 to 15 nt is expected (Fig. 1).
5. Follow the order of addition indicated.
6. The optimal temperature for transcription initiation assay involving synthetic promoter templates maybe different depending on the length of the upstream promoter region. The optimal temperature for the transcription assay involving -40 LSP template is 36 °C (Fig. 2b).

Acknowledgements

We thank past and present members of the Temiakov laboratory. This work was funded by NIH R35 GM131832.

References

1. Clayton D (2000) Transcription and replication of mitochondrial DNA. Hum Reprod Embryol 15:11–17
2. Morozov YI, Parshin AV, Agaronyan K et al (2015) A model for transcription initiation in human mitochondria. Nucleic Acids Res 43:3726–3735
3. Agaronyan K, Morozov YI, Anikin M, Temiakov D (2015) Replication-transcription switch in human mitochondria. Science 347:548–551

4. Falkenberg M, Gaspari M, Rantanen A et al (2002) Mitochondrial transcription factors B1 and B2 activate transcription of human mtDNA. Nat Genet 31:289–294
5. Sologub M, Litonin D, Anikin M et al (2009) TFB2 is a transient component of the catalytic site of the human mitochondrial RNA polymerase. Cell 139:934–944
6. Lodeiro MF, Uchida AU, Arnold JJ et al (2010) Identification of multiple rate-limiting steps during the human mitochondrial transcription cycle in vitro. J Biol Chem 285:16387–16402
7. Morozov YI, Agaronyan K, Cheung ACM et al (2014) A novel intermediate in transcription initiation by human mitochondrial RNA polymerase. Nucleic Acids Res 42:3884–3893
8. IDT https://www.idtdna.com/pages/education/decoded/article/annealing-oligonucleotides. Accessed 25 Sep 2018
9. Shi Y, Dierckx A, Wanrooij PH et al (2012) Mammalian transcription factor A is a core component of the mitochondrial transcription machinery. Proc Natl Acad Sci 109:16510–16515

Chapter 4

Investigating Mitochondrial Transcriptomes and RNA Processing Using Circular RNA Sequencing

Irina Kuznetsova, Oliver Rackham, and Aleksandra Filipovska

Abstract

Transcriptomic technologies have revolutionized the study of gene expression and RNA biology. Different RNA sequencing methods enable the analyses of diverse species of transcripts, including their abundance, processing, stability, and other specific features. Mitochondrial transcriptomics has benefited from these technologies that have revealed the surprising complexity of its RNAs. Here we describe a method based upon cyclization of mitochondrial RNAs and next generation sequencing to analyze the steady-state levels and sizes of mitochondrial RNAs, their degradation products, as well as their processing intermediates by capturing both 5′ and 3′ ends of transcripts.

Key words Next generation sequencing, RNA processing, Mitochondria, RNA-Seq

1 Introduction

Next generation sequencing has advanced our understanding of gene regulation by providing unprecedented coverage of transcriptomes. In particular RNA sequencing has revolutionized organelle gene expression in diverse organisms by defining transcriptome organization, the discovery of new transcripts and bringing to light multiple different layers of gene regulation. The mitochondrial transcriptome has been revealed to be far more complex than previously thought [1], especially in animals, despite the small and compact nature of the mitochondrial genome. Mitochondrial gene expression is intimately linked to energy production, since the 13 polypeptides encoded by the mitochondrial genome are essential components of the oxidative phosphorylation (OXPHOS) system [2, 3]. Mitochondrial gene expression is required for energy production and changes in response to different physiological demands and environmental challenges [4, 5]. Consequently, investigating mitochondrial transcriptomes provides insight into

Michal Minczuk and Joanna Rorbach (eds.), *Mitochondrial Gene Expression: Methods and Protocols*, Methods in Molecular Biology, vol. 2192, https://doi.org/10.1007/978-1-0716-0834-0_4,

the regulation of energy metabolism at the RNA level under varied conditions and in response to stress.

We have used RNA sequencing technologies to reveal new features of the mitochondrial transcriptome in mammals including the existence of mitochondrial DNA (mtDNA)-derived small RNAs and long noncoding RNAs [1, 6], beyond the 11 mRNAs, 22 tRNAs, and 2 rRNAs that were originally annotated as being encoded by mtDNA [7]. The diverse size and unique features of mitochondrial RNAs have necessitated the use of several different types of RNA sequencing to study mitochondrial (mt) RNAs [1, 8–11]. We have used canonical RNA sequencing (RNA-Seq) to measure the steady-state levels of mitochondrial mRNAs and rRNAs [9, 10, 12] as well as the precursor transcripts that contain tRNAs [8, 10] in a strand-specific manner, as the mitochondrial genome is transcribed as two polycistronic transcripts from the heavy and light strand of the mtDNA [13]. Since the RNA-Seq method does not effectively capture RNAs smaller than 90 nt, we have used small RNA sequencing (sRNA-Seq) to investigate the steady-state levels of mt-tRNAs and small RNAs [1, 10, 14] to selectively capture and enrich these species. We have used parallel analyses of RNA ends (PARE) [15] to specifically capture the 5′ ends of mitochondrial RNAs and define processing sites within the mitochondrial transcriptome as well as to identify new transcripts [1, 8, 11, 16]. Although all of these techniques are valuable, they provide knowledge that is specific to each method necessitating them to be performed individually which can often be prohibitively expensive.

Recently we developed a new technique that can capture all mtRNAs to provide information on their steady-state levels, new transcripts and processing intermediates in a single library and sequencing reaction without the need to carry out several different RNA-Seq methods. This approach takes advantage of circularization of RNA prior to library construction [17, 18] (Fig. 1), to preserve the identities of their 5′ and 3′ termini followed by deep sequencing, which we describe below. We have used this method to identify steady-state levels of mtRNAs as well as rare processing intermediates in normal mitochondria and stalled intermediates produced when mitochondrial RNase P function is lost [19].

2 Materials

All reagents for RNA work are prepared in DEPC-treated ultrapure water and the equipment used is treated with RNaseZap (Ambion) and rinsed in DEPC-treated ultrapure water before use. Sterile RNase-free filter pipette tips and other disposable plasticware should be used to prevent contamination and degradation of RNA samples. All RNA samples should be stored at −80 °C.

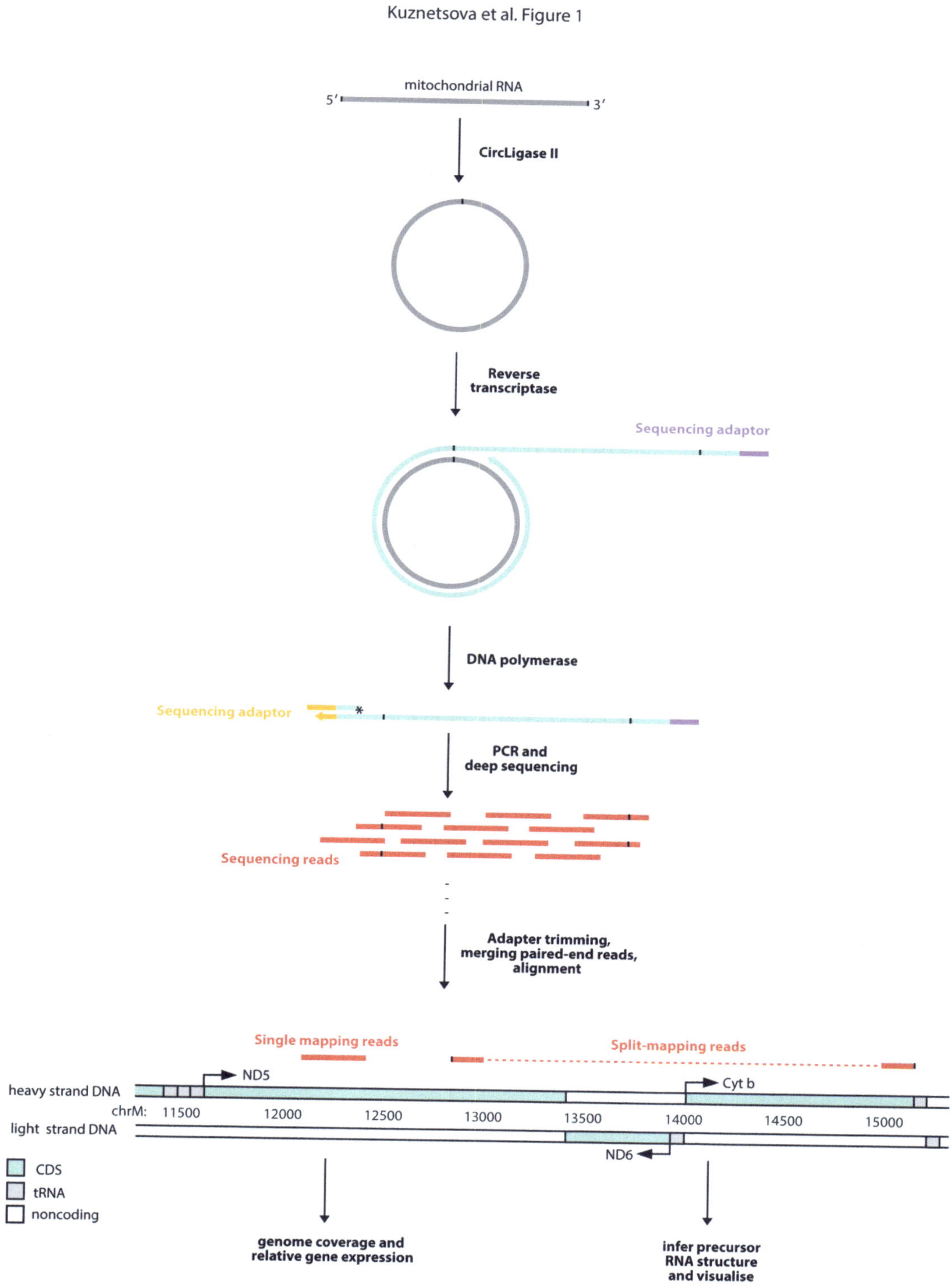

Fig. 1 Schematic showing the method for circularized RNA sequencing

2.1 Molecular Biology Reagents

1. Agencourt AMPure XP magnetic beads (Beckman Coulter).
2. 3 M sodium acetate (NaOAC) (pH 5.2).
3. 70% ethanol.
4. 100% ethanol.
5. CircLigase II ssDNA Ligase (Epicentre).
6. FailSafe PCR 2× PreMix E (Epicentre).
7. Glycoblue (Ambion).
8. Glycogen (Invitrogen), RiboMinus kit (Invitrogen).
9. RNase OUT (Invitrogen).
10. RNase R (Epicentre).
11. Oligo Clean & Concentrator (Zymo).
12. DNA Clean & Concentrator-5 (Zymo).
13. Superscript II (Invitrogen).
14. Klenow DNA polymerase I (NEB).

2.2 Primers

1. cDNA primer "RC-Seq-cDNA": GACGTGTGCTCTTCCG ATCTNNNNNN
2. 3′-end extension primer "RC-Seq-ex": ACACGACG CTCTTCCGATCTNNNNNNNN/3Phos/
3. Forward PCR primer "RC-Seq-PCRfwd" (Illumina): AATGA TACGGCGACCACCGAGATCTACACTCTTTCCCTACAC GACGCTCTTCCGATCT
4. Reverse PCR primer "RC-Seq-PCRrev1" (Illumina, index sequence is bold): CAAGCAGAAGACGGCATACGAGAT**C GTGAT**GTGACTGGAGTTCAGACGTGTGCTCTTCCGA TCT
5. Reverse PCR primer "RC-Seq-PCRrev2" (Illumina, index sequence is bold): CAAGCAGAAGACGGCATACGAGAT **ACATCG**GTGACTGGAGTTCAGACGTGTGCTCTTCCG ATCT
6. Reverse PCR primer "RC-Seq-PCRrev3" (Illumina, index sequence is bold): CAAGCAGAAGACGGCATACGAGA T**GCCTAA**GTGACTGGAGTTCAGACGTGTGCTCTTCC GATCT
7. Reverse PCR primer "RC-Seq-PCRrev4" (Illumina, index sequence is bold): CAAGCAGAAGACGGCATACGAG AT**TGGTCA**GTGACTGGAGTTCAGACGTGTGCTCTTC CGATCT
8. Reverse PCR primer "RC-Seq-PCRrev5" (Illumina, index sequence is bold): CAAGCAGAAGACGGCATACGAGAT **CACTGT** GTGACTGGAGTTCAGACGTGTGCTCTTCCG ATCT

9. Reverse PCR primer "RC-Seq-PCRrev6" (Illumina, index sequence is bold): CAAGCAGAAGACGGCATACGAGAT**ATTGGC**GTGACTGGAGTTCAGACGTGTGCTCTTCCGATCT

3 Methods

3.1 RNA Preparation

1. Isolate RNA from mitochondria using the miRNeasy kit, incorporating on-column DNase digest, according to the manufacturer's instructions.
2. Perform rRNA depletion reactions with the Ribo-Zero rRNA Removal Kit (Human/Mouse/Rat) and use between 500 ng and 1 μg of mtRNA.
3. Precipitate the RNA by adding 2 μL of 3 M NaOAc, pH 5.2, 2 μL glycogen (20 μg/μL), and 60 μL 100% ethanol and incubate at −80 °C for 30 min or overnight.
4. Collect the RNA by centrifugation at 20,200 × *g* for 25 min at 4 °C.
5. Carefully remove the ethanol with a pipette without disrupting the RNA pellet.
6. Wash the pellet with 300 μL of 70% ethanol, removing as much 70% ethanol as possible with a pipette.
7. Air dry the pellet for 10 min at room temperature.
8. Resuspend the RNA in 13 μL of RNase-free DEPC-treated water.

3.2 RNA Circularization

1. Add the following to a sterile, RNase-free 1.5 mL microcentrifuge tube:
   (a) ~500 ng of the prepared RNA.
   (b) 1 μL CircLigase II ssDNA Ligase.
   (c) 2 μL 10× reaction buffer.
   (d) 1 μL 50 mM $MnCl_2$.
   (e) 4 μL 5 M Betaine.
   (f) DEPC-treated ultrapure water to 20 μL.
2. Incubate the reaction at 60 °C for 1 h.

3.3 RNase R Digestion

1. To remove the remaining linear RNA, add 2.3 μL of 10× RNase R buffer and 1 μL of RNase R (20 U) to the reaction mixture from above.
2. Incubate the reaction at 37 °C for 10 min.

3. Following the digestion isolate the circularized RNA using Oligo Clean & Concentrator columns following the manufacturer's instructions.
4. Elute the RNA with 11 μL nuclease-free water.

3.4 RC-Seq Library Preparation

1. To generate cDNA from the circularized RNA, in a RNase-free 1.5 mL microcentrifuge tube, add the following:
   (a) Entire circularized RNA solution.
   (b) 0.5 μL "RC-Seq-cDNA" cDNA primer (100 μM).
   (c) 1 μL 10 mM dNTP solution (containing 10 mM dATP, 10 mM dGTP, 10 mM dCTP, and 10 mM dTTP).
2. Incubate the reaction at 65 °C for 5 min in a thermal cycler, then cool directly on ice for at least 1 min.
3. Add the following to the reaction:
   (a) 4 μL 5× Superscript II reaction buffer.
   (b) 2 μL 0.1 M DTT.
   (c) 1 μL RNase Out.
   (d) 1 μL Superscript II.
4. Mix the reaction gently and place in a thermal cycler at 25 °C for 15 min, then 42 °C for 30 min.
5. Add 2 μL of 1 M KOH and heat to 95 °C for 15 min, then cool to room temperature and neutralize by adding 2 μL 1 M HCl.
6. Purify the cDNA with DNA Clean & Concentrator columns and elute with 20 μL H_2O.
7. To extend the cDNA add:
   (a) 0.5 μL 0.1 M DTT.
   (b) 1 μL 10 mM dNTP.
   (c) 0.5 μL 100 μM 3′-end extension primer.
   (d) 2.5 μL 5× NEB Buffer 2.
   (e) 0.5 μL Klenow DNA polymerase I.
8. Incubate the reaction at 25 °C for 15 min, and then at 95 °C for 3 min to deactivate the enzyme.
9. Purify the tagged cDNA with DNA Clean & Concentrator columns and elute with 23.5 μL H_2O.
10. To amplify the cDNA prepare the following reaction:
    (a) purified cDNA solution.
    (b) 25 μL Failsafe PCR Premix E.
    (c) 0.5 μL forward PCR primer ("RC-Seq-PCRfwd") (40 μM).

(d) 0.5 μL reverse PCR primer ("RC-Seq-PCRrev1" or another for indexing) (40 μM).

(e) 1 μL Failsafe PCR enzyme.

11. Heat the reaction at 95 °C for 1 min, followed by 18 cycles (or 12–24 cycles depending on the quantity of RNA input) of 95 °C for 30 s, 55 °C for 30 s, and 68 °C for 3 min with a final extension step at 68 °C for 7 min.
12. Purify the crude PCR product on Agencourt AMPure XP magnetic beads using a 1:1 volume ratio (50 μL beads: 50 μL PCR, use 200 G tips for all bead pipetting, air dry for 5 min after 2 × 300 μL 70% ethanol washes) (*see* **Note 1**).
13. Elute the final PCR product in 28 μL ultrapure water.
14. Analyze library size distribution using a Bioanalyzer and quantitate by qPCR (*see* **Note 2**).
15. Sequence the products using an Illumina MiSeq in paired-end mode (2 × 150 nt) with the standard Illumina sequencing primers: HP10 read 1, HP12 i7 index seq primer, HP11 read 2. Use only 0.5% of the PhiX control library spiked into the sequencing run.

4 Bioinformatic Analysis Workflow for Circularized RNA Sequencing Data

The bioinformatic work flow analysis was developed specifically for the RNA circularization procedure and the work flow is schematically shown in Fig. 2.

4.1 Software Used for Data Analyses

Input data: High-throughput data in FASTQ format.

Summary of all software used for the analyses is shown in Table 1.

4.2 Workflow

The Illumina MiSeq output data is produced as FASTQ format files where the length of paired-end reads is 250 bp. The workflow is schematically represented in Fig. 2.

4.2.1 Quality Check

Check the quality of the raw data. The output is presented in HTML format.

Input: *input_file_R1.fastq*
input_file_R2.fastq

Example: *fastqc input_file_R1.fastq input_file_R2.fastq*

4.2.2 Adapter Trimming

Search for the presence of the adapter sequence in the read sequence and remove them if any are found.

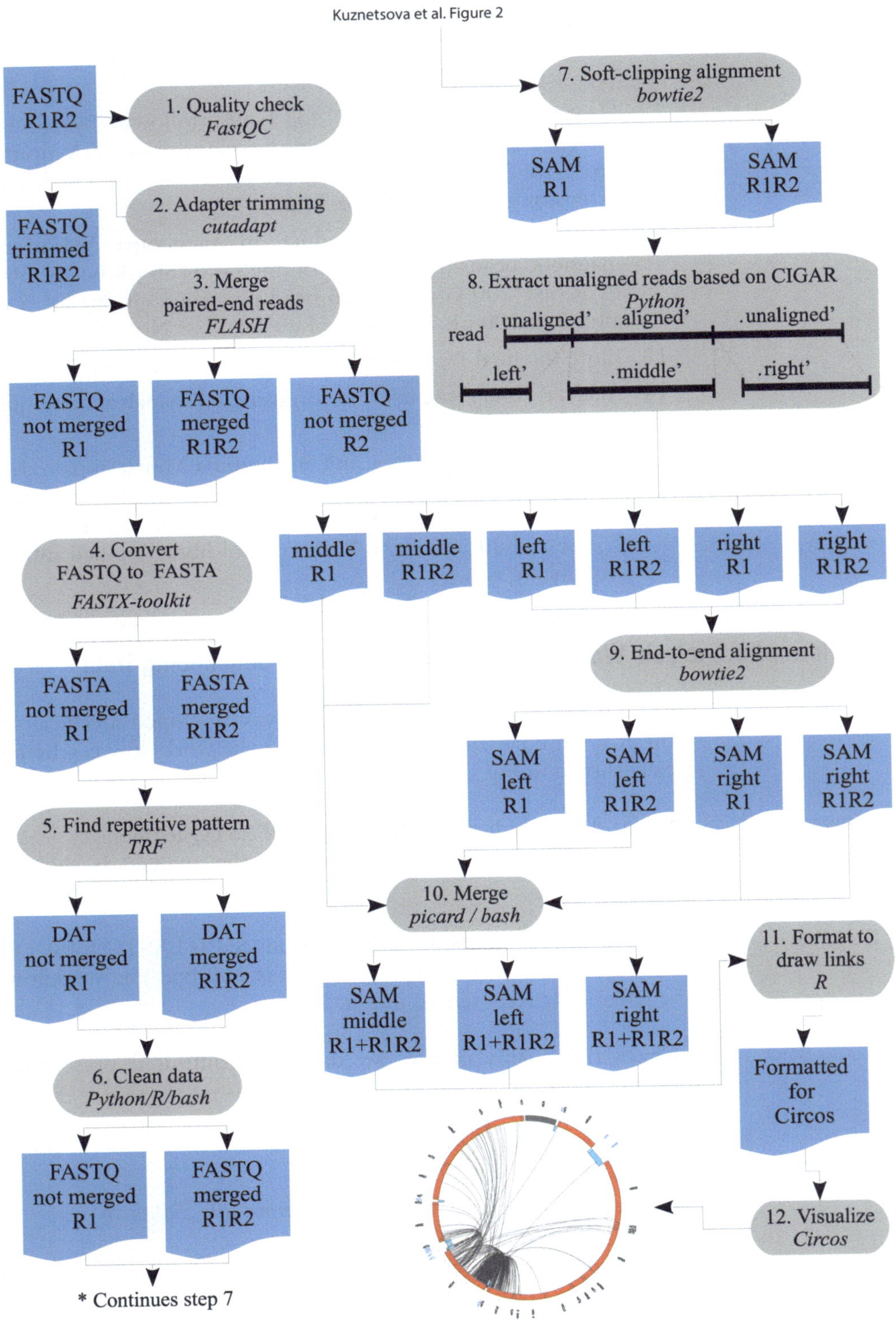

Fig. 2 Bioinformatics analysis workflow for circularized RNA

Table 1
Software used for analyses of circular RNA sequencing datasets

Software	Description	Reference
FastQC	High-throughput quality control.	[20]
Cutadap	Adapter trimming software.	[21]
FLASH	Merges paired-end reads into single-end reads.	[22]
FASTX-toolkit	Set of command line tools for high-throughput data (fastq_to_fasta).	[23]
TRF	Searches for tandem repeats in DNA sequences.	[24]
bowtie2	Aligner software.	[25]
picard	Set of command line tools for high-throughput data (MergeSamFiles, SamFormatConverter).	https://broadinstitute.github.io/picard/
Circos	Visualization software.	[26]
bedtools	Set of command line tools for high-throughput data (genomecov).	[27]
R	Data processing, manipulation.	[28]
Python	Data processing, manipulation.	[29]
bash	Data processing, manipulation.	

Input: *input_file_R1.fastq*
input_file_R2.fastq

Adapters: *-a adapt_fwd, adapter from forward reads*
-A adapt_rev, adapter from revers reads

Parameters: *-m 20, removes trimmed reads that have length less than 20 bp*
-p, for paired-output

Example: *cutadapt –m 20 –a adapt_fwd –A adapt_rev –o out_-file_trimmed_R1.fastq –p out_file_trimmed_R2.fastq input_fi-le_R1.fastq input_file_R2.fastq*

4.2.3 Fast Length Adjustment of Short Reads (FLASH)

Merge paired-end reads into one long sequence. The software outputs three files. One file contains paired-end reads that should be merged into a single sequence. The other two files contain the first and second read pairs that could not be merged. Merged reads and only first read pair of not merged by FLASH files should be used for further analysis.

Input: *input_file_trimmed_R1.fastq*
input_file_trimmed_R2.fastq

Parameters: *-m, minimum overlapping length. This parameter was left as default, which is 10 bp.*

-M, maximum overlapping length. This parameter was set to 245 bp.

Example: *flash input_file_R1.fastq input_file_R2.fastq -M 245*

4.2.4 Convert FASTQ to FASTA (FASTX-toolkit)

Convert the FASTQ file to FASTA format.

Input: *input_file_merged_reads.fastq*
input_file_not_merged_R1.fastq

Example: *fastq_to_fasta –i input_file_merged_reads.fastq –o input_file_merged_reads.fasta*

fastq_to_fasta –i input_file_merged_R1.fastq –o input_file_merged_R1.fasta

4.2.5 Tandem Repeats Finder (TRF)

Find if repetitive sequences are present within a read. The TRF output file is represented in a text format as dat.

Input: *input_file_merged_reads.fasta*
input_file_not_merged_R1.fasta

Parameters: *match, matching weight*
mismatch, mismatching penalty
delta, indel penalty
pm, match probability (whole number)
pi, indel probability (whole number)
minscore, minimum alignment score to report
maxperiod, maximum period size to report
-h, output as html
-d, data file

Example: ***trf*** *input_file_merged_reads.fasta 2 7 7 80 10 50 200 –h –d*
trf *input_file_not_merged_R1.fasta 2 7 7 80 10 50 200 –h –d*

4.2.6 Data Refinement

Remove unnecessary noise, such as empty rows and software-related information, that are produced by TRF tool. There are several options in presenting TRF results:

1. "None" is assigned if no repetitive patterns are found within a read.
2. One sequence is displayed if only one repetitive pattern sequence is found within a read.
3. Several sequences are displayed if multiple repetitive patterns are found within a read. Move multiple repetitive patterns of the read to one line.

Select the longest sequence from multiple repetitive sequences found by TRF. Remove repetitive sequence patterns with the length less than 20 bp. However, keep reads where a repetitive pattern has not been found. Use TRF processed data and information from a file generated by FLASH to extract information related to the same read such: read ID, read sequence, repetitive pattern sequence, and quality sequence. Find where a repetitive sequence starts in the related read and extract a double size of the repetitive sequence. If a read has "None" found repetitive patterns use the entire read length. Generate FASTQ format.

4.2.7 Soft-Clipping Alignment

Align prepared data to the mitochondrial genome with selected soft-clipping or local mode. This option aligns part of the read rather than aligning a read from end-to-end. Results are presented in SAM format.

Input: *clean_TRF_merged_reads.fastq*
clean_TRF_not_merged_R1.fastq

Parameters: *-x, the basename of the index for the reference genome*
--sensitive-local, soft-clipping mode
-U, input file
-S, alignment output in SAM format

Example: *bowtie2 –x bt2_indx --very-sensitive-local -U clean_TRF_-merged_reads.fastq –S soft_clipping_merged_reads.sam*
bowtie2 –x bt2_indx --very-sensitive-local -U clean_TRF_not_-merged_R1.fastq –S soft_clipping_not_merged_R1.sam

4.2.8 CIGAR Field

Extract aligned and unaligned parts of the read sequences based on CIGAR filed. A read can have partially aligned region which for simplicity is called "middle," and/or two unaligned regions "left" and/or "right." Extract "left" and/or "right" unaligned read sequences, convert to FASTQ format.

4.2.9 End-to-End Alignment

Align extracted and converted to FASTQ format "right" and "left" regions of the read to the mitochondrial reference genome this time with the end-to-end mode, which is default option in bowtie2. Results are represented in SAM format.

Input: *left_unaligned_merged_reads.fastq*
right_unaligned_merged_reads.fastq
left_unaligned_not_merged_R1.fastq
right_unaligned_not_merged_R1.fastq

Parameters: *-x, the basename of the index for the reference genome*
-U, input file
-S, alignment output in SAM format

Example: *bowtie2 –x bt2_indx -U left_unaligned_merged_reads.fastq –S left_aligned_merged_reads.sam*

bowtie2 –x bt2_indx -U right_unaligned_merged_reads.fastq –S right_aligned_merged_reads.sam

bowtie2 –x bt2_indx -U left_unaligned_not_merged_R1.fastq –S left_aligned_not_merged_R1.sam

bowtie2 –x bt2_indx -U right_unaligned_not_merged_R1.fastq –S right_aligned_not_merged_R1.sam

4.2.10 Merge Aligned Reads

Combine merged reads and first pair not merged by FALSH that align according to soft-clip (-local) mode into one file. Combine "left" merged reads and the first pair not merged by FALSH that align according to end-to-end mode. Combine "right" merged reads and first pair not merged by FALSH that align according to end-to-end mode.

Input: *soft_clipping_merged_reads.sam*
soft_clipping_not_merged_R1.sam
right_aligned_merged_reads.sam
right_aligned_not_merged_R1.sam
left_aligned_merged_reads.sam
left_aligned_not_merged_R1.sam

Example: *java –jar picard.jar mergeSamFiles I=soft_clipping_merged_reads.sam I=soft_clipping_not_merged_R1.sam O=soft_clipping_middle.sam*
java –jar picard.jar mergeSamFiles I=right_aligned_merged_reads.sam I=right_aligned_not_merged_R1.sam O=soft_clipping_right.sam
java –jar picard.jar mergeSamFiles I=left_aligned_merged_reads.sam I=left_aligned_not_merged_R1.sam O=soft_clipping_left.sam

4.2.11 Data Preparation for Visualization

Follow the Circos software manual to prepare all required files for visualization. Briefly, Circos requires configuration file (.conf), mitochondrial karyotype file, information for both strands, gene names, and formatted data for drawing links. Use data created in previous step for generating links. Find reads that share the same read ID between the three files. There are several possible scenarios:

1. The same read ID is shared between all three files, "middle"-"right" and "middle"-"left."
2. The same read ID is shared only between "middle"-"right" files, but not present at "left" file.
3. The same read ID is shared only between "middle"-"left" files, but not present at "right" file.

Table 2
Data format for visualizing links in Circos

mmM	Link start (middle)	Link start (middle)	Mmm	Link end (left/right)	Link end (left/right)
mmM	100	100	mmM	734	734
mmM	199	199	mmM	925	925
...	...	...	...	...	...

Reads that come from the "middle" file are considered as a starting point of the link and is located within a region in the gene of interest. Reads from the "left" and "right" files are considered as the end point of the link and represent unprocessed transcript intermediates. To visualize transcript intermediates for specific mitochondrial gene:

1. Select a gene of interest.
2. Find the 5′–3′ coordinates for the gene.
3. Extract reads coordinates that fall into 5′–3′ region of the selected gene from the "middle" file.
4. Extract reads that share the same read ID between "middle" file and "left" and/or "right" files.
5. Create links information in Circos format (Table 2). The coordinate that comes from the "middle" part of the read is used to build a link with the coordinate that comes from the "right" or "left" part of the read.

4.2.12 Visualization

Visualize with Circos.

Input: *rna_visual.conf*

Parameters: *-mitochondrial karyotype file*
-minus and plus strands information
-gene information
-data for building links
-configuration file

Example: *circos –conf rna_visual.conf –debug_group summary, timer*

5 Notes

1. Agencourt AMPure XP magnetic beads change performance over time and should ideally be used within a month of purchase for optimal performance.
2. The library size should be greater than 200 bp after purification.

Acknowledgements

The work was supported by fellowships and project grants from the National Health and Medical Research Council (APP1159594, APP1154932, APP1154646 to AF and OR), Australian Research Council (to AF and OR), the Cancer Council of Western Australia (to OR and AF). IK is supported by a UWA Postgraduate Scholarship.

References

1. Mercer TR et al (2011) The human mitochondrial transcriptome. Cell 146:645–658
2. Rackham O, Mercer TR, Filipovska A (2012) The human mitochondrial transcriptome and the RNA-binding proteins that regulate its expression. WIREs RNA 3:675–695
3. Hallberg BM, Larsson N-G (2014) Making proteins in the powerhouse. Cell Metab 20:226–240
4. Ferreira N, Rackham O, Filipovska A (2018) Regulation of a minimal transcriptome by repeat domain proteins. Semin Cell Dev Biol 76:132. https://doi.org/10.1016/j.semcdb.2017.08.037
5. Lee RG, Rudler DL, Rackham O, Filipovska A (2018) Is mitochondrial gene expression coordinated or stochastic? Biochem Soc Trans 46:1239–1246
6. Rackham O et al (2011) Long noncoding RNAs are generated from the mitochondrial genome and regulated by nuclear-encoded proteins. RNA 17:2085–2093
7. Montoya J, Ojala D, Attardi G (1981) Distinctive features of the 5′-terminal sequences of the human mitochondrial mRNAs. Nature 290:465–470
8. Rackham O et al (2016) Hierarchical RNA processing is required for mitochondrial ribosome assembly. Cell Rep 16:1874–1890
9. Perks KL et al (2018) PTCD1 is required for 16S rRNA maturation complex stability and mitochondrial ribosome assembly. Cell Rep 23:127–142
10. Siira SJ et al (2018) Concerted regulation of mitochondrial and nuclear non-coding RNAs by a dual-targeted RNase Z. EMBO Rep 19: e46198. https://doi.org/10.15252/embr.201846198
11. Siira SJ, Shearwood A-MJ, Bracken CP, Rackham O, Filipovska A (2017) Defects in RNA metabolism in mitochondrial disease. Int J Biochem Cell Biol 85:106–113. https://doi.org/10.1016/j.biocel.2017.02.003
12. Kühl I et al (2017) Transcriptomic and proteomic landscape of mitochondrial dysfunction reveals secondary coenzyme Q deficiency in mammals. elife 6:1494
13. Gustafsson CM, Falkenberg M, Larsson N-G (2016) Maintenance and expression of mammalian mitochondrial DNA. Annu Rev Biochem 85:133–160
14. Kuehl I et al (2016) POLRMT regulates the switch between replication primer formation and gene expression of mammalian mtDNA. Sci Adv 2:e1600963
15. German MA et al (2008) Global identification of microRNA-target RNA pairs by parallel analysis of RNA ends. Nat Biotechnol 26:941–946
16. Rackham O, Filipovska A (2014) Methods in molecular biology, vol 1125. Humana Press, Totowa, NJ, pp 263–275

17. Acevedo A, Brodsky L, Andino R (2015) Mutational and fitness landscapes of an RNA virus revealed through population sequencing. Nature 505:686–690
18. Chu Y et al (2015) Intramolecular circularization increases efficiency of RNA sequencing and enables CLIP-Seq of nuclear RNA from human cells. Nucleic Acids Res 43:e75–e75
19. Kuznetsova I et al (2017) Simultaneous processing and degradation of mitochondrial RNAs revealed by circularized RNA sequencing. Nucleic Acids Res 5:5487–5500
20. Wingett SW, Andrews S (2018) FastQ Screen: a tool for multi-genome mapping and quality control. F1000Res 7:1338
21. Martin M (2011) Cutadapt removes adapter sequences from high-throughput sequencing reads. EMBnet J 17:10–12
22. Magoč T, Salzberg SL (2011) FLASH: fast length adjustment of short reads to improve genome assemblies. Bioinformatics 27:2957–2963
23. Gordon A (2010) Unpublished. G. H. F. A. S.-R. P. T. Fastx-toolkit
24. Benson G (1999) Tandem repeats finder: a program to analyze DNA sequences. Nucleic Acids Res 27:573–580
25. Langmead B, Salzberg SL (2012) Fast gapped-read alignment with Bowtie 2. Nat Methods 9:357–359
26. Krzywinski M et al (2009) Circos: An information aesthetic for comparative genomics. Genes Dev 19:1639–1645
27. Quinlan AR, Hall IM (2010) BEDTools: a flexible suite of utilities for comparing genomic features. Nat Commun 26:841–842
28. Ihaka R, Gentleman R (2012) R: a language for data analysis and graphics. J Comput Graph Stat 5:299–314
29. Rossum G (1995) Python reference manual. CWI, Amsterdam

Chapter 5

Detection of 5-formylcytosine in Mitochondrial Transcriptome

Lindsey Van Haute and Michal Minczuk

Abstract

Posttranscriptional RNA modifications have recently emerged as essential posttranscriptional regulators of gene expression. Here we present two methods for single nucleotide resolution detection of 5-formylcytosine (f^5C) in RNA. The first relies on chemical protection of f^5C against bisulfite treatment, the second method is based on chemical reduction of f^5C to hm^5C. In combination with regular bisulfite treatment of RNA, the methods allow for precise mapping of f^5C. The protocol is used for f^5C detection in mtDNA-encoded RNA, however, it can be straightforwardly applied for transcriptome-wide analyses.

Key words 5-formylcytosine, Next-generation sequencing, RNA modification, RedBS RNA-Seq, fCAB RNA-Seq, epitranscriptome

1 Introduction

Posttranscriptional RNA modifications, often referred to as epitranscriptome, can influence RNA folding, structure, and function. As such, they play a role in accuracy, efficiency, and regulation of translation, have been associated with mRNA decay and circadian clock speed and seem to play a role in early embryo development and cancer [1, 2]. Over 140 different RNA modifications have been identified so far, but little is known about the exact role and most studies focus on the function of the most abundant modifications, such as N1-methyladenosine (m^1A), pseudouridine (Ψ), and 5-methylcytidine (m^5C) [3].

The function and biogenesis of 5-formyldeoxycytosine (f^5dC) in nuclear DNA, as an oxidative derivative of highly abundant 5-methyldeoxycytosine (m^5dC), have been studied extensively and many different techniques are available to detect this modification [4–6]. The presence of 5-formylcytosine in RNA (f^5C) has been shown over 25 years ago [7]. However, until recently, very little was known about the biogenesis of this RNA modification. In

Michal Minczuk and Joanna Rorbach (eds.), *Mitochondrial Gene Expression: Methods and Protocols*, Methods in Molecular Biology, vol. 2192, https://doi.org/10.1007/978-1-0716-0834-0_5,

cytoplasmic RNA, f^5C has been detected at position 34 (wobble base) of mammalian ct-tRNA$^{Leu(CAA)}$ [8, 9]. In mitochondrial RNA, f^5C has been found on the wobble base of mt-tRNA^{Met}. A series of recent papers have shown that initially a methyl group is added to the cytosine at position 34 of these tRNAs, which is then converted to a formyl group [10–15].

We describe two methods for f^5C detection based upon next generation RNA-Seq, which can be applied simultaneously. Both methods rely on differences in bisulfite RNA conversion of chemically modified or protected f^5C. RNA bisulfite sequencing (BS) is a well-established method to detect m^5C and hm^5C. Since bisulfite does convert f^5C, this method cannot distinguish f^5C from unmodified C. Our first method, reduced bisulfite RNA sequencing (RedBS RNA-Seq), relies on the chemical reduction of f^5C to hm^5C by $NaBH_4$, with the resulting hm^5C being subsequently detected by RNA BS. The second protocol, 5-formylcytosine chemically assisted bisulfite RNA sequencing (fCAB RNA-Seq) is based upon *O*-ethylhydroxylamine protection of f^5C from bisulfite conversion (Fig. 1).

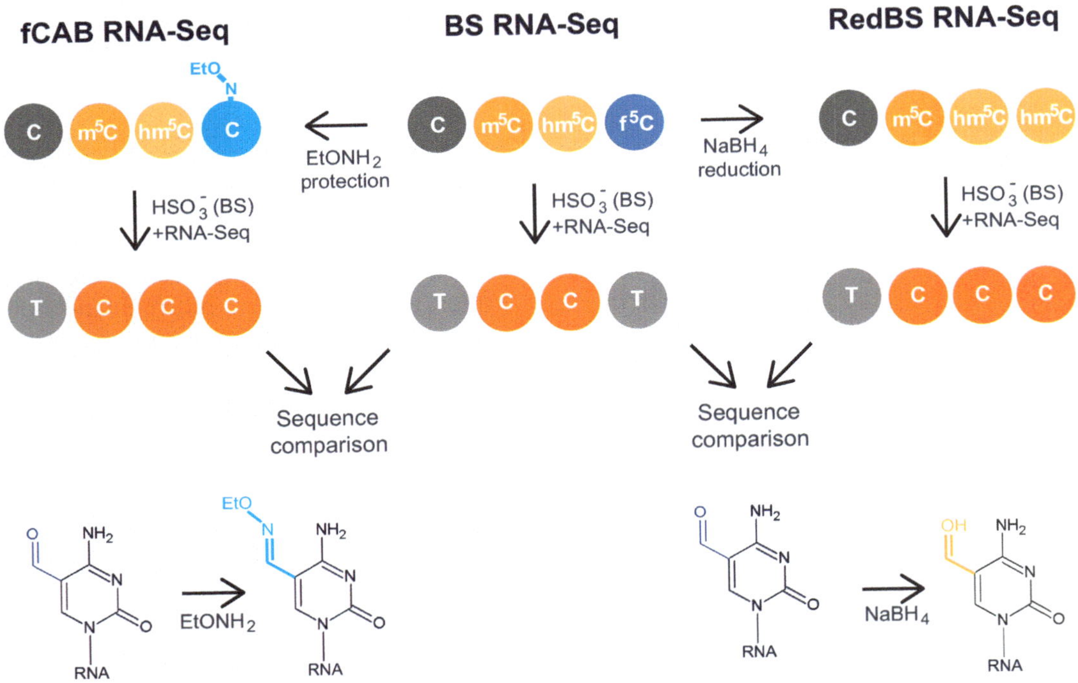

Fig. 1 Outline of chemically assisted bisulfite sequencing (fCAB RNA-Seq) and reduced bisulfite RNA sequencing (RedBS RNA-Seq) to map f^5C in RNA. In f^5C chemically assisted bisulfite sequencing (fCAB RNA-Seq), *O*-ethylhydroxylamine is used to protect f^5C against deamination to uracil (left). In reduced bisulfite RNA sequencing (RedBS RNA-Seq) f^5C is chemically reduced to hm^5C by $NaBH_4$; hm^5C is then detected in the same manner as m^5C in a standard bisulfite sequencing (BS) procedure (right). Sequence comparison, using a BS RNA-Seq of untreated sample (middle) as a reference, reveals f^5C RNA sites

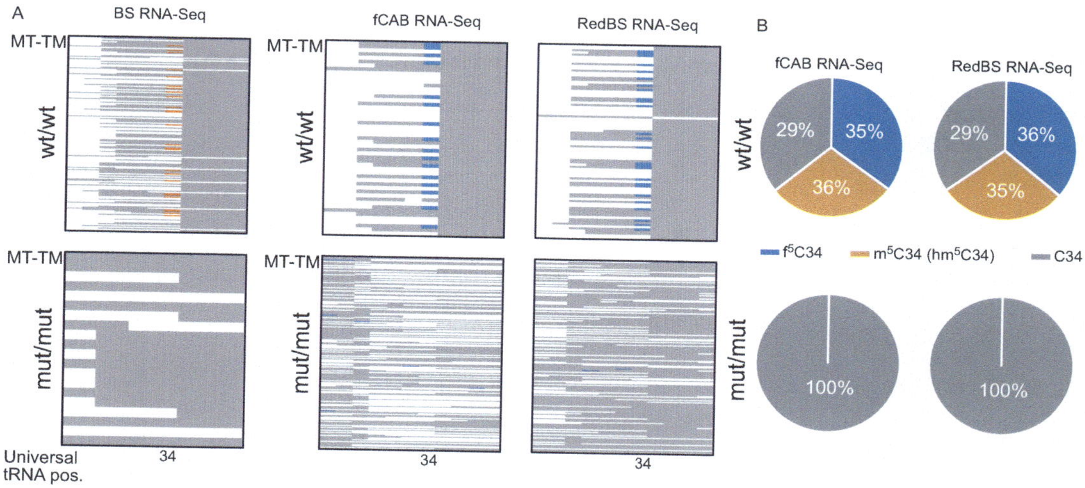

Fig. 2 Example of reduced bisulfite RNA sequencing (RedBS RNA-Seq) and chemically assisted bisulfite sequencing (fCAB RNA-Seq) on nucleotide level. Levels of f^5C in mitochondrial $tRNA^{Met}$ (MT-TM) are analyzed in wild type (wt/wt) fibroblasts and in fibroblast carrying a mutation in the NSUN3 gene (mut/mut). NSUN3 is responsible for the formation of m^5C on position 34, which is further converted to f^5C by ALKBH1 [12–14, 18]. (**a**) Heatmaps of BS RNA-Seq, fCAB RNA-Seq and RedBS RNA-Seq reads for MT-TM for wild type (wt/wt) and NSUN3 mutant (mut/mut) fibroblasts. Unconverted cytosines are shown in dark gray, while unmodified cytosines are shown in light gray. (**b**) Summary of the fCAB RNA-Seq and RedBS RNA-Seq results for wt/wt and mut/mut fibroblasts

These two newly developed approaches allow for detection of f^5C transcriptome-wide with individual nucleotide resolution (Fig. 2). Other current methods can detect only global levels of f^5C, for example, fluorogenic labeling [16], or require extensive mass spectrometry expertise to analyze f^5C in a sequence context [13]. Therefore, these two protocols may facilitate the search for new 5-formylated cytosines, reveal their functional role in both cytoplasmic and mitochondrial RNA, consequently assisting further expansion of epitranscriptomic research.

2 Materials

2.1 RNA Preparation (See Note 1)

1. TriZol reagent (Thermo Fisher Scientific).
2. Chloroform.
3. 2-propanol.
4. 70% Ethanol in DEPC treated water.
5. Nuclease free water (Ambion).
6. TURBO DNA-free Kit (Ambion).
7. Ribo Zero Gold (Illumina).
8. Magnetic rack for eppendorf tubes.

2.2 Conversion of Modifications

2.2.1 Hydroxylamine Protection for fCAB RNA-Seq

1. 100 mM MES buffer, pH = 5.
2. 10 mM *O*-ethylhydroxylamine (Sigma Aldrich).
3. RNasin Ribonuclease Inhibitor (Promega).

2.2.2 $NaBH_4$ Reduction for RedBS RNA-Seq

1. $NaBH_4$ (Sigma Aldrich).
2. Anhydrous methanol (Sigma Aldrich).
3. Injection needle and syringe.

2.2.3 RNA Precipitation

1. 3 M sodium acetate.
2. 100% ethanol.
3. GlycoBlue Coprecipitant (15 mg/mL) (Thermo Fisher).
4. 70% ethanol in DEPC-treated water.
5. Nuclease-free H_2O.

2.2.4 Bisulfite Treatment

1. Imprint DNA Modification Kit (Sigma Aldrich).
2. Micro Bio-Spin 6 columns in Tris buffer (BioRad).
3. 1 M Tris-Cl, pH 9.

2.3 Library Preparation

2.3.1 Sample Preparation

1. T4 PNK (NEB).
2. DNA ligase buffer (NEB).
3. Nuclease-free H_2O.

2.3.2 Library Preparation

1. TruSeq Small RNA Library Preparation Kit (Illumina).
2. T4 RNA Ligase 2, Deletion Mutant (200 U/μL).
3. 15% TBE-Urea gel.
4. RNA Gel Loading Dye (2×) (ThermoFisher).
5. RNase free TBE buffer.
6. Sybr Gold Nucleic Acid Gel Stain (ThermoFisher).
7. Dark reader/UV transilluminator.
8. RNasin Ribonuclease Inhibitor (Promega).
9. Superscript III (ThermoFisher).

2.3.3 Clean Up

1. Agencourt AMPure XP beads.
2. Magnetic stand.
3. Freshly prepared 80% ethanol.
4. Nuclease free water.

3 Methods

3.1 RNA Preparation (See Note 2)

OPTIONAL: In order to enrich for mtRNA, mitochondria could be isolated from the analyzed cells or tissue, according to published protocols [17]. For whole-transcriptome analysis, total RNA is extracted from the analyzed material.

3.1.1 RNA Extraction

1. Add 1 mL TriZol reagent to the cell pellet (up to 1×10^7 cells) or mitochondrial enriched fraction.
2. Incubate 5 min at RT.
3. Add 200 μL chloroform + vortex at least 10 s.
4. Incubate 5 min at RT.
5. Centrifuge 11,000 rcf 15 min 4 °C.
6. Transfer aqueous phase to new tube.
7. Precipitate RNA with 500 μL 2-propanol, leave at RT for 20 min.
8. Centrifuge 11,000 rcf 15 min 4 °C.
9. Discard supernatant, wash pellet with 70% ethanol.
10. Discard supernatant, remove as much ethanol as possible and air-dry pellet for 5 min.
11. Resuspend in nuclease-free H_2O.

3.1.2 DNase Treatment

1. Take 20 μg RNA in 70 μL nuclease-free water (*see* **Note 3**).
2. Add 8 μL 10× DNase Buffer, 7 μL DNase.
3. Incubate at 37 °C for 30 min.
4. Add 12 μL of DNase Inactivation reagent and mix well by vortex.
5. Incubate 5 min at RT mixing occasionally (2–3 times).
6. Centrifuge at 10,000 rcf for 2 min and transfer 90 μL into a new tube. Keep on ice.

3.1.3 Ribosomal RNA Depletion (See Note 4)

1. Deplete RNA samples from rRNA with Ribo Zero Gold (Illumina) as described by the manufacturer.

3.2 Conversion of Modifications

RedBS RNA-Seq and fCAB RNA-Seq could be used individually; however, it is advantageous to use both methods simultaneously. In that case, each experimental RNA sample from Subheading 3.1.3 has to be divided in three parts (one for RedBS RNA-Seq, one for fCAB RNA-Seq, and one for BS RNA-Seq).

1. Add 1 μg RNA to 10 mM *O*-ethylhydroxylamine in 100 mM MES buffer (pH 5.0) (total volume 100 μL).
2. Add 5 μL RNasin Ribonuclease Inhibitor.

3.2.1 O-ethylhydroxylamine Protection for fCAB RNA-Seq

3. Incubate at 37 °C for 2 h.
4. Continue to Subheading 3.2.3 RNA precipitation.

3.2.2 $NaBH_4$ Reduction for RedBS RNA-Seq

1. Denature 1 μg RNA (in 20 μL H_2O) at 100 °C for 10 min.
2. Chill on ice for 10 min.
3. Add 20 μL freshly prepared 40 μM $NaBH_4$ solution and incubate at 25 °C for 15 min (*see* **Note 5**).
4. Add another 20 μL freshly prepared 40 μM $NaBH_4$ solution and incubate for a further 15 min at 25 °C.
5. Continue immediately to Subheading 3.2.3 RNA precipitation (*see* **Note 6**).

3.2.3 RNA Precipitation

This step applies to *O*-ethylhydroxylamine protected RNA (Subheading 3.2.1), $NaBH_4$ reduced RNA (Subheading 3.2.2) and untreated RNA (Subheading 3.1.3).

1. Adjust volume of the RNA samples resulting from the previous steps to 200 μL with nuclease-free water.
2. Add 1 μL GlycoBlue Coprecipitant.
3. Add 18.5 μL 3 M sodium acetate.
4. Add 600 μL 100% ethanol.
5. Incubate at −20 °C overnight.
6. Centrifuge at maximum speed for 15 min at 4 °C.
7. Briefly rinse pellet with ice cold 70% ethanol.
8. Centrifuge max speed for 2 min.
9. Remove supernatant and allow pellet to air-dry.
10. Resuspend in 10 μL nuclease free H_2O.

3.2.4 Bisulfite Treatment

This step also applies to *O*-ethylhydroxylamine protected RNA (Subheading 3.2.1), $NaBH_4$ reduced RNA (Subheading 3.2.2) and untreated RNA (Subheading 3.1.3) that were precipitated as described in the preceding Subheading 3.2.3.

1. To prepare the "Bisulfite Solution Mix", add 1.1 mL of "DNA Modification Solution" to a vial of "DNA Modification Powder" and vortex 2 min or until clear. Next, add 40 μL of "Balance Solution and vortex briefly" (*see* **Note 7**).
2. Add 2 μg of RNA to a PCR tube, add 110 μL of "Bisulfite Solution Mix" and vortex briefly.
3. Perform deamination reaction in PCR machine. The conditions used are:
   (a) Three cycles of: 90 °C for 5 min and 60 °C for 60 min.
   (b) Hold 20 °C.

4. Desalt by passaging through micro bio-spin column (*see* **Note 8**):
   (a) Invert the column sharply several times before snapping of the tip.
   (b) Place in 2 mL tube and remove the cap (column begins to flow).
   (c) Allow buffer to drain by gravity (about 2 min) and discard buffer.
   (d) Centrifuge for 2 min at 1000 × *g* and discard remaining buffer.
   (e) Place column in a clean 1.5 mL tube and carefully apply the sample to the column.
   (f) Centrifuge 2 min at 1000 × *g*.
   (g) Apply the eluate to a new column.
   (h) Centrifuge 4 min at 1000 × *g*.
5. Desulfonate by adding equal volume of 1 M Tris-Cl (pH 9) and incubate 1 h at 37 °C.
6. Precipitate the RNA as described in Subheading 3.2.3.

3.3 Library Preparation for Next Generation Sequencing

3.3.1 Sample Preparation

1. T4 PNK treatment: To 10 μL bisulfite treated RNA add:
   (a) 5 μL 10× T4 DNA Ligase buffer (*see* **Note 9**).
   (b) 5 μL T4 PNK.
   (c) Add water up to 50 μL.
2. Keep at 37 °C for 30 min, followed by heat inactivation at 65 °C for 20 min.
3. Precipitate the RNA as described in Subheading 3.2.3, but resuspend in 6 μL nuclease-free H_2O.

3.3.2 Library Preparation

1. Ligate 3′ end adapters according to the manufacturer's recommendations.
2. Ligate 5′ end adapters according to the manufacturer's recommendations.
3. Run samples on 15% TBE-Urea gel in TBE buffer:
   (a) Add RNA gel loading dye and denature samples for 10 min at 70 °C (immediately put on ice) and run until separated enough to distinguish between "adapter only" fragments (~120 nt) and "RNA ligated with adapters" (*see* **Note 10**).
   (b) Stain with Sybr Gold Nucleic Acid Gel Stain for 2–4 min. Cut bands that are larger than 140 nt on a dark reader/UV transilluminator (*see* **Note 11**).
   (c) Add equal volume 1× TBE buffer + RNasin Ribonuclease Inhibitor and leave overnight at 4 °C with mixing.

(d) Centrifuge max speed and collect supernatant.

(e) Precipitate the RNA as described in Subheading 3.2.3. Elute in 7 μL nuclease free water.

4. Reverse transcribe according to the Illumina TruSeq Small RNA Library Prep Guide.
5. Perform PCR amplification according to the manufacturer's recommendations (11–15 cycles).

3.3.3 Library Cleanup

Adjust sample volume to 100 μL and clean the PCR product with AMPure XP beads (1.8:1 ratio) following the manufacturer's recommendations.

3.3.4 Library Validation and Next Generation Sequencing

Validate the quality and size of the library and submit the library for sequencing on an Illumina platform. Check the requirements of your next generation sequencing facility for the correct concentration.

3.4 Bioinformatic Analysis

1. Adapter and quality trim (Phred score 20) the reads and remove short fragments (<20) (Trim_galore).
2. Align reads to a computationally bisulfite-converted reference genome (GRCh38) with Bismark (using Bowtie2).
3. Compare conversion rate of fCAB RNA-Seq and RedBS RNA-Seq with conversion levels of standard bisulfite-treated sample.

4 Notes

1. It is crucial that all buffers and reagents are RNase free. Diethylpyrocarbonate (DEPC)-treated ultrapure water should be used. All equipment is treated with RNaseZap (Ambion) before use. Sterile RNase-free filter tips should be used to prevent degradation of RNA.
2. Care should be taken that all procedures are performed in an RNase-free environment (*see* also **Note 1**). Thaw all reagents on ice. Experiments are performed on room temperature unless otherwise specified.
3. Approximately 80% of the total RNA in rapidly growing mammalian cells is rRNA. Unless specific studies of rRNA are intended, rRNA depletion is highly recommended. Although the protocol works with a lower RNA input, a higher input gives a better-quality library after treatment.
4. The amount of total RNA per tube should not exceed 5 μg. For each sample we perform three individual rRNA depletion reactions (rather than one reaction combining all samples) and pool the remaining RNA back together (to avoid variation between the tubes). Alternatively, other rRNA depletion kits can be used e.g. NEBNext rRNA Depletion Kit (NEB).

5. $NaBH_4$ solution is prepared by adding 1.5 mg of $NaBH_4$ in 1 mL of anhydrous methanol, with vortexing until the entire solid dissolved. Bubbles can be observed; open lid regularly to release any pressure.
6. Since sodium acetate (used for RNA precipitation) quenches the reaction, it is important to immediately continue with the RNA precipitation after incubation.
7. The names of the buffers, products, and mixes used here are the names used in the Imprint DNA Modification Kit (Sigma Aldrich).
8. One column might not be enough to fully desalt the sample. Therefore, two micro bio-spin columns per sample could be needed.
9. Alternatively, T4 PNK buffer could be used, if extra ATP is added.
10. Bisulfite treatment tends to fragment RNA, so there will be a faint smear with sometimes, but not always, some faint but distinct bands. Use the entire region above 140 nt in size to capture all RNA, while removing adaptor only fragments that are 120 nt in size.
11. Since elution is diffusion-based, it is crucial that the fragments are cut into tiny pieces (max 1 mm^3).

Acknowledgements

Medical Research Council, UK (MC_UU_00015/4) is acknowledged for the support of our work.

References

1. Rebelo-Guiomar P, Powell CA, Van Haute L et al (2018) The mammalian mitochondrial epitranscriptome. Biochim Biophys Acta Gene Regul Mech 1862:429
2. Delaunay S, Frye M (2019) RNA modifications regulating cell fate in cancer. Nat Cell Biol 21:552–559
3. Boccaletto P, Machnicka MA, Purta E et al (2018) MODOMICS: a database of RNA modification pathways. 2017 update. Nucleic Acids Res 46:D303–D307
4. Booth MJ, Marsico G, Bachman M et al (2014) Quantitative sequencing of 5-formylcytosine in DNA at single-base resolution. Nat Chem 6:435–440
5. Plongthongkum N, Diep DH, Zhang K (2014) Advances in the profiling of DNA modifications: cytosine methylation and beyond. Nat Rev Genet 15:647–661
6. Song CX, Szulwach KE, Dai Q et al (2013) Genome-wide profiling of 5-formylcytosine reveals its roles in epigenetic priming. Cell 153:678–691
7. Moriya J, Yokogawa T, Wakita K et al (1994) A novel modified nucleoside found at the first position of the anticodon of methionine tRNA from bovine liver mitochondria. Biochemistry 33:2234–2239
8. Pais de Barros JP, Keith G, El Adlouni C et al (1996) 2′-O-methyl-5-formylcytidine (f5Cm), a new modified nucleotide at the 'wobble' of two cytoplasmic tRNAs Leu (NAA) from bovine liver. Nucleic Acids Res 24:1489–1496
9. Brzezicha B, Schmidt M, Makalowska I et al (2006) Identification of human tRNA:m5C methyltransferase catalysing intron-dependent m5C formation in the first position of the

anticodon of the pre-tRNA Leu (CAA). Nucleic Acids Res 34:6034–6043
10. Blanco S, Dietmann S, Flores JV et al (2014) Aberrant methylation of tRNAs links cellular stress to neuro-developmental disorders. EMBO J 33:2020–2039
11. Trixl L, Amort T, Wille A et al (2018) RNA cytosine methyltransferase Nsun3 regulates embryonic stem cell differentiation by promoting mitochondrial activity. Cell Mol Life Sci 75:1483–1497
12. Haag S, Sloan KE, Ranjan N et al (2016) NSUN3 and ABH1 modify the wobble position of mt-tRNAMet to expand codon recognition in mitochondrial translation. EMBO J 35:2104–2119
13. Nakano S, Suzuki T, Kawarada L et al (2016) NSUN3 methylase initiates 5-formylcytidine biogenesis in human mitochondrial tRNA (Met). Nat Chem Biol 12:546–551
14. Van Haute L, Dietmann S, Kremer L et al (2016) Deficient methylation and formylation of mt-tRNA(Met) wobble cytosine in a patient carrying mutations in NSUN3. Nat Commun 7:12039
15. Van Haute L, Powell CA, Minczuk M (2017) Dealing with an unconventional genetic code in mitochondria: the biogenesis and pathogenic defects of the 5-formylcytosine modification in mitochondrial tRNA(Met). Biomolecules 7:E24
16. Samanta B, Seikowski J, Hobartner C (2016) Fluorogenic labeling of 5-formylpyrimidine nucleotides in DNA and RNA. Angew Chem Int Ed Eng 55:1912–1916
17. Minczuk M, He J, Duch AM et al (2011) TEFM (c17orf42) is necessary for transcription of human mtDNA. Nucleic Acids Res 39:4284–4299
18. Kawarada L, Suzuki T, Ohira T et al (2017) ALKBH1 is an RNA dioxygenase responsible for cytoplasmic and mitochondrial tRNA modifications. Nucleic Acids Res 45:7401–7415

Chapter 6

Visualization of Mitochondrial RNA Granules in Cultured Cells Using 5-Bromouridine Labeling

Vanessa Joanne Xavier and Jean-Claude Martinou

Abstract

The incorporation of nucleoside analogs is a useful tool to study the various functions of DNA and RNA. These analogs can be detected directly by fluorescence or by immunolabeling, allowing to visualize, track, or measure the nucleic acid molecules in which they have been incorporated. In this chapter, methodologies to measure human mitochondrial transcription are described. The nascent RNA that is transcribed from mitochondrial DNA (mtDNA) has been shown to assemble into large ribonucleoprotein complexes that form discrete foci. These structures were called mitochondrial RNA granules (MRGs) and can be observed in vitro by the incorporation of a 5-Bromouridine (BrU), which is subsequently visualized by fluorescent immunolabeling. Here, a combined protocol for the MRGs detection is detailed, consisting of BrU labeling and visualization of one of their *bona fide* protein components, Fas-activated serine-threonine kinase domain 2 (FASTKD2). Based on immunodetection, the half-life and kinetics of the MRGs under various experimental conditions can further be determined by chasing the BrU pulse with an excess of Uridine.

Key words Mitochondrial RNA Granules (MRGs), Mitochondrial transcription, Mitochondrial DNA, Nascent RNA, 5-Bromouridine, Uridine, Immunofluorescence, Pulse-chase, Half-life

1 Introduction

The human mitochondrion contains its own, highly compacted 16.5 kb genome which codes for 22 tRNAs, two ribosomal RNAs, and 13 polypeptides that form subunits of the electron transport chain complexes and ATP synthase. The mtDNA is transcribed into two long polycistronic RNA molecules that are further processed into functional transcripts. Endonucleolytic processing and maturation of these transcripts are likely to occur within MRGs since many of the enzymes required for these processes are localized within these structures. The MRGs are membraneless subvikely displaying physical properties of liquid-like droplets [7]. They can be detected microscopically, by either immunolabeling of one of its protein components, or using BrU immunolabeling. Unlike 5-Bromouridine triphosphate (BrUTP), BrU can be added directly to the

Michal Minczuk and Joanna Rorbach (eds.), *Mitochondrial Gene Expression: Methods and Protocols*, Methods in Molecular Biology, vol. 2192, https://doi.org/10.1007/978-1-0716-0834-0_6,

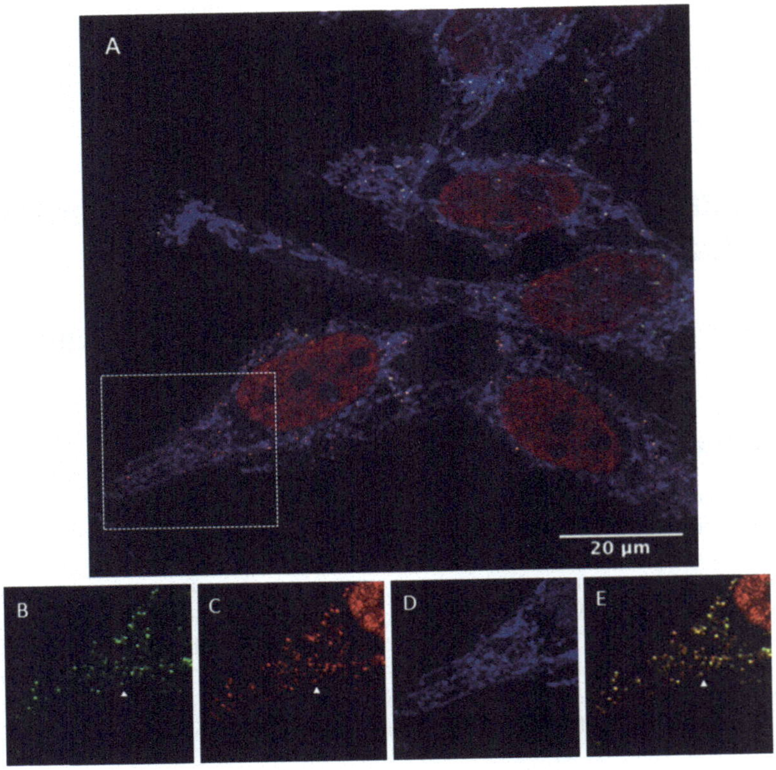

Fig. 1 Confocal analysis of MRGs in HeLa cells. (**a**) Composite image of MRGs labeled with FASTKD2 in green colocalizing with BrU in red, within the mitochondrial network stained with MitoTracker DeepRed in blue. (**b**–**d**) Zoomed image of FASTKD2, BrU, and Mitochondria, respectively. (**e**) Zoomed image of the colocalization between FASTKD2 and BrU. White arrowheads indicate a single MRG

culture media, where it is readily taken up by growing cells. The ribonucleotide salvage pathway in cells ensures that the BrU is included into the pool of nucleotide phosphates that is primed for nucleic acid synthesis [8]. For most cultured cancer cell lines, an hour pulse of BrU, followed by immunolabeling is sufficient for MRG foci to be observed along the mitochondrial network in a characteristic "beads on a string" formation (Fig. 1).

The BrU appears to be incorporated into nascent RNA as long as it is present in the culture medium and is in excess over endogenous uridine. Following its removal from the culture medium or addition of an excess of unlabeled uridine, the latter is preferentially used for transcription. This technique called pulse-chase labeling allows to measure the half-life of nascent transcripts. The half-lives of MRGs in T24 cells [1] and in 143B [2] have been shown to be approximately 43 min and 50 min, respectively. A perturbation in the mitochondrial transcription machinery has been previously shown to result in a longer half-life of MRGs, implying that the rate of transcription and degradation of RNA are tightly linked [2].

2 Materials

2.1 Cell Culture

1. 10% DMEM Cell culture media for HeLa cells: Dulbecco's modified Eagle medium (DMEM) supplemented with 10% heat-inactivated fetal bovine serum, 100 μg/mL of streptomycin, 100 U/mL of penicillin and 2 mM L-glutamine.
2. Trypsin-EDTA.
3. Sterile Phosphate Buffered Saline (PBS).
4. Coverslips (12 mm in diameter).

2.2 Incorporation of 5-Bromouridine (BrU) and Uridine

1. 0.25 M, 50× stock solution of 5-Bromouridine dissolved in PBS, sterile filtered.
2. 1.25 M, 50× stock solution of uridine dissolved in PBS, sterile filtered.

2.3 Immunofluorescence

1. 4% Paraformaldehyde (PFA) solution, pH 6.9.
2. IF buffer: 0.1% Triton X-100, 5% Normal Goat Serum in PBS.
3. Mitotracker DeepRed FM (Thermo Fisher M22426).
4. Primary Antibodies: Anti-FASTKD2 Rabbit polyclonal (Proteintech 17464-1-AP), Anti-Bromodeoxyuridine mouse IgG_1 (Merck Clone: BMC93189).
5. Fluorescent tag conjugated Secondary Antibodies: Goat anti-Rabbit IgG (H+L) Highly Cross-Adsorbed Secondary Antibody conjugated with Alexa Fluor 488 (Invitrogen A-11034), Goat anti-Mouse IgG (H+L) Cross-Adsorbed Secondary Antibody conjugated with Alexa Fluor 594 (Invitrogen A-11005).
6. Mounting Reagent.
7. Opaque Humidifying Chamber lined with parafilm.

3 Methods

3.1 Visualization of MRGs by Immunofluorescence

1. Culture HeLa cells in 10% DMEM within an incubator supplied with 5% CO_2 at 37 °C and harvest them by trypsinization when they are 60% confluent. Count and adjust the cell number so that 0.3×10^5 cells are seeded on each coverslip. Allow cells to attach overnight (*see* **Note 1**).
2. The next day, aspirate the spent media and refresh cells with a 1:50 dilution of the 0.25 M stock of BrU in 10% DMEM, at the final concentration of 5 mM. Return the cells to the incubator for 1 h (*see* **Note 2**).
3. After 40 min, add MitoTracker DeepRed to the cells at the final working concentration of 200 nM. Return the cells to the incubator to complete the final 20 min of the BrU pulse.

4. At the end of the BrU pulse, aspirate the medium.
5. Immediately add pre-warmed (37 °C) 4% PFA to the cell monolayer and incubate for 15 min at room temperature (*see* **Note 3**).
6. Remove the PFA and wash the cell monolayer with room temperature PBS, 3 times.
7. Place the coverslips in a humidifying chamber and add IF buffer onto the coverslips for 30 min at room temperature to block and permeabilize the sample.
8. Dilute the primary antibodies in the IF buffer. Use the anti-Bromodeoxyuridine antibody at a dilution of 1:200 and the anti-FASTKD2 antibody at a dilution of 1:300. Apply this solution onto the coverslips for 1.5 h at room temperature (*see* **Note 5**).
9. Wash the coverslip with PBS, 3 times for 5 min each.
10. Dilute the secondary antibodies in the IF buffer at a dilution of 1:1000 and apply it onto the coverslips for 1 h at room temperature.
11. Wash the coverslips with PBS, 3 times for 5 min each.
12. Rinse the coverslips in water, blot dry, and mount onto a glass slide and leave to set overnight before microscopic analysis.

3.2 5-Bromouridine Pulse: Uridine Chase Experiments

1. Perform **steps 1** and **2** of Subheading 3.1 for quadruplicate coverslips.
2. After the BrU pulse, wash cells twice with culture medium before refreshing with culture medium containing a 1:50 dilution of 1.25 M uridine. This will bring the final concentration of uridine to 25 mM.
3. Incubate the cells individually with uridine for 0, 30, 90, and 180 min.
4. At the end of the pulse-chase, stain the cells with Mitotracker, fix, and immunolabel for BrU as described in **steps 5–12** of Subheading 3.1 before microscopic analysis.
5. Count the number of BrU foci within the mitochondrial network at each time point of the Uridine chase. Determine the half-life of the granules by the time it takes 50% of the original number of granules to disaggregate.

4 Notes

1. Cells for MRG labeling should be seeded such that a confluency of 60% can be achieved before sample preparation. This is to ensure that there is sufficient surface area for the

mitochondrial network of each cell to be spread out clearly within the cell body. In addition, cell confluency may alter mitochondrial activity.

2. The BrU solution often precipitates out when thawed from −20 °C. It should be warmed up to 37 °C and vortexed before use.
3. Add the appropriate amount of PFA for culture dish, ensuring that the cell monolayer is fully covered.
4. A clean, specific labeling of the mitochondria is useful in distinguishing BrU-labeled MRGs. Therefore, using a mitochondrial dye, such as MitoTracker or immunolabeling the mitochondria in conjunction with BrU is recommended.
5. Another MRG protein, G-rich sequence factor 1 (GRSF1) can be used effectively for immunolabeling MRG foci as well (Sigma HPA036985).
6. This protocol was not effective in labeling the MRGs in Mouse Embryonic Fibroblasts and therefore is not optimized for use in murine cells.
7. Performing a "Z stack" step-wise image acquisition with confocal microscopy is more suitable for imaging the MRGs which lie on various planes along the mitochondrial network.

References

1. Iborra FJ, Kimura H, Cook PR (2004) The functional organization of mitochondrial genomes in human cells. BMC Biol 2(1):9
2. Jourdain A, Koppen M, Wydro M, Rodley C, Lightowlers R, Chrzanowska-Lightowlers Z, Martinou J (2013) GRSF1 regulates RNA processing in mitochondrial RNA granules. Cell Metab 17(3):399–410
3. Antonicka H, Sasarman F, Nishimura T, Paupe V, Shoubridge E (2013) The mitochondrial RNA-binding protein GRSF1 localizes to RNA granules and is required for posttranscriptional mitochondrial gene expression. Cell Metab 17(3):386–398
4. Jourdain A, Koppen M, Rodley C, Maundrell K, Gueguen N, Reynier P, Martinou J (2015) A mitochondria-specific isoform of FASTK is present in mitochondrial RNA granules and regulates gene expression and function. Cell Rep 10(7):1110–1121
5. Antonicka H, Shoubridge E (2015) Mitochondrial RNA granules are centers for posttranscriptional RNA processing and ribosome biogenesis. Cell Rep 10(6):920–932
6. Tu Y, Barrientos A (2015) The human mitochondrial DEAD-box protein DDX28 resides in RNA granules and functions in mitoribosome assembly. Cell Rep 10(6):854–864
7. Jourdain AA, Boehm E, Maundrell K, Martinou J (2016) Mitochondrial RNA granules: compartmentalizing mitochondrial gene expression. J Cell Biol 212(6):611–614
8. Jao CY, Salic A (2008) Exploring RNA transcription and turnover in vivo by using click chemistry. PNAS 105(41):15779–15784

Chapter 7

Quantitative Proteomics in *Drosophila* with Holidic Stable-Isotope Labeling of Amino Acids in Fruit Flies (SILAF)

Florian A. Schober, Ilian Atanassov, Christoph Freyer, and Anna Wredenberg

Abstract

Protein-focused research has been challenging in *Drosophila melanogaster* due to few specific antibodies for Western blotting and the lack of effective labeling methods for quantitative proteomics. Herein, we describe the preparation of a holidic medium that allows stable-isotope labeling of amino acids in fruit flies (SILAF). Furthermore, in this chapter, we provide a protocol for mitochondrial enrichments from *Drosophila* larvae and flies together with a procedure to generate high-quality peptides for further analysis by mass spectrometry. Samples obtained following this protocol can be used for various functional studies such as comprehensive proteome profiling or quantitative analysis of posttranslational modifications upon enrichment. SILAF is based on standard fly routines in a basic wet lab environment and provides a flexible and cost-effective tool for quantitative protein expression analysis.

Key words Drosophila, Proteomics, Stable-isotope labeling, SILAC, Mitochondria

1 Introduction

Stable-isotope labeling of amino acids in cell culture (SILAC) has been a powerful method to quantitatively assess protein content by high-resolution mass spectrometry (MS). In its original application, cells are grown in a medium that contains one or more non-radioactive isotopes of amino acids [1], typically leucine, lysine, and/or arginine. Upon incorporation of a heavy amino acid isotope during translation, a protein gains discrete mass and its peptides can be distinguished from light isotopic counterparts during an MS analysis. This allows the measurement of two or more differently labeled samples at the same time. Although protein quantification in single-shot experiments can now be performed cheaper and easier by label-free quantification, a broad range of experiments are typically performed with or require SILAC, among

Michal Minczuk and Joanna Rorbach (eds.), *Mitochondrial Gene Expression: Methods and Protocols*, Methods in Molecular Biology, vol. 2192, https://doi.org/10.1007/978-1-0716-0834-0_7, © The Author(s) 2021

those deep quantitative proteome profiling using fractionation, differential posttranslational modification quantification, immunoprecipitation, and turnover studies [2].

SILAC has been adapted to a range of multicellular models, including worms [3] and mice [4]. For *Drosophila melanogaster*, the fruit fly, a SILAC method was proposed in 2010 [5] and subsequently developed further [6, 7]. It relied on labeling of yeast cells with a lysine isotope, which is then fed to flies. To decrease costs and increase labeling efficiency, we developed stable-isotope labeling of amino acids in fruit flies (SILAF) that is based on a holidic medium with purified ingredients [8, 9]. By replacing "light" L-Lysine-$^{12}C_6$ (lysine-0) with "heavy" L-Lysine-$^{13}C_6$ (lysine-6), we achieve full labeling already at larval stage 2, which, when combined with peptide fractionation, allows differential quantification of more than 4500 proteins. This is due to the high accuracy of SILAC as samples are combined early on in the experiment. Furthermore, it is possible to measure protein turnover rates in whole adult flies with a labeling pulse. Combined with mitochondrial enrichment, this technique allows deep insights into the mitochondrial fly proteome across a wide dynamic range, comprising nuclear-encoded proteins and mitochondrial-encoded subunits of the oxidative phosphorylation system.

2 Materials

2.1 Yeast Medium

Drosophila are grown on standard yeast medium prior to labeling on holidic food. Media are prepared in deionized water.

1. Stove and a large pot.
2. Plastic tubes, clear, flat bottom.
3. Cotton balls to fit the size of the plastic tubes.
4. Cotton blanket.
5. Gum agar.
6. Sucrose.
7. Powdered yeast.
8. Preservatives: 100 g/L methylparaben in 100% ethanol, propionic acid. Protect from light.

2.2 Holidic Lysine-0 and Lysine-6 Media

Stock solutions are prepared in purified, deionised water, such as Milli-Q® grade water, if not indicated differently (*see* **Note 1**). The provided amounts of stock solutions are best for preparations of

100 mL media at a time. All stock solutions should be renewed at least every 3 months.

1. Heating block with shaking function.
2. Autoclave.
3. 100 mL autoclavable glass bottle with lid.
4. Small stirrer and stirring plate.
5. Plastic tubes, clear, flat bottom, for fly husbandry.
6. Cotton balls to fit the size of the plastic tubes.
7. Syringe filters for sterile filtering.
8. Fine balance with 0.1 mg accuracy.
9. Difco™ agar.
10. Sucrose.
11. Cholesterol at 20 g/L in 100% ethanol, prepare fresh.
12. Metal ions: $CaCl_2 \cdot 6H_2O$ (250 g/L), anhydrous $MgSO_4$ (250 g/L), $CuSO_4 \cdot 5H_2O$ (2.5 g/L), $FeSO_4 \cdot 7H_2O$ (25 g/L), $MnCl_2 \cdot 4H_2O$ (1 g/L), $ZnSO_4 \cdot 7H_2O$ (25 g/L). Aliquot individually 110 μL into PCR strips and store at −20 °C (*see* **Note 2**).
13. Acetate buffer: 3% acetic acid, KH_2PO_4 (30 g/L), $NaHCO_3$ (10 g/L), pH 4.0 (*see* **Notes 3** and **4**). Filter sterilize through a syringe filter and store aliquots of 11 mL at 4 °C.
14. Essential amino acid stock: L-Arginine (26.92 g/L), L-Histidine (10.79 g/L), L-Methionine (9.96 g/L), L-Phenylalanine (16.65 g/L), L-Threonine (18.27 g/L), L-Tryptophan (5.30 g/L), L-Valine (19.81 g/L). Titrate to pH 4.5, filter sterilize and store aliquots of 6.5 mL at 4 °C (*see* **Note 5**).
15. Nonessential amino acid stock: L-Alanine (18.18 g/L), L-Asparagine (16.99 g/L,), L-Aspartic acid (19.34 g/L), L-Glutamine (18.50 g/L), Glycine (12.66 g/L), L-Proline (16.14 g/L), L-Serine (22.74 g/L). Titrate to pH 4.5, filter sterilize and store aliquots of 6.5 mL at 4 °C (*see* **Note 5**).
16. Vitamin stock: Thiamine (0.067 g/L), Riboflavin (0.033 g/L), Nicotinic acid (0.399 g/L), Calcium pantothenate (0.516 g/L), Pyridoxine (0.083 g/L), Biotin (0.007 g/L). Store aliquots of 2.2 mL at −20 °C away from light.
17. Folic acid solution: folic acid (0.5 g/L). Aliquot to 110 μL in PCR strips and store at −20 °C (*see* **Note 6**).
18. Nucleic acids/lipids: choline chloride (6.25 g/L), myo-inositol (0.63 g/L), inosine (8.13 g/L), uridine (7.5 g/L). Filter sterilize and store aliquots of 750 μL at 4 °C.
19. L-Glutamic acid (100 g/L). Filter sterilize and store aliquots of 1.6 mL at 4 °C.

20. Additional amino acids as powders: L-Isoleucine, L-Leucine, L-Tyrosine, L-Cysteine.
21. Preservatives: 100 g/L methylparaben in 100% ethanol, propionic acid. Protect from light.
22. Lysine isotopes as powders: L-Lysine-$^{12}C_6$ · HCL ("light lysine-0"), L-Lysine-[$^{13}C[4/_6]^{15}N[0/_0]$] · HCL ("heavy lysine-6") (*see* **Note 7**).

2.3 Mitochondrial Enrichment

1. Petri dishes.
2. Soft paint brush with about 4 mm top diameter.
3. Pasteur pipettes.
4. STE buffer: 250 mM Sucrose, 2 mM EGTA, 5 mM Tris. Titrate to pH 7.4 and store at 4 °C (*see* **Note 8**).
5. Powdered bovine serum albumin (BSA).
6. 2 mL round-bottom glass homogenizers with tightly fitting Teflon-coated pestle.
7. Electrical homogenizer with adjustable speed.
8. 1.5 and 2.0 mL protein low-binding tubes.
9. Bench-top high-speed centrifuge with adjustable temperature and fixed-angle rotor for 1.5 and 2 mL tubes for up to 9000 × *g*.

2.4 Peptide Sample Preparation

1. Sterile inoculation needle.
2. Liquid nitrogen.
3. Petri dishes.
4. 6 M guanidine hydrochloride (GuHCl), fresh in 100 mM ammonium bicarbonate, pH 8.0.
5. Homogenizer and pestles, fitting to the inner shape of a 1.5 mL tube.
6. Sonicator.
7. Protein quantification assay that has been tested insensitive to <1 M GuHCl, for example BCA.
8. Dithiothreitol.
9. 2-chloroacetamide, protected from light.
10. 100 mM ammonium bicarbonate, pH 8.0.
11. Lysyl endopeptidase LysC, MS grade.
12. Formic acid.
13. Disposable 3 mL cartridges with a C18 disk.
14. Syringe prepared to fit the 3 mL C18 cartridge (*see* **Note 9**).

15. Methanol.
16. 40% acetonitrile in water.
17. SpeedVac or similar.
18. NanoDrop™ spectrophotometer or similar.

3 Methods

3.1 Preparation of Yeast Medium for Fly Husbandry Prior to Labeling

1. 10 g of agar are stirred in 1 L of room temperature deionised water and brought to boil in a large pot.
2. 50 g of sucrose and 100 g of yeast powder are added while stirring with a whisk and boiled for 5 min.
3. The liquid medium is allowed to cool down to 40–45 °C. Stir at least once per hour to prevent the yeast from setting.
4. Add 30 mL methylparaben stock solution and 3 mL propionic acid to the yeast medium and stir.
5. With a 25 mL serological pipette, 6 mL food is dispersed into round, clear, flat-bottom plastic vials. Stir the food in the pot several times while aliquoting. After aliquoting, the filled plastic vials are covered with a cotton blanket and left to solidify overnight.
6. The vials are plugged with cotton balls that fit the size of the vials.
7. Food is stored at 4 °C for up to 2 weeks.

3.2 Preparation of Holidic SILAF Medium

In order to prepare holidic SILAF medium, take measures to work in a semi-sterile lab environment (*see* **Note 10**). A flowchart of the procedure is shown in Fig. 1a.

1. Thaw one 100 μL aliquot of each metal solution ($CaCl_2$, $MgSO_4$, $CuSO_4$, $FeSO_4$, $MnCl_2$, and $ZnSO_4$).
2. Prepare 1.5–2 mL of a 20 mg/mL cholesterol solution in 100% ethanol and heat to 50 °C while shaking at 1000 rpm.
3. Measure 69.1 g of room temperature deionised water in a 100 mL autoclavable glass bottle with a small magnetic stirrer and mark the top liquid height with a pen on the glass. Decant about 30% of the water. Place the bottle on a magnetic stirring plate.
4. Add 112 mg L-isoleucine, 203 mg L-leucine, and 93 mg L-tyrosine to the bottle while the stirrer is rotating, as well as 1.71 g sucrose and 2 g agar.
5. Add 100 μL of each metal solution, as well as 1.5 mL of cholesterol in ethanol (*see* **Note 11**).

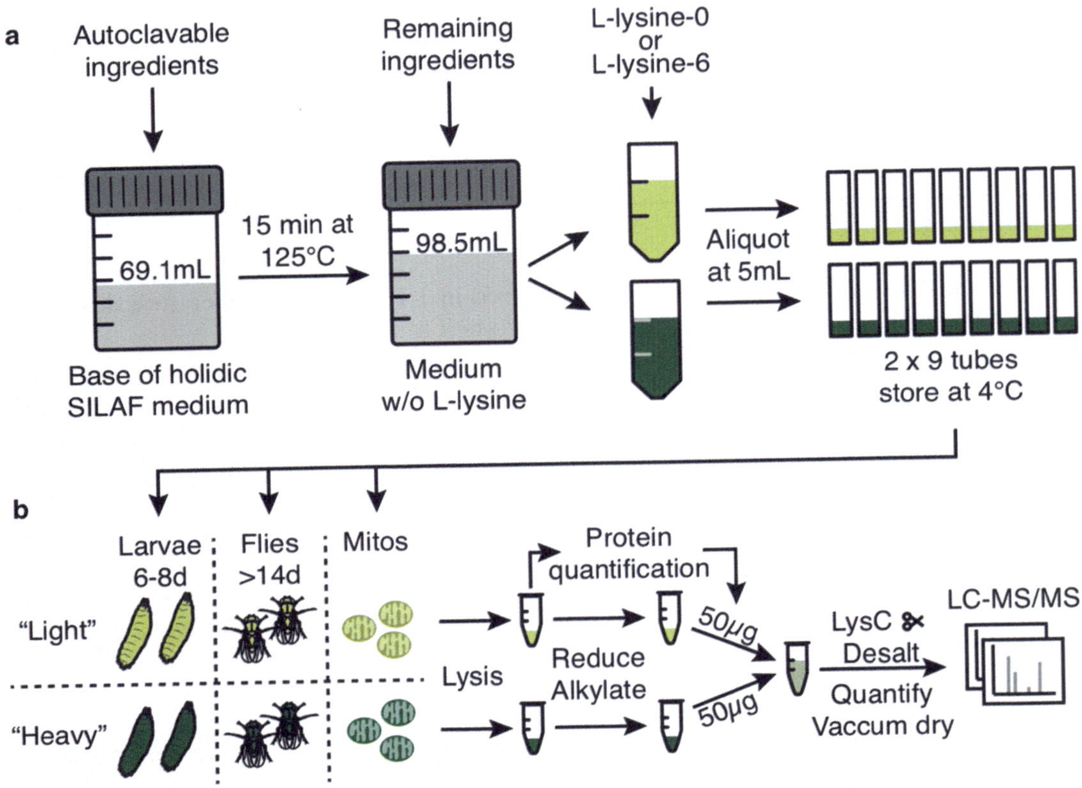

Fig. 1 A typical workflow for (**a**) the preparation of "light" and "heavy" holidic food and (**b**) the generation of SILAF peptide samples after larvae or flies have been grown to a fully labeled state from larval stage 2 or mitochondria (mitos) have been enriched

6. Stop stirring and fill the buffer to the mark with room temperature deionized water.
7. Autoclave the food base at 125 °C for 15 min after the final pressure has been reached, then switch off the autoclave and wait until the food base is cooled to about 80 °C.
8. In the meanwhile, prepare further required solutions: thaw vitamins and folic acid protected from light; weigh 6.815 mg per 5 mL of food of lysine-0 and 8.793 mg per 5 mL of food of lysine-6, and suspend each in 75 μL of deionized water per 5 mL of food (*see* **Note 12**); make a 50 mg/mL solution of L-cysteine in deionized water.
9. Heat a water bath to 50 °C with two 50 mL tubes required for final mixing.
10. Place the 80 °C warm holidic food base on a stirrer and let it cool to 50–60 °C. Add 10 mL of acetate buffer (*see* **Note 13**), 800 μL of nucleic acid/lipid solution, 6.05 mL of essential amino acids and nonessential amino acid solution each,

1.52 mL L-glutamate solution, 683 μL L-cysteine solution, 2.1 mL vitamins, 100 μL folic acid, 600 μL propionic acid, and 1.5 mL methylparaben solution (*see* **Note 14**).

11. Add 75 μL per 5 mL final food volume of lysine-0 or lysine-6 to one of the labeled 50 mL tube in the water bath. Using the graduation, fill up to the required final volume with holidic medium (*see* **Note 15**), cap and shake vigorously. Place the tube back in the water bath for 1 min to remove bubbles.
12. Aliquot 5 mL each into pre-labeled vials. Protect those with a piece of paper tissue and let them cool down for 90 min to overnight. Plug with cotton balls and store at 4 °C for up to 1 week (*see* **Note 16**).

3.3 Fly Husbandry for Quantitative Proteomics

1. Set the relevant crosses first on yeast medium (*see* **Note 17**). When maximum fecundity is expected, put flies to lay on either light or heavy SILAF medium for the desired amount of time (*see* **Note 18**) at a temperature and humidity of choice (*see* **Note 19**), typically 25 °C and 60% humidity with a 12/12-h light/dark cycle.
2. Grow larvae until at least larval stage 2 to achieve >95% to complete labeling (*see* **Note 20**) with lysine-6. We typically choose day 7 for collecting larval samples as larvae are not climbing yet but in L3 stage and are labeled close to the lysine-6 purity extent. Flies hatch at 2 weeks after egg lay.
3. Either perform a mitochondrial enrichment as described in Subheading 3.4 or collect samples for whole tissue proteomics. For the latter, pick larvae with a sterile inoculation needle and gloves. Rinse off food remnants in a Petri dish with distilled water and dry larvae with a corner of paper tissue. Anesthetize flies with carbon dioxide. When performing full-body proteomics we prefer to analyze male, nonvirgin flies in order to avoid any bias caused by egg-carrying females. Transfer to a 1.5 mL low-binding tube, conveniently five to ten insects per tube, snap freeze in liquid nitrogen and store at −80 °C until further processing.

3.4 Mitochondrial Enrichment

Mitochondria are best prepared from larvae as their tissue is softer than flies and thus easier to homogenize. Further, mitochondrial enrichments from flies are more difficult to clean as cuticles and wing fragments tend to float and co-enrich with mitochondria (*see* **Note 21**).

1. Solubilize 5% BSA in STE buffer (STE + BSA buffer), calculating 10 mL per sample. This buffer should always be freshly prepared.
2. Place the glass homogenizer, an aliquot of STE buffer (10 mL per sample), and the STE + BSA buffer in an ice bucket.

3. Layer 3 cm of room temperature, deionized water onto food in vials with larvae and wait for 5 min. Then use a soft paint brush to swirl off larvae from the food. Swirl the tube and pour larvae and liquid into a Petri dish.
4. Pick 10–30 larvae of each label (*see* **Note 22**) with the brush into a precooled, labeled 2 mL glass homogenizer with 2 mL of cold STE + BSA buffer (*see* **Note 23**). Swirl larvae using the brush and take off most of the liquid with a Pasteur pipette. Subsequently add 1 mL of cold, fresh STE-BSA.
5. Place a Teflon-coated pestle into the glass vessel and gently homogenize larvae with 14 strokes at 700 rpm. Keep cold on ice before, during and after homogenization.
6. Pipette the homogenate into a precooled 2 mL protein low-binding tube and centrifuge at 1000 × *g* for 5 min at 4 °C.
7. Nuclei, not disrupted cells and larger larval fragments will be collected in the pellet at the bottom. Without disrupting this pellet, transfer the supernatant containing mitochondria into a new, cold 1.5 mL protein low-binding tube. Centrifuge at 3000 × *g* for 10 min at 4 °C.
8. Discard the supernatant and gently wash the mitochondrial pellet with 1 mL of cold STE + BSA (*see* **Note 24**). Centrifuge again at 3000 × *g* for 10 min at 4 °C.
9. Discard the supernatant and gently wash the mitochondrial pellet with 1 mL of cold STE buffer *without* BSA. Centrifuge at 9000 × *g* for 5 min at 4 °C.
10. Discard the supernatant and spin down remaining liquid with a short pulse at 9000 × *g* and 4 °C. Take of the remaining supernatant with a 10/20 μL tip and freeze the pellet at −80 °C.

3.5 Peptide Sample Preparation

We appreciate that there are multiple ways of preparing peptides from frozen samples, including 1D SDS-PAGE fractionation and in-gel digestion. For this, a comprehensive pipeline can be found in [10]. We find good protein coverage of mitochondrial, larval and fly samples using the herein provided protocol, sketched in Fig. 1b. The mixing strategy can be modified to fit the experimental needs (*see* **Note 25**), below we present the simplest approach.

1. Move samples from −80 °C to a room temperature rack and cover with 200 μL 6 M GuHCl in 100 mM ammonium bicarbonate, pH 8.0. If working with larvae or flies, then homogenize all samples for about 10 s with Teflon pestles that fit the conical shape of a 1.5 mL tube. If working with mitochondria, resuspend the mitochondrial pellet in GuHCl buffer until it turns clear without any remaining clumps. Incubate samples at room temperature for 10 min.

2. Sonicate four times at a 10 s on/off cycle in cold water and incubate for further 10 min at room temperature.
3. Centrifuge tubes for 5 min at maximum speed >10,000 × *g* for 5 min. Transfer 180 μL of supernatant to a new 1.5 mL low-binding tube. Make sure not to take wings or cuticles when working with flies. If unavoidable, centrifuge again or remove larger particles with a 10 μL tip.
4. Dilute 2 μL of transferred supernatant in water and quantify with BCA protein assay (*see* **Note 26**) so that quantification results can be obtained after 45 min.
5. Reduce the remaining protein-containing supernatant with 9 μL of freshly prepared 100 mM dithiothreitol in water for 30 min at 55 °C with mild shaking. Place the tube on ice for 10 s to cool to room temperature, add 10 μL of fresh 300 mM 2-chloroacetamide in water and alkylate at room temperature without light for 15 min.
6. Calculate the volume needed for 50 μg of protein in each sample and mix 50 μg of each light and heavy fraction in a new 2.0 mL tube. Fill up to 1.8 mL with 100 mM ammonium bicarbonate buffer pH 8.0 to reduce the GuHCl concentration to <1 M. Add 1–2 μg of mass-spectrometry grade lysyl endopeptidase LysC in the manufacturer's recommended resuspension buffer and incubate at 37 °C overnight for a maximum of 18 h and mild shaking.
7. Next day, some white precipitates may have formed. Acidify samples by adding 1.2% formic acid (*see* **Note 27**) in a hood and spin at 3000 × *g* and room temperature for 10 min to pellet the precipitates.
8. Desalt the supernatant on a 3 mL cartridge containing a C18 disk according to the manufacturer's recommendations (*see* **Note 28**). Typically, we condition the column with 200 μL of methanol and equilibrate with 500 μL water. The sample is applied and the flowthough is collected in the original tube. Washes include: first wash 1 mL of acidified sample buffer (100 mM ammonium bicarbonate), second wash 500 μL of water, and third wash 500 μL 0.5% formic acid in water. Peptides are eluted with 300 μL 40% acetonitrile in water two times by pushing all of the acetonitrile/water solution through the disk into a new 1.5 mL low-binding tube.
9. The eluate of 600 μL is dried in a SpeedVac at room temperature. Be careful to not over-dry the peptide pellets.

10. Pellets are dissolved in 20 μL 0.5% formic acid for 10 min at room temperature and 1 μL is quantified on a NanoDrop photospectrometer. The shape of the curve is inspected (*see* **Note 29**) and the peptide amount in the remaining 19 μL is calculated. An anticipated amount with 100 μg of input material for light plus heavy is 20–30 μg. The solution is dried in a SpeedVac again and stored at −80 °C until sent to a proteomics facility on dry ice.

4 Notes

1. We use the holidic FLYAA food composition described by Piper et al. [9].
2. $FeSO_4$ oxidizes rapidly in liquid water and precipitates as rust. Freeze quickly and use directly after thawing.
3. Use a vessel much larger than the anticipated amount of buffer and add $NaHCO_3$ slowly to the buffer. CO_2 release might make liquid spill.
4. The acetate buffer should reach its pH after addition of all reagents and we normally do not titrate it. If profoundly off, an ingredient might be wrong or missing.
5. We usually prepare 50 mL of non-/essential amino acid stocks, which is sufficient for 700 mL holidic food. Allow sufficient time for weighing and dissolving.
6. Folic acid can require dropwise addition of 1 M NaOH in order to dissolve.
7. The price of lysine-6 can be quite high. We found that custom bulk orders of up to 1 mg were usually much cheaper than default prices with a lower price limit of 8 € per 99.5% pure lysine-6 per fly vial of holidic food.
8. A 1 L stock of STE buffer is most convenient. The pH of the buffer can be readily adjusted after the initial preparation. Note that the buffer capacity deceases rapidly below 7 and the pH of 7.4 will have to be re-measured and eventually adjusted before every mitochondrial preparation. Use a pH meter with a glass electrode and not paper strips as the colorimetric readout would be off by orders of magnitude due to the buffer composition.
9. We use 10 mL disposable plastic syringes with a smooth-going rubber pestle and two 2.5 mL tips that are inversely put together and cut in a way to seal the top of a 3 mL cartridge air-tight. Wash the top of the finished syringe in acetonitrile before use to clean away potential contaminants.

10. Although it is recommended to work as clean as possible on ethanol-wiped surfaces with previously frozen or filtered substances, a sterile environment is not required to achieve complete incorporation of lysine-6. However, the cooking procedures should be re-evaluated for every other metabolite being changed.
11. The cholesterol tends to precipitate easily on rough surfaces. Either add the 1.5 mL of cholesterol in ethanol at once with a <5 mL serological pipette or change plastic tip while pipetting 2×750 μL. Add the cholesterol slowly with the tip submerged in liquid. Small clumps of cholesterol might appear after autoclaving, which can be avoided by careful emulsion and constant stirring.
12. Make sure to use the same molar amounts and not weight per volume for both lysine-0 and lysine-6, which is a final of 9.32 mM and a stock of 620 mM.
13. The original recipe by Piper et al. [8] suggests to add the acetate buffer before autoclaving. However, the food did not solidify well in our hands. This could be solved by adding the buffer after autoclaving.
14. Add the buffer and amino acid stocks slowly to the still liquid food base as the cold solutions can cause clumping.
15. 100 mL of food will not be enough for 50 mL of both light and heavy aliquots. Calculate with maximum 45 mL instead, i.e., nine tubes each.
16. Vials dry quickly, which is visible by cracks between food and plastic vial. If observed, add one to two drops of water to rehydrate the food.
17. The parent fly generation does not have to be pre-labeled to achieve full incorporation of lysine-6 into the larval L2/L3 proteome.
18. Flies lay well on holidic food. Aim for a medium egg density as too populated vials tend to give smaller larvae that climb ahead of time without pupating. Therefore, monitor the egg density during egg lay every 2 h.
19. Take into account that larvae grow differently on holidic food compared to yeast medium. For instance, climbing of wild-type white Dahomey flies at 25 °C and 60% humidity is delayed to 8 days after egg lay compared to standard yeast medium, and hatching occurs after approximately 2 weeks. Furthermore, weak crosses might not be able to develop well on holidic SILAF medium. However, at 18 °C, we found some weak fly stocks to be able to cope better with holidic SILAF medium

than yeast medium. Precise growth conditions have to be evaluated before the actual experiment on light SILAF medium. We did not observe any developmental and proteomic differences between light and heavy flies.

20. If SILAF is to be established in a *Drosophila* laboratory, make sure to run tests on incorporation efficiency by picking larvae from only lysine-6 containing food every 2 days as well as pupae and hatched flies and check the lysine-6/lysine-0 ratio by mass spectrometry.
21. If required, mitochondria can also be enriched from adult flies. In that case, start Subheading 3.4 with **step 4** and perform **step 6** twice. Additionally, we found that a larger tube surface-area-to-volume ratio during differential centrifugation as in a 1.5 mL tube would further help in cleaning the sample.
22. For instance, if control and treated/mutant insects are expected to have the same size and protein content, light and heavy insects can be mixed already at the picking step. The earlier in the process samples are mixed, the more powerful SILAF will be at reducing technical variability.
23. The amount of larvae can be chosen depending on the size of the treated/mutant phenotype so that the amount of control and treated/mutant will be approximately similar at the end of the mitochondrial enrichment.
24. BSA is included in the buffer to reduce the amount of free fat from larvae during mitochondrial enrichment. However, BSA will likely contribute to the most abundant peptide contaminants and it is therefore crucial to wash the mitochondrial pellet at least once with buffer without BSA. When working with flies, which contain less fat than larvae, it is advisable to omit BSA in all steps.
25. Be as gentle as possible while washing the mitochondrial pellet. Do not wash the pellet off the wall directly and try to avoid breaking it at the pipette tip. However, one should obtain an even suspension, which might take up to 2 min per sample.
26. Not all protein assays are suitable for quantifying protein in GuHCl. Perform sensitivity tests on a range of GuHCl-dilutions the first time this protocol is performed. We get sufficient accuracy by diluting the protein solution 1:10 in water.
27. The pH after formic acid addition should be between 2 and 3. It is advisable to test this on pH paper the first time the experiment is performed.

28. Make sure to never dry the column and always leave a small amount of liquid on top of the disk. The only exception are the two elution steps, in which acetonitrile in water is completely passed through the disk each time.
29. Expect a high absorption toward UV range and a smaller peak at 280 nm.

Acknowledgements

This project has received funding from the European Research Council (ERC) under the European Union's Horizon 2020 research and innovation program (grant agreement no. 715009 for AW). AW is supported by the Swedish Research Council (VR2016-02179), the Knut & Alice Wallenberg Foundation (KAW 2013.0026). IA receives support from the Max Planck Society. FAS is a scholar of the Studienstiftung des deutschen Volkes.

References

1. Ong S-E, Blagoev B, Kratchmarova I et al (2002) Stable isotope labeling by amino acids in cell culture, SILAC, as a simple and accurate approach to expression proteomics. Mol Cell Proteomics 1:376–386
2. Ong S-E (2012) The expanding field of SILAC. Anal Bioanal Chem 404:967–976
3. Fredens J, Engholm-Keller K, Giessing A et al (2011) Quantitative proteomics by amino acid labeling in C. elegans. Nat Publ Group 8:845–847
4. Krüger M, Moser M, Ussar S et al (2008) SILAC mouse for quantitative proteomics uncovers kindlin-3 as an essential factor for red blood cell function. Cell 134:353–364
5. Sury MD, Chen J-X, Selbach M (2010) The SILAC fly allows for accurate protein quantification in vivo. Mol Cell Proteomics 9:2173–2183
6. Xu P, Tan H, Duong DM et al (2012) Stable isotope labeling with amino acids in drosophila for quantifying proteins and modifications. J Proteome Res 11:4403–4412
7. Chang Y-C, Tang H-W, Liang S-Y et al (2013) Evaluation of drosophila metabolic labeling strategies for in vivo quantitative proteomic analyses with applications to early pupa formation and amino acid starvation. J Proteome Res 12:2138–2150
8. Piper MDW, Blanc E, Leitão-Gonçalves R et al (2014) A holidic medium for Drosophila melanogaster. Nat Publ Group 11:100–105
9. Piper MDW, Soultoukis GA, Blanc E et al (2017) Matching dietary amino acid balance to the in silico-translated exome optimizes growth and reproduction without cost to lifespan. Cell Metab 25:610–621
10. Schmidt C, Urlaub H (2009) iTRAQ-labeling of in-gel digested proteins for relative quantification. In: Proteomics. Humana Press, Totowa, NJ, pp 207–226

Chapter 8

Mass Spectrometric Analysis of Mitochondrial RNA Modifications

Yuma Ishigami, Tsutomu Suzuki, and Takeo Suzuki

Abstract

Mitochondrial RNAs are modified posttranscriptionally. These modifications are required for proper functioning of RNA molecules, and thereby contribute to essential mitochondrial processes. Herein, we describe our latest mass spectrometry-based platform for analysis of posttranscriptional modifications of mitochondrial tRNAs, and measuring the in vitro activity of mitochondrial RNA-modifying enzymes.

Key words Mitochondrial tRNA, RNA modification, Mass spectrometry

1 Introduction

Human mitochondrial DNA (mtDNA) encodes 37 genes. These include: 11 mRNAs for 13 protein subunits of the respiratory chain complexes, 22 tRNAs, and 2 rRNAs [1, 2]. Both mtDNA strands are transcribed by mitochondrial RNA polymerase, assisted by mitochondrial transcription factors, to yield long polycistronic precursor RNAs comprising rRNAs, tRNAs, and mRNAs [3]. These transcripts are folded into distinct secondary and tertiary structures, and processed into individual RNAs. Since tRNAs are located between mRNAs and rRNAs without any intervening sequences in precursor RNAs, the 5′ and 3′ ends of tRNAs are cleaved by RNA endonucleases, resulting in the separation of mRNAs and rRNAs. Thus, tRNAs are said to "punctuate" mRNAs encoded in mtDNAs [4]. During RNA processing, posttranscriptional modifications are enzymatically introduced in regions of tRNAs and rRNAs. These modifications are required for the proper functioning of tRNAs and mitoribosomes [2, 5]. In addition, epitranscriptome mapping detected the 1-methyladenosine (m^1A) modification at a single site in ND5 mRNA [6].

Posttranscriptional modifications are critical structural components of RNA molecules, as well as regulatory elements [7, 8]. We

Michal Minczuk and Joanna Rorbach (eds.), *Mitochondrial Gene Expression: Methods and Protocols*, Methods in Molecular Biology, vol. 2192, https://doi.org/10.1007/978-1-0716-0834-0_8,

previously reported that a lack of tRNA modification results in pathological consequences [2]. This was the first reported instance of human disease caused by aberrant RNA modification, and yielded the term "RNA modopathy" as a new category of human disease [9].

To map posttranscriptional modifications of RNAs, we established a platform for RNA isolation and analysis. To isolate individual RNAs, we developed chaplet column chromatography [10, 11] and reciprocal circulating chromatography [12]. For direct analysis of RNAs, we devised a capillary liquid chromatography (LC) nano electrospray ionization (ESI) mass spectrometry (MS) method for RNA-MS analysis [13, 14]. This system allows us to analyze complex mixtures of RNA fragments digested by RNases, and to map the species and positions of modifications in each fragment. Previously, we successfully isolated 22 mt-tRNAs from bovine liver and human placenta, and mapped 15 types of modifications at 118 positions in bovine mt-tRNAs [14], as well as 18 types of modifications at 137 positions in human mt-tRNAs [23].

In the present work, we describe our updated MS-based protocol for analysis of post-transcriptional modifications of human mt-tRNAs (Fig. 1), and measuring the in vitro activity of m^1A methyltransferase TRMT61B (Fig. 2) [15, 16].

2 Materials

2.1 Cyanoethylation of Pseudouridine in mt-tRNA

For reagents 1 and 2, LC-MS grade or analytical grade is recommended.

1. Triethylamine.
2. Acetic acid.
3. Ethanol.
4. Ethylenediaminetetraacetic acid (EDTA), prepare a 0.5 M EDTA-Na (pH 8.0) stock solution.
5. Acrylonitrile.

2.2 In Vitro Reconstitution of m^1A in mt-rRNA Fragments

1. An in vitro transcribed human mitochondrial 16S rRNA segment (positions 866–979) with the following sequence:
   5′-GGCACCGCCUGCCCAGUGACACAUGUUUAAC GGCCGCGGUACCCUAACCGUGCAAAGGUAGCAUAA UCACUUGUUCCUUAAAUAGGGACCUGUAUGAAU GGCUCCACGAGGGUU-3′ [16].
2. Recombinant TRMT61B protein without a mitochondrial targeting sequence (MTS) [15, 16].
3. *S*-adenosyl-L-methionine (AdoMet).
4. Potassium chloride.

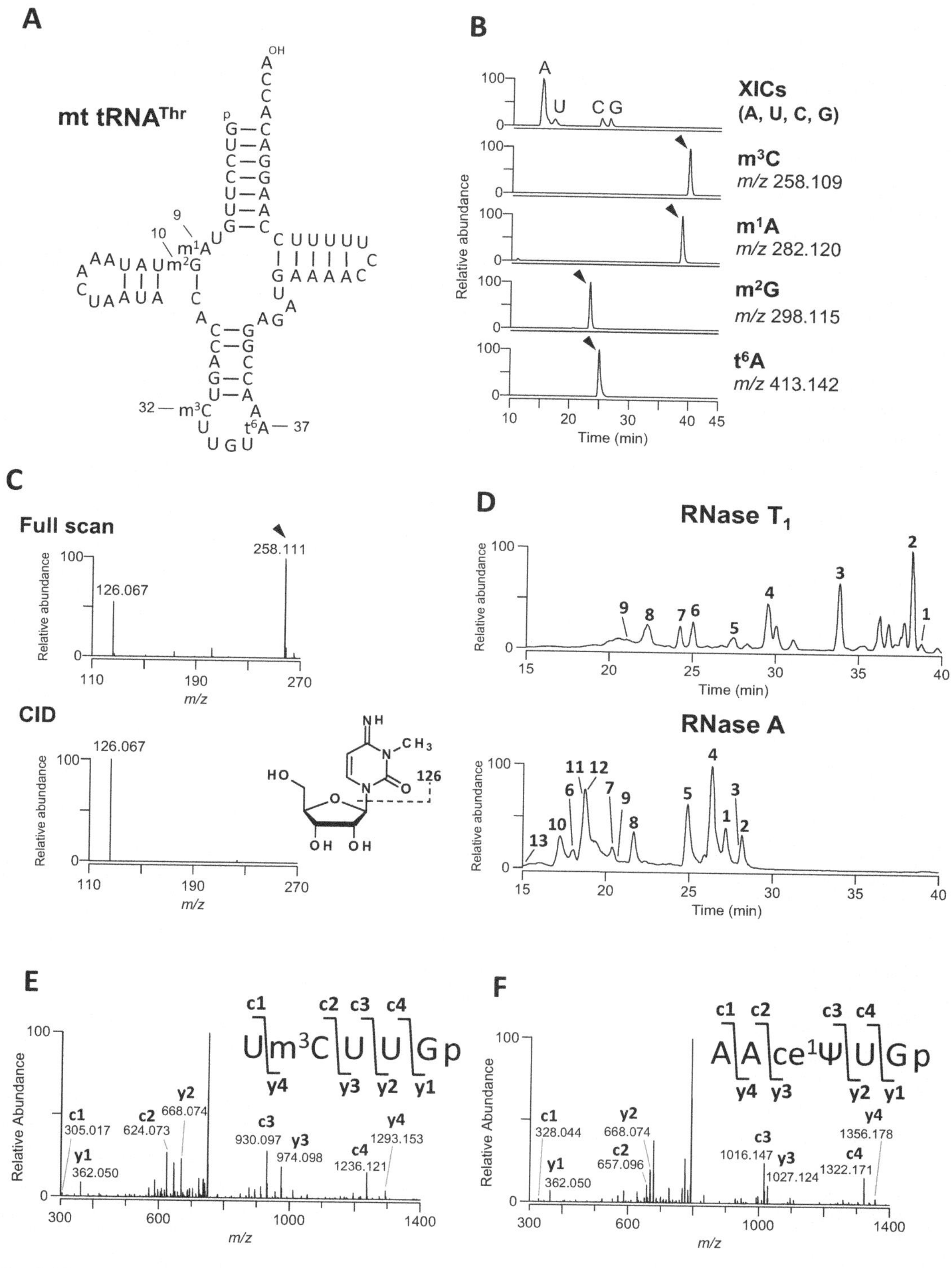

Fig. 1 Mass spectrometric analysis of posttranscriptional modifications in human mt-tRNA^{Thr}. (**a**) Secondary structure of human mt-tRNA^{Thr} with modifications [21]. Modified sites are numbered as in the MODOMICS and tRNAdb 2009 databases [8, 22]. Symbols for each modification are as follows: *m^1A* 1-methyladenosine, *m^2G*

5. Magnesium chloride.
6. HEPES-KOH (pH 7.5).
7. Dithiothreitol.
8. Phenol/chloroform/isoamyl alcohol (PCI; 25:24:1, pH 7.5).

2.3 RNA Cleanup by Drop Dialysis

1. Isolated mt-tRNA (*see* **Note 1**).
2. Ultrapure water (ddH_2O, Milli-Q water, etc.).
3. MF-Millipore membrane filter, 0.025 μm, cut into appropriate size and shape (e.g., ~2 cm diameter disks).
4. Sterile vessel of appropriate size, such as a microplate-sized reservoir or a disposable dish for culturing cells.

2.4 Nuclease Digestion of mt-tRNA and LC-MS Analysis

1. RNase T_1, recombinant.
2. RNase A, affinity purified or recombinant.
3. Nuclease P1. Prepare a 1 U/μL stock solution after desalting and cleanup by drop dialysis (*see* **Note 2**).
4. *Escherichia coli* C75 alkaline phosphatase (TaKaRa, 2120A). Prepare a 0.1 U/μL stock solution after desalting and cleanup by drop dialysis (*see* **Note 2**).

   For reagents 5–12, LC-MS grade (at least analytical grade) is recommended.
5. Ammonium acetate.
6. Ammonium bicarbonate.
7. Acetonitrile.
8. 1,1,1,3,3,3-hexafluoro-2-propanol (HFIP).

Fig. 1 (continued) N^2-methylguanosine, *m^{3}C* 3-methylcytidine, *t^{6}A* *N^6*-threonylcarbamoyladenosine. Their chemical structures are available in the MODOMICS database of RNA modifications [8]. (**b**) HILIC/MS nucleoside analysis of human mt-tRNA^{Thr}. Extracted ion chromatograms (XICs) showing protonated nucleoside ions (M + H$^+$) of unmodified nucleosides (A, *m*/*z* 268.105; U, *m*/*z* 245.077; C, *m*/*z* 244.093; G, *m*/*z* 284.099; top panel) overlaid on a trace, m^{3}C (second panel), m^{2}G (third panel), m^{1}A (fourth panel), and t^{6}A (bottom panel). Monoisotopic *m*/*z* values are indicated on the right of each panel. (**c**) Full-scan mass spectrum (top panel) showing detection of the protonated m^{3}C nucleoside (*m*/*z* 258.111, indicated by an arrowhead) and its base-related ion (*m*/*z* 126.067) that is generated by spontaneous cleavage of the N-glycoside bond (dotted line in the chemical structure) during ionization. The lower panel shows a CID spectrum of m^{3}C (the precursor ion is *m*/*z* 258). A base-related ion was detected as a product ion. (**d**) RNA-MS mapping of RNA fragments of human mt-tRNA^{Thr} digested by RNase T_1 (upper panel) and A (lower panel) represented by base peak chromatograms. All detected fragments are numbered as listed in Table 1. (**e**) CID spectrum of the RNase T_1-digested fragment of human mt-tRNA^{Thr} (Fragment No. 6). c- and y-series product ions in the CID spectrum are assigned on the fragment sequence. The nomenclature of product ions is illustrated in Scheme 1. (**f**) RNA-MS mapping of Ψ. A CID spectrum of the RNA fragment containing ce^{1}Ψ (RNase T_1-digested fragment at positions 30–34 of human mt-tRNA^{Cys}). c- and y-series product ions in the CID spectrum are assigned on the fragment sequence. The nomenclature of product ions is illustrated in Scheme 1

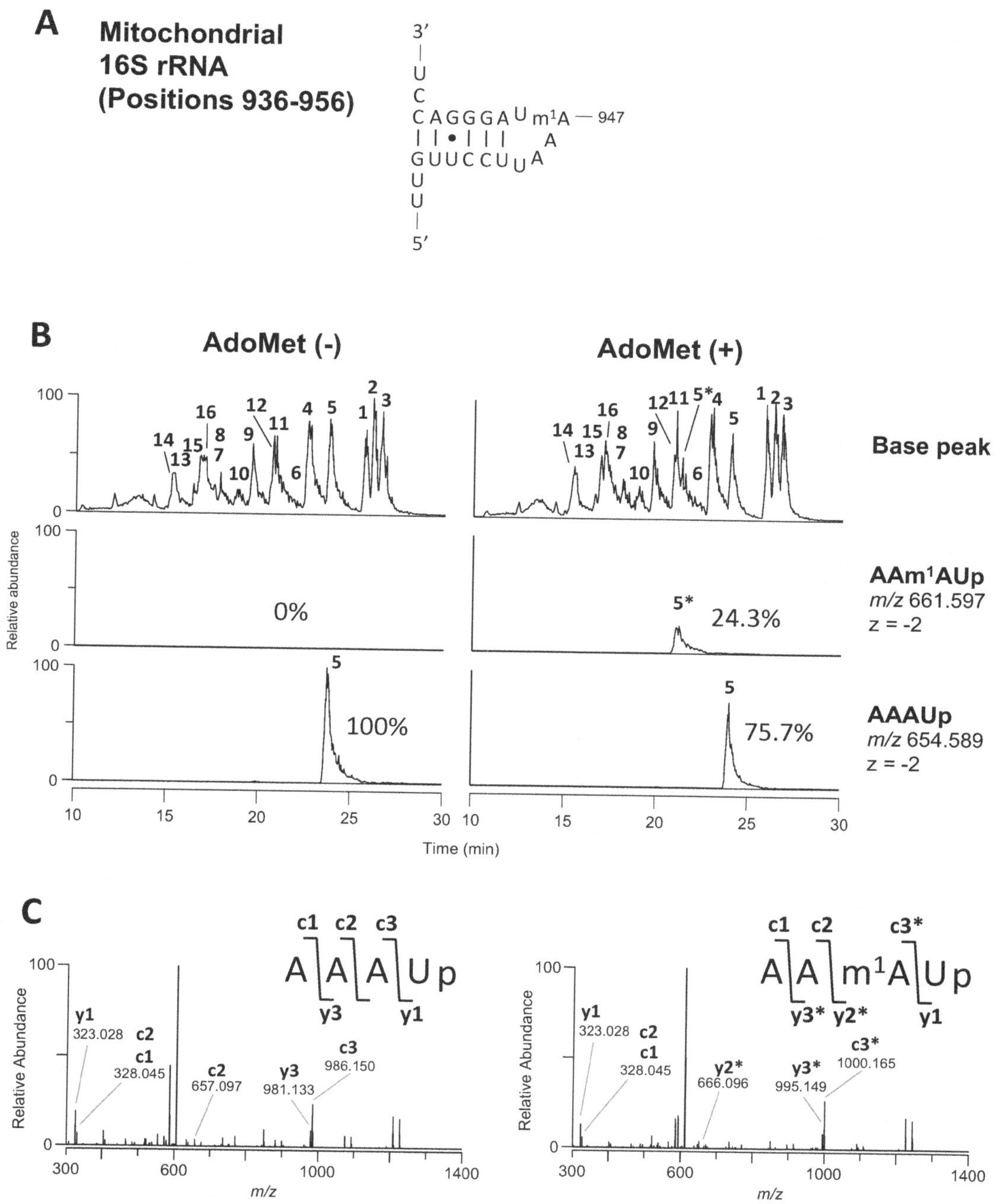

Fig. 2 In vitro activity of TRMT61B measured by RNA-MS. (**a**) Partial secondary structure of human mitochondrial 16S rRNA surrounding the m^{1}A947 site [16]. (**b**) In vitro reconstitution of m^{1}A947 catalyzed by TRMT61B in the presence (right panels) or absence (left panels) of AdoMet. RNA-MS analysis of RNase A-digested fragments of the substrate RNA are shown as base peak chromatograms (top panels), mass chromatograms for the methylated fragment (AAm^{1}AUp, middle panels), and unmethylated fragment (AAAUp, bottom panels). Detected fragments indicated on the trace are numbered as listed in Table 2. (**c**) CID spectra of AAAUp (left panel) and AAm^{1}AUp (right panel). c- and y-series product ions in the CID spectrum are assigned on the fragment sequence. The nomenclature of product ions is illustrated in Scheme 1

Table 1
Lists of RNase-digested fragments of human mt-tRNA^{Thr}

No.	Fragment sequence	Molecular mass	Calculated *m/z*	Observed *m/z*	Charge state
RNase T_1					
1	UAUAAACUAAUACACCAGp	5768.797	720.092	720.095	−8
2	AAAACCUUUUUCCAAGp	5087.665	634.950	634.954	−8
3	$Ut^6AAACCGp$	2411.361	1204.673	1204.672	−2
4	UCCUUGp	1891.216	944.600	944.601	−2
5	ACACCA (3′ terminal)	1840.326	919.155	919.154	−2
6	Um^3CUUGp	1600.191	799.088	799.087	−2
7	Um^1Am^2Gp	1026.167	1025.159	1025.159	−1
8	AUGp	998.136	997.128	997.128	−1
9	AGp	692.111	691.103	691.102	−1
RNase A					
1	GGAGAUp	2017.283	1007.634	1007.645	−2
2	AAGGACp	2000.304	999.144	999.145	−2
3	GAAAACp	1984.309	991.147	991.149	−2
4	t^6AAACp	1455.247	726.616	726.618	−2
5	AAACp	1310.209	654.097	654.098	−2
6	m^1Am^2GUp	1026.167	1025.159	1025.159	−1
7	AGUp	998.136	997.128	997.129	−1
8	AAUp	982.141	981.133	981.135	−1
9	pGUp (5′ terminal)	749.050	748.042	748.042	−1
10	GUp	669.083	668.075	668.075	−1
11	AUp	653.088	652.081	652.085	−1
12	ACp	652.104	651.097	651.097	−1
13	m^3CUp	643.093	642.085	642.085	−1

Representative observed *m/z* values are indicated ("p" represents phosphate group)

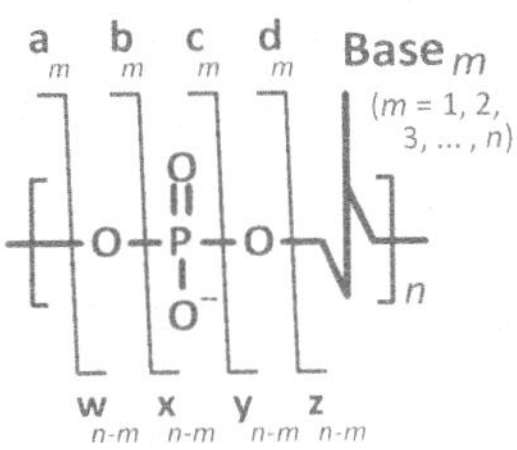

Scheme 1 The nomenclature of product ions (related to Figs. 1e, f, 2c)

9. Methanol.
10. Triethylamine.
11. Acetic acid.
12. Ultrapure water or similar.

In addition to the LC-MS systems described here and in previous publications [13, 14, 17], any equivalent systems can be adapted for RNA-MS analysis.

Table 2
List of RNase A-digested fragments of the RNA segment of human mitochondrial 16S rRNA

No.	Fragment sequence	Molecular mass	Calculated *m/z*	Observed *m/z*	Charge state
1	GAGGGUp	2033.278	1015.631	1015.633	−2
2	AGGGACp	2016.299	1007.142	1007.144	−2
3	AAAGGUp	2001.288	999.636	999.640	−2
4	GAAUp	1327.188	662.586	662.590	−2
5*	AAm^1AUp	1325.209	661.597	661.597	−2
5	AAAUp	1311.193	654.589	654.593	−2
6	pGGCp (5′ terminal)	1093.113	1092.105	1092.106	−1
7	GGUp	1014.131	1013.123	1013.130	−1
8	GGCp	1013.147	1012.139	1012.142	−1
9	AGUp	998.136	997.128	997.133	−1
10	AGCp, GACp	997.152	996.144	996.146	−1
11	AAUp	982.141	981.133	981.140	−1
12	AACp	981.157	980.149	980.153	−1
13	GUp	669.083	668.075	668.077	−1
14	GCp	668.099	667.091	667.091	−1
15	AUp	653.088	652.081	652.083	−1
16	ACp	652.104	651.097	651.098	−1

Representative observed *m/z* values are indicated

13. A nano-flow LC-MS system, composed of a DiNa splitless nano high-performance LC (HPLC) system (KYA Technologies) with a Nanovolume Valve (Valco Instruments) and an LTQ Orbitrap XL (Thermo Fisher Scientific) or Q Exactive (Thermo Fisher Scientific) equipped with a nano-ESI interface.
14. A HiQ sil ODS capillary column (C18W-3, 50 × 0.15 mm; KYA Technologies) and a HiQ sil ODS trapping column (1 × 0.5 mm; KYA Technologies) for nano-flow separation.
15. A micro-flow LC-MS system composed of an Ultimate 3000 LC system (Dionex) and a Q Exactive (Thermo Fisher Scientific) with an ESI source.
16. A SeQuant ZIC-cHILIC hydrophilic interaction LC (HILIC) column (3 μm particle size, 150 × 2.1 mm; Merck Millipore) with a SeQuant ZIC-cHILIC guard kit pre-column cartridge (3 μm particle size, 20 × 2.1 mm; Merck Millipore) for micro-flow separation.

17. An InertSustain C18 reversed-phase chromatography (RPC) column (250 × 2.1 mm, 5 μm particle size; GL Sciences, 5020-07316) with an InertSustain C18 cartridge guard column E pre-column cartridge (5 μm particle size, 10 × 3 mm; GL Sciences) for micro-flow separation.

3 Methods

3.1 Cyanoethylation of Pseudouridine (Ψ) in mt-tRNA (See Note 3)

1. Prepare a 1 μL solution of mt-tRNA (5 pmol/μL) in a new microtube (Fig. 1a).
2. Add 30 μL of 50% (v/v) ethanol/1.1 M trimethylammonium acetate (TEAA; pH 8.6) and mix thoroughly [18].
3. Add 0.5 M EDTA at a final concentration of 1 mM and mix thoroughly.
4. Add 4 μL of acrylonitrile, mix thoroughly, and incubate at 70 °C for 2 h (*see* **Note 4**).
5. Transfer the reaction mixture to a new microtube.
6. Collect the cyanoethylated mt-tRNA via two rounds of conventional ethanol precipitation to completely remove acrylonitrile.
7. Dissolve the tRNA pellet in a small amount of water.
8. Desalt and clean up tRNAs by drop dialysis (*see* Subheading 3.3).

3.2 In Vitro Reconstitution of m^1A in the mt-rRNA Fragment

1. Prepare enzyme solution (25 μL) composed of 1 μM TRMT61B, 300 mM KCl, 4 mM $MgCl_2$, 2 mM dithiothreitol, and 40 mM HEPES-KOH (pH 7.5).
2. Prepare substrate solution (25 μL) composed of 4 μM 16S rRNA segment and 2 mM AdoMet. In parallel, use solution without AdoMet as a negative control.
3. Mix the two solutions and incubate at 37 °C for 1 h.
4. Add 150 μL of water and 200 μL of PCI, and mix vigorously to extract RNA.
5. Transfer the aqueous phase to a new tube and perform ethanol precipitation.
6. Dissolve the RNA pellet in a small amount of water.
7. Desalt and clean up the RNA by drop dialysis (*see* Subheading 3.3).

3.3 Drop Dialysis of RNA Solution (See Note 5)

1. Float membrane filters on the surface of a sufficient amount of water in a sterile vessel.
2. Gently place 10–50 μL of RNA solution on the membrane filter.

3. Incubate for 30–60 min at room temperature for dialysis.
4. Carefully collect RNA solution from the membrane filter.
5. Collect residual solution on the membrane filter with 10 μL of water.
6. Repeat **step 5** to ensure complete recovery.
7. Combine samples, dry, and then dissolve in a small amount of water.

3.4 Nuclease Digestion of mt-tRNA and Nucleoside Analysis by LC-MS

1. Digest isolated tRNA (5–10 pmol) at 37 °C for 30–60 min in a 9 μL reaction mixture containing 10 mM ammonium acetate (pH 5.3) and 0.0033 U/μL nuclease P1.
2. Add 0.5 μL of 1 M ammonium bicarbonate and 0.5 μL of 0.03 U/μL alkaline phosphatase and incubate at 37 °C for 30–60 min (*see* **Note 6**).
3. For HILIC/MS analysis, after the reaction, dry the reaction mixture and dissolve in 40 μL of 90% (v/v) acetonitrile solution (*see* **Note 7**).
4. Subject the digested nucleosides to a micro-flow LC-MS/Q Exactive system in positive and/or negative ion mode combined with data-dependent tandem MS (MS/MS) mode coupled to an Ultimate 3000 LC with a HILIC column at a flow rate of 100 μL/min (Fig. 1b). The mobile phase is composed of 5 mM ammonium acetate (pH 5.3; solvent A) and acetonitrile (solvent B). A multistep gradient is performed as follows: 90–40% B in 0–30 min, 40% B in 30–40 min, 40–90% B in 40–45 min, and 90% B in 45–60 min.
5. For RPC/MS analysis, after the reaction, adjust the volume of the reaction mixture to ~20 μL with water (*see* **Note 6**).
6. Subject the digested nucleosides to a micro-flow LC-MS/Q Exactive system in positive and/or negative ion mode coupled to an Ultimate 3000 LC with a RPC column at a flow rate of 100 μL/min. The mobile phase is composed of 5 mM ammonium acetate (pH 5.3; solvent A) and acetonitrile (solvent B). A multistep gradient is performed as follows: 2% B in 0–5 min, 2–20% B in 5–30 min, 20–95% B in 30–40 min, 95% B in 40–45 min, and 2% B in 45–60 min.
7. Analyze the data (*see* Subheading 3.6). Representative results are shown in Fig. 1b, c.

3.5 Ribonuclease Digestion of RNA and Fragment Analysis by LC-MS

1. For RNase T_1 digestion, 1–2 pmol of RNA sample (cyanoethylated RNA or modified RNA segment) in 10 μL of reaction mixture containing 25 mM ammonium acetate (pH 5.3) and 2 U/μL RNase T_1 (*see* **Note 8**) is incubated at 37 °C for 30–60 min (*see* **Note 9**).

2. For RNase A digestion, 1–2 pmol of RNA sample (cyanoethylated RNA or modified RNA segment) in 10 μL of reaction mixture containing 25 mM ammonium acetate (pH 7.7) and 1 ng/μL RNase A (*see* **Note 10**) is incubated at 37 °C for 30–60 min (*see* **Note 9**).
3. After **steps 1** and **2**, add an equal volume of 0.1 M TEAA (pH 7.0) to the reaction mixture and mix thoroughly.
4. Subject RNA fragments digested by RNase T_1 or A to a capillary LC nano-ESI MS system (negative ion scan and data-dependent MS/MS mode) at a flow rate of 300 nL/min. The mobile phase is composed of 0.4 M HFIP (pH 7.0, adjusted with triethylamine; solvent A) and 0.4 M HFIP (pH 7.0) with 50% methanol (solvent B). A linear gradient is performed as follows: 5–100% B in 0–35 min, 100% B in 35–40 min, and 0% B in 40–50 min.
5. Analyze the data (*see* Subheading 3.6). A typical example of tRNA modification mapping is shown in Fig. 1d. MS analysis of RNA methyltransferase is shown in Fig. 2b.

3.6 MS Data Analyses for RNA Modifications

1. Identify types of modified nucleosides in LC-MS nucleoside analysis of target RNAs in Subheading 3.4 (Fig. 1b). Each modified nucleoside is detected as a positively charged proton adduct ($M + H^+$) in mass chromatograms and spectra using the Qual Brower tool within Xcalibur 4.2 software (Thermo Fisher Scientific). Typical elution profiles of modified nucleosides are available in our previous publications [13, 14]. To confirm the chemical structure of each modification, the nucleoside ion ($M + H^+$) is decomposed by collision-induced dissociation (CID) and the resultant product ions are assigned in the deduced chemical structure (Fig. 1c).
2. List RNA fragment sequences and nucleotide composition, including modifications of target RNAs, and calculate their m/z values from the exact atomic composition, as detailed in Tables 1 and 2 (*see* **Note 11**).
3. Assign mass chromatograms and spectra for unmodified RNA fragments using the calculated m/z values from the LC-MS dataset obtained in Subheading 3.4 (Figs. 1d and 2b; Tables 1 and 2; *see* **Note 12**). RNA fragments are detected as negatively charged deprotonated ions.
4. Assign mass chromatograms and spectra for RNA fragments containing modified nucleosides detected in Subheading 3.6, **step 1** using calculated m/z values (Figs. 1d and 2b; Tables 1 and 2; *see* **Note 13**).
5. Sequence each RNA fragment (especially modified fragments) by assigning product ions in CID spectra (Figs. 1e and 2c). As pseudouridine (Ψ) is derivatized to 1-cyanoethylpseudourine

($ce^1\Psi$) by cyanoethylation in Subheading 3.1, an RNA fragment containing Ψ is detected as an ion with a 53 Da increase in molecular mass in mass chromatograms. The position of $ce^1\Psi$ can be determined using CID spectra (Fig. 1f).

4 Notes

1. To isolate mitochondrial tRNA species of interest, refer to our previous publications [10, 12].
2. Some constituents of enzyme storage buffers can interfere with LC-MS analysis. We usually clean up the enzyme solution by drop dialysis as described in Subheading 3.3.
3. This step can be ignored if there is no need to determine Ψ sites.
4. To avoid vaporization, heating by a thermal cycler equipped with a heated lid is highly recommended.
5. Drop dialysis is performed to further clean up samples for LC-MS analysis with high sensitivity.
6. Reacted samples can be stored at −80 °C for a few weeks.
7. Dried samples can be stored at −80 °C for a few weeks. Before LC-MS analysis, dissolve samples in 90% acetonitrile.
8. RNase T_1 cleaves RNA at the 3′ side of G residues, leaving 3′-phosphate and 5′-hydroxyl forms, which produces fragments represented by HnGp (H = A, C, or U) except for terminal fragments. Note that some modified guanosines such as 1-methylguanosine (m^1G) are resistant to RNase T_1 digestion.
9. Reacted samples can be stored at −80 °C for a few weeks. TEAA is added just before LC-MS analysis (as described in Subheading 3.5, **step 3**).
10. RNase A cleaves RNA at the 3′ side of Y (Y = C or U), leaving 3′-phosphate and 5′-hydroxyl forms, which produces fragments represented by RnYp (R = A or G) except for terminal fragments. Note that some modified pyrimidines, such as 3-methylcytidine (m^3C), are resistant to RNase A digestion.
11. Useful tools are available for calculation and assignment, including Mongo Oligo Mass Calculator [19] and RNAModMapper [20].
12. Fragment No. 1 (Table 1) is detected as an octaply charged deprotonated ion with m/z 720.095, consistent with the calculated m/z (720.092).

13. Fragment No. 6 (Table 1) is detected as a doubly charged deprotonated ion with *m/z* 799.087, which is 7.07 larger *m/z* than that of UCUUGp (792.080), indicating the presence of a single methyl group (14.016 Da) in this fragment.

Acknowledgments

We thank Yuriko Sakaguchi and Yuka Yashiro for technical support, and Dr. Yohei Kirono (Thomas Jefferson University) for providing materials. This work was funded by Grants-in-Aid for Scientific Research on Priority Areas from the Ministry of Education, Culture, Sports, Science, and Technology of Japan (MEXT), and the Japan Society for the Promotion of Science (JSPS; grant no. 26702035 and 18H02094 to Ta. S., and 26113003, 26220205, and 18H05272 to Ts. S.).

References

1. Barrell BG, Bankier AT, Drouin J (1979) A different genetic code in human mitochondria. Nature 282(5735):189–194. https://doi.org/10.1038/282189a0
2. Suzuki T, Nagao A, Suzuki T (2011) Human mitochondrial diseases caused by lack of taurine modification in mitochondrial tRNAs. Wiley Interdiscip Rev RNA 2(3):376–386. https://doi.org/10.1002/wrna.65
3. Hallberg BM, Larsson NG (2014) Making proteins in the powerhouse. Cell Metab 20 (2):226–240. https://doi.org/10.1016/j.cmet.2014.07.001
4. Ojala D, Montoya J, Attardi G (1981) tRNA punctuation model of RNA processing in human mitochondria. Nature 290 (5806):470–474. https://doi.org/10.1038/290470a0
5. Rebelo-Guiomar P, Powell CA, Van Haute L, Minczuk M (2019) The mammalian mitochondrial epitranscriptome. Biochim Biophys Acta Gene Regul Mech. 1862(3):429–446. https://doi.org/10.1016/j.bbagrm.2018.11.005
6. Safra M, Sas-Chen A, Nir R, Winkler R, Nachshon A, Bar-Yaacov D, Erlacher M, Rossmanith W, Stern-Ginossar N, Schwartz S (2017) The m1A landscape on cytosolic and mitochondrial mRNA at single-base resolution. Nature 551(7679):251–255. https://doi.org/10.1038/nature24456
7. Suzuki T (2005) Biosynthesis and function of tRNA Wobble modifications. In: Grosjean H (ed) Fine-tuning of RNA functions by modification and editing, Topics in current genetics, vol 12. Springer, Berlin, pp 23–69
8. Boccaletto P, Machnicka MA, Purta E, Piatkowski P, Baginski B, Wirecki TK, de Crecy-Lagard V, Ross R, Limbach PA, Kotter A, Helm M, Bujnicki JM (2018) MODOMICS: a database of RNA modification pathways. 2017 update. Nucleic Acids Res 46(D1):D303–D307. https://doi.org/10.1093/nar/gkx1030
9. Asano K, Suzuki T, Saito A, Wei FY, Ikeuchi Y, Numata T, Tanaka R, Yamane Y, Yamamoto T, Goto T, Kishita Y, Murayama K, Ohtake A, Okazaki Y, Tomizawa K, Sakaguchi Y, Suzuki T (2018) Metabolic and chemical regulation of tRNA modification associated with taurine deficiency and human disease. Nucleic Acids Res 46(4):1565–1583. https://doi.org/10.1093/nar/gky068
10. Suzuki T, Suzuki T (2007) Chaplet column chromatography: isolation of a large set of individual RNAs in a single step. Methods Enzymol 425:231–239. https://doi.org/10.1016/S0076-6879(07)25010-4
11. Suzuki T, Suzuki T, Wada T, Saigo K, Watanabe K (2002) Taurine as a constituent of mitochondrial tRNAs: new insights into the functions of taurine and human mitochondrial diseases. EMBO J 21(23):6581–6589. https://doi.org/10.1093/emboj/cdf656
12. Miyauchi K, Ohara T, Suzuki T (2007) Automated parallel isolation of multiple species of non-coding RNAs by the reciprocal circulating chromatography method. Nucleic Acids Res

35(4):e24. https://doi.org/10.1093/nar/gkl1129

13. Sakaguchi Y, Miyauchi K, Kang BI, Suzuki T (2015) Nucleoside analysis by hydrophilic interaction liquid chromatography coupled with mass spectrometry. Methods Enzymol 560:19–28. https://doi.org/10.1016/bs.mie.2015.03.015
14. Suzuki T, Suzuki T (2014) A complete landscape of post-transcriptional modifications in mammalian mitochondrial tRNAs. Nucleic Acids Res 42(11):7346–7357. https://doi.org/10.1093/nar/gku390
15. Chujo T, Suzuki T (2012) Trmt61B is a methyltransferase responsible for 1-methyladenosine at position 58 of human mitochondrial tRNAs. RNA 18 (12):2269–2276. https://doi.org/10.1261/rna.035600.112
16. Bar-Yaacov D, Frumkin I, Yashiro Y, Chujo T, Ishigami Y, Chemla Y, Blumberg A, Schlesinger O, Bieri P, Greber B, Ban N, Zarivach R, Alfonta L, Pilpel Y, Suzuki T, Mishmar D (2016) Mitochondrial 16S rRNA is methylated by tRNA methyltransferase TRMT61B in all vertebrates. PLoS Biol 14 (9):e1002557. https://doi.org/10.1371/journal.pbio.1002557
17. Ohira T, Suzuki T (2016) Precursors of tRNAs are stabilized by methylguanosine cap structures. Nat Chem Biol 12(8):648–655. https://doi.org/10.1038/nchembio.2117
18. Mengel-Jorgensen J, Kirpekar F (2002) Detection of pseudouridine and other modifications in tRNA by cyanoethylation and MALDI mass spectrometry. Nucleic Acids Res 30(23):e135. https://doi.org/10.1093/nar/gnf135
19. Cantara WA, Crain PF, Rozenski J, McCloskey JA, Harris KA, Zhang X, Vendeix FA, Fabris D, Agris PF (2011) The RNA modification database, RNAMDB: 2011 update. Nucleic Acids Res 39(Database issue):D195–D201. https://doi.org/10.1093/nar/gkq1028
20. Yu N, Lobue PA, Cao X, Limbach PA (2017) RNAModMapper: RNA modification mapping software for analysis of liquid chromatography tandem mass spectrometry data. Anal Chem 89 (20):10744–10752. https://doi.org/10.1021/acs.analchem.7b01780
21. Lin H, Miyauchi K, Harada T, Okita R, Takeshita E, Komaki H, Fujioka K, Yagasaki H, Goto YI, Yanaka K, Nakagawa S, Sakaguchi Y, Suzuki T (2018) CO_2-sensitive tRNA modification associated with human mitochondrial disease. Nat Commun 9 (1):1875. https://doi.org/10.1038/s41467-018-04250-4
22. Juhling F, Morl M, Hartmann RK, Sprinzl M, Stadler PF, Putz J (2009) tRNAdb 2009: compilation of tRNA sequences and tRNA genes. Nucleic Acids Res 37(Database issue): D159–162F. https://doi.org/10.1093/nar/gkn772
23. Suzuki T, Yashiro Y, Kikuchi I, Ishigami Y, Saito H, Matsuzawa I, Okada S, Mito M, Iwasaki S, Ma D, Zhao X, Asano K, Lin H, Kirino Y, Sakaguchi Y, Suzuki T (2020) Complete chemical structures of human mitochondrial tRNAs. Nat Commun in press

Chapter 9

mito-Ψ-Seq: A High-Throughput Method for Systematic Mapping of Pseudouridine Within Mitochondrial RNA

Aldema Sas-Chen, Ronit Nir, and Schraga Schwartz

Abstract

RNA modifications are present in most cellular RNAs and are formed posttranscriptionally by enzymatic machineries that involve hundreds of enzymes and cofactors. RNA modifications impact the life cycle of the RNA, its stability, folding, cellular localization, as well as interactions with RNA and protein partners. RNA modifications are important for mitochondrial function and are required for proper processing and function of mitochondrial (mt) tRNA and rRNA. Underscoring their importance, several mitochondrial diseases are caused by defects in mt-RNA modifications, stemming from mutations in mtDNA at or near mt-RNA modification sites or in nuclear-encoded mt-RNA modifying enzymes. A highly abundant RNA modification, involved in mitochondrial physiology and pathology is pseudouridylation (Ψ), which is catalyzed by enzymes of the Pseudouridine Synthase (PUS) family. Although some Ψ sites in mt-rRNA and mt-tRNA have been identified, little is known about the functional role of these modifications. Furthermore, it is unknown which enzyme facilitates the modification of each site and it is likely that many yet undiscovered mt-RNA modifications exist, as is evidenced by recent work showing some Ψ sites on mRNA. Here, we present mito-Ψ-Seq, a high-throughput method for semiquantitative mapping of Ψ in mt-RNA.

Key words Pseudouridine, Next-generation sequencing, RNA modification, Epitranscriptome, Misincorporation signatures, Reverse-transcription arrest, Mitochondria

1 Introduction

Key functions of mitochondria include: generation of ATP by oxidative phosphorylation (OXPHOS), production and detoxification of reactive oxygen species, involvement in calcium homeostasis [1], and certain types of apoptosis [2]. The relatively small and compact mitochondrial genome (mtDNA) comprises genes encoding mitochondrial (mt-) tRNAs, mRNAs, and rRNAs, which are transcribed as precursor polycistrons [3]. The polycistrons undergo posttranscriptional endonucleolytic processing to produce individual transcripts, with distinct steady state levels within the mitochondria [4]. The precursor mitochondrial transcripts are also known to undergo posttranscriptional nucleotide modifications [5]. Recent

Michal Minczuk and Joanna Rorbach (eds.), *Mitochondrial Gene Expression: Methods and Protocols*, Methods in Molecular Biology, vol. 2192, https://doi.org/10.1007/978-1-0716-0834-0_9,

screens have found several RNA-modifying genes to be essential for OXPHOS [6], but little is known about the function(s) and the loci of the modifications that they catalyze. Among these mt-RNA modifying enzymes are pseudouridine synthases (PUSs) that catalyze the conversion of uridine into pseudouridine. This conversion is thought to confer structural stability through formation of an extra hydrogen bond in the nucleotide [7, 8]. A well-known mitochondrial pseudouridine synthase is PUS1, which catalyzes the modification of specific nucleotides in mt-tRNA molecules [9]. Mutations in PUS1 lead to human disease, clinical features of which include lactic acidosis, myopathy, and sideroblastic anemia [10, 11]. More recent research identified three previously uncharacterized, putative PUS enzymes—RPUSD3, RPUSD4, and TRUB2—as being essential for mitochondrial translation. RPUSD4 was proposed to introduce the only pseudouridine of 16S mt-rRNA [6, 12, 13]. However, further research is required to determine the exact functional role of this pseudouridylation. PUSL1 is another PUS enzyme that has been localized in mammalian mitochondria, but its targets and function have not been characterized [14].

The vast majority of studies of RNA modifications in mitochondria have focused on modifications in tRNA and rRNA. This is primarily due to technical limitations, which have hampered the ability to detect and quantify modifications in mRNAs present at relatively low steady-state levels. Yet, it is becoming clear that RNA modifications, in particular pseudouridines, are present on mitochondrial mRNAs. These changes can be dynamically regulated and potentially impact mitochondrial physiology [15]. Thus, for example, recent data on putative mitochondrial PUS enzymes suggested the presence of pseudouridine in mitochondrial mRNA of the COXI and COXIII genes [12, 13]. Despite these pre-existent examples there is a lack of a detailed, systematic understanding of the nature and location of the modifications on mt-mRNA substrates, as well as of the enzymes that catalyze their formation. Establishing such an enzyme–substrate relationship will be indispensable in elucidating the function of the epitranscriptomic modifications in mt-mRNA in human health and disease.

As part of our efforts to systematically explore and functionally characterize the pseudouridine epitranscriptome landscape, we have developed Ψ-seq, a methodology dedicated to high-throughput mapping of pseudouridine at single base resolution [16, 17]. Closely related approaches were developed by other groups [18–20]. Ψ-seq has proved prolific in identifying pseudouridine in nuclear-encoded ncRNAs and mRNAs, starting with total or poly(A)-enriched RNA. However, since mt-mRNAs are dramatically less abundant than rRNAs and tRNAs (of both the nuclear and mitochondrial genomes) identifying single nucleotide modifications of such molecules using our original Ψ-seq protocol presents an experimental and computational challenge, which requires high sequencing depth. Here we describe mito-Ψ-seq, an adaptation of Ψ-seq for specific interrogation of pseudouridines in mitochondrial RNA (Fig. 1). By adding a mitochondrial isolation step prior to RNA purification (adapted from [21, 22]), mito–Ψseq enables high-throughput identification of pseudouridine in mt-mRNA, at a dramatically lower sequencing depth than before. Additional adjustments to the original Ψ-seq protocol allow simultaneous capturing of small RNAs, such as tRNAs. In addition, the protocol was adapted for 96-well plates, substantially increasing the scale at which it can be applied. Overall, mito-Ψ-seq contributes to our understanding pertaining to mechanisms governing regulation of gene expression in mitochondria, and may shed light on potentially novel mechanisms of pathogenesis.

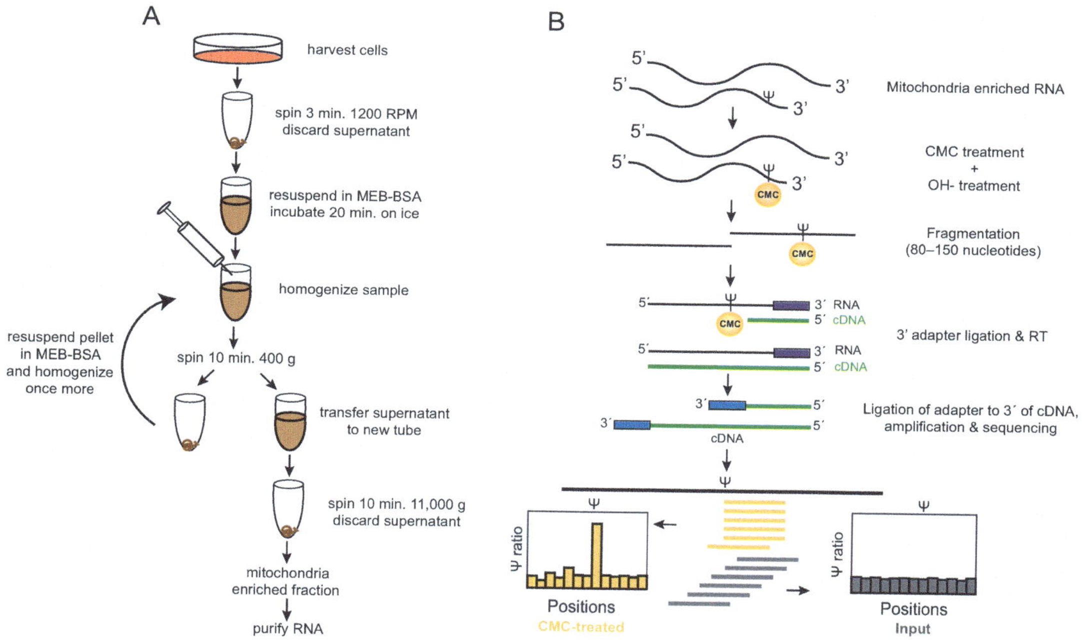

Fig. 1 Scheme of mito-Ψ-Seq protocol. (**a**) Mitochondria isolation. Whole cells are collected and resuspended in mitochondria extraction buffer (MEB-BSA). After a 20 min incubation on ice, cells are homogenized (it is recommended to repeat the homogenization step once more) and undergo a series of low- and high-speed centrifugations. The resulting pellet, representing the mitochondria-enriched fraction, is used as input for RNA purification. An optional treatment of the pellet with benzonase may precede RNA purification of the mitochondrial-enriched fraction (not shown). (**b**) Library preparation. Mitochondrial-enriched RNA is treated with CMC followed by incubation at alkaline pH, leading to Ψ-CMC adducts. RNA is then fragmented to a size range of 80–150 nt. Next, an adaptor is ligated to the 3′ end of the RNA (purple), followed by reverse transcription, which is expected to lead to premature termination one base pair immediately downstream of pseudouridylated sites. A second adaptor is ligated to the 3′ end of the cDNA (blue). Libraries are amplified and sequenced in paired end mode. A Ψ ratio is calculated as the ratio between reads starting at a position and reads overlapping it for both treatment (yellow) and input (gray) samples

2 Materials

2.1 Mitochondria Extraction Buffer (MEB)

1. Mitochondria Extraction Buffer (MEB): in a graduated cylinder or a glass beaker mix 5 mL of 1 M Tris-EDTA, pH 7.4 and 1 mL of 0.5 M EDTA with 400 mL water. Weigh 54.6 g Mannitol and transfer to the cylinder. Mix well and make up to 500 mL with water. Store at 4 °C.
2. MEB-BSA: 0.1% BSA in MEB.

2.2 RNA Purification

1. TRI Reagent (Sigma).
2. Chloroform.
3. 2-Propanol.
4. 75% Ethanol (EtOH), diluted in nuclease-free water.

2.3 CMC Treatment

1. 1 M Bicine (pH 8.5).
2. 8 M Urea.
3. 10× Sodium Bicarbonate buffer (pH 10.4), 2.105 g in 50 mL of water, titrated with NaOH.

   Prepare these solutions freshly whenever preparing a library.
4. Bicine Buffer (1 mL): 50 μL 1 M Bicine (pH 8.5), 8 μL 0.5 M EDTA (Sigma), 0.875 mL 8 M urea, add water to 1 mL.
5. Sodium Bicarbonate Buffer (1 mL): Dilute 10× Sodium Bicarbonate buffer (pH 10.4) 1:10 in water.
6. 0.34 M CMC in Bicine buffer; weigh a few grains of CMC (Sigma) in a 50 mL tube, and calculate how much Bicine buffer to add, vortex. For instance for 50 mg, 346.7 μL Bicine buffer are required.

2.4 RNA Washes

1. Silane beads—Dynabeads™ MyOne™ Silane (Thermo Fisher).
2. RLT buffer (QIAGEN).
3. 100% EtOH, prepare 75% EtOH.
4. Water Molecular Biology Reagent (Sigma).
5. DynaMag™-96 Side Magnet (Thermo Fisher).

2.5 RNA Fragmentation

1. RNA Fragmentation Reagents (Ambion).

2.6 DNAse Treatment and Phosphorylation

1. RNase Inhibitor, Murine (NEB).
2. Turbo DNAse (Life technologies).
3. Fast AP Thermosensitive Alkaline phosphatase (Fermentas).

4. T4 PNK (NEB).
5. FNK buffer; 300 μL PNK buffer (NEB), 300 μL Fast AP buffer (Fermentas) and 600 μL water.

2.7 Ligations

1. 10 μM RNA adapter for first ligation 5′—/5Phos/rArG rArUrC rGrGrA rArGrA rGrCrA rCrArC rGrUrC/3ddC/—3′.
2. 100 μM DNA adaptor for second ligation 5′—/5Phos/AG ATC GGA AGA GCG TCG TGT AG/3ddC/—3′.
3. DMSO 100%.
4. T4 RNA Ligase 1 (ssRNA Ligase) high conc. (NEB), includes ATP, PEG 800, ligase buffer.

2.8 First Strand cDNA Synthesis

1. Primer 5′—AGA CGT GTG CTC TTC CG—3′ (10 μM stock, 10 pmol final concentration).
2. SuperScript™ III Reverse Transcriptase (Invitrogen), includes the buffer and DTT.
3. dNTP Mix—10 mM Solution (Jena Bioscience).
4. RNase Inhibitor, Murine (NEB).
5. ExoSap-it PCR Product Cleanup Reagent (Affymetrix).

2.9 RNA Hydrolysis

1. 0.5 M Ethylenediaminetetraacetic acid disodium salt solution for molecular biology in H_2O (Sigma-Aldrich).
2. 10 M Sodium hydroxide solution BioUltra, for molecular biology, in H_2O (Sigma).
3. 1.0 N Hydrochloric acid solution, BioReagent, suitable for cell culture (Sigma).
4. 1 M dilution of the NaOH.

2.10 PCR Enrichment

1. 2× KAPA HiFi HotStart ReadyMix PCR Kit (KAPA Biosystems).
2. 100 μM stocks of the following primers. Combine the 2P_universal primer with one of the barcoded primers, in a concentration of 25 μM each.

   2P_universal primer: AATGATACGGCGACCACCGAGATCTACACTCTTTCC
   CTACACGACGCTCTTCCGATCT

   Barcoded primers are as published before [23]. Examples of two possible barcoded primers:

CAAGCAGAAGACGGCATACGAGAT***CCTGGTAG***GTGAC TGGAGTTCAGACGTGTGCTCTTCCGATCT	2P_504
CAAGCAGAAGACGGCATACGAGAT***TAAGCATG***GTGAC TGGAGTTCAGACGTGTGCTCTTCCGATCT	2P_375

3. SPRI Beads—Ampure XP Agencourt (Beckman Coulter).

3 Methods

3.1 Mitochondrial Isolation

Carry out all procedures on ice unless otherwise specified.

1. Harvest cells: aspirate growth medium and wash cells with cold PBS (*see* **Note 1**). Scrape the cells and transfer into 15 mL tubes. Alternatively, use trypsin to detach cells and transfer trypsinized cells into 15 mL tubes. Centrifuge cells at 1200 rpm (250 rcf) for 3 min. Aspirate PBS/trypsin and resuspend in 1 mL PBS and transfer to a 1.5 mL tube. Centrifuge at 1200 rpm for 3 min. Aspirate PBS and keep the pellet on ice (*see* **Note 2**).
2. Resuspend cell pellet in 0.7 mL MEB-BSA.
3. Incubate on ice for 20 min.
4. Homogenize the sample by running through a 25-G needle 15 times (*see* **Note 3**).
5. Centrifuge at 400 × *g* for 10 min.
6. Transfer the mitochondria containing supernatant to a new tube.
7. RECOMMENDED: Resuspend the pellet in MEB-BSA and repeat **steps 4–6** for the pellet containing tube (*see* **Note 4**). Combine the mitochondria containing supernatant with the supernatant from **step 6**.
8. Centrifuge the supernatant (total volume ~1.4 mL, if **step 7** was conducted) at 11,000 × *g* for 10 min.
9. Keep the mitochondria-enriched pellet and discard the supernatant.
10. OPTIONAL: To further enrich for mitochondrial RNA, the pellet from **step 9** can be further treated with benzonase, an endonuclease, which will degrade cytoplasmic RNA carried over with the mitochondrial pellet. If benzonase treatment is not needed continue to **step 17** (*see* **Note 5**).
11. Resuspend pellet in 1 mL MEB supplemented with 50 U/mL of benzonase.
12. Incubate on ice for 15 min.
13. Centrifuge at 11,000 × *g* for 10 min.
14. Discard supernatant and resuspend pellet in 1 mL MBE.
15. Centrifuge at 11,000 × *g* for 10 min to remove remaining benzonase.
16. Discard supernatant.
17. Store mitochondria-enriched pellet at −80 °C or continue to RNA purification.

3.2 RNA Purification

The mitochondria isolation stage enriches the sample for mitochondrial RNA. Thus, for the purpose of pseudouridine detection in mt-rRNA, mt-tRNA, and mt-mRNA, isolation of total RNA from the resulting pellets is sufficient for achieving proper representation of these RNA types in downstream analysis. However, if desired, further enrichment of specific RNA species can be obtained by various methods (e.g., poly(A) selection, size selection, etc.). RNA purification is carried out using TRI Reagent (Sigma T9424) according to manufacturer's instructions.

3.3 Preparation of cDNA Libraries for Next-Generation Sequencing

The library preparation protocol can be conveniently carried out for multiple samples in parallel using multi-pipettors in PCR strips or 96-well PCR plates.

3.3.1 Pseudouridine Tagging by CMC

1. Libraries are typically prepared from 200 ng of mitochondrial-enriched RNA. The sample volume should be brought to 20 μL.
2. To pre-clean Silane Beads wash 20 μL of Silane Beads as follows. Place beads on magnet and remove supernatant. Add 50 μL RLT buffer, place on magnet and remove supernatant. Resuspend beads in 3× the sample volume (60 μL RLT) (*see* **Note 6**).
3. Add resuspended beads to sample, and then fill tube to capacity (150 μL) with 100% EtOH. Mix and incubate for 1 min. Place on magnet and remove supernatant.
4. Add 100 μL of 75% EtOH, wash by transferring from side to side of the magnet, remove supernatant. Repeat 75% EtOH wash.
5. Dry beads for 1 min.
6. Resuspend sample in 15 μL Bicine buffer.
7. Place on magnet and elute into a new well. Add either 15 μL of 0.34 M CMC in Bicine Buffer or 15 μL of Bicine Buffer as control.
8. Incubate at 37 °C for 20 min.
9. To remove excess CMC wash 20 μL beads as in **step 2**, except resuspension should be carried out in 90 μL (3× the reaction volume).
10. Repeat **steps 3–5** of this section.
11. Add 30 μL of Sodium Bicarbonate Buffer to beads, mix well, place on magnet and elute into a new well.
12. Incubate at 37 °C for 3 h.
13. Wash 20 μL beads as in **step 1**, except resuspension should be carried out in 90 μL (3× the reaction volume).

14. To elute, add 19 μL of water to beads, mix well, place on magnet and transfer 18 μL into a new well.

The library preparation protocol is based on previously published protocols [16, 24–26], with small changes. For the sake of completeness, we provide the full protocol below.

3.3.2 RNA Fragmentation

1. To 18 μL of sample add 2 μL of zinc fragmentation buffer (Life Technologies).
2. Heat at 70 °C for 2 min in a thermocycler.
3. Immediately place on ice/cold block and add 2 μL EDTA stop solution.
4. Wash 20 μL of beads as in **step 2** in Subheading 3.3.1, except resuspension of beads is in 66 μL RLT (3× the reaction volume).
5. Repeat **steps 3–5** from Subheading 3.3.1.
6. Resuspend beads in 16.5 μL of water, mix well, place on magnet and elute by transferring 15.5 μL of the sample into a new well.

3.3.3 DNAse Treatment and Dephosphorylation

1. To each sample of 15.5 μL add 6 μL 5× FNK buffer, 0.5 μL RNAse inhibitor, 1 μL Turbo DNAse, 3 μL FastAP, 4 μL T4 PNK.
2. Incubate for 30 min at 37 °C.
3. Wash 20 μL beads as in Subheading 3.3.1, except resuspend beads in 90 μL RLT. To elute, add 7 μL water to beads, mix well, place on magnet and elute by transferring 6 μL of the sample into a new well.

3.3.4 First Ligation: Adapter Ligation to the RNA

1. To 6 μL of the RNA add 1 μL of 10 μM RNA adapter 5′—/5Phos/rArG rArUrC rGrGrA rArGrA rGrCrA rCrArC rGrUrC/3ddC/—3′.
2. Incubate at 70 °C for 2 min and place directly on ice or a cold block.
3. Add the following materials: 2 μL 10× T4 RNA ligase buffer, 1.8 μL DMSO, 0.2 μL ATP (100 mM), 8 μL PEG 8000 (50%), 0.3 μL RNAse inhibitor, 1.2 μL (36 U) T4 RNA Ligase 1, high concentration.
4. Incubate the mix at 23 °C for 90 min. It is possible to stop here and freeze in −80 °C.
5. Wash 15 μL of Silane Beads as follows: Place beads on magnet and remove supernatant. Add 50 μL RLT buffer, place on magnet, and remove supernatant. Resuspend beads in 3× the sample volume (60 μL RLT).

6. Add resuspended beads to sample, and then add 100% EtOH to create a selection against the smaller, to remove unattached adaptors. In case smaller RNA molecules are of interest (e.g., tRNAs) use 0.8× of the reaction and RLT combined volume (64 μL), or else use 0.6× (48 μL). Mix and incubate for 1 min. Place on magnet and remove supernatant.
7. Add 100 μL of 75% EtOH, wash by transferring from side to side of the magnet, remove supernatant. Repeat 75% EtOH wash.
8. Dry beads for 1 min.
9. To elute, add 13.5 μL of water to beads, mix well, place on magnet, and elute by transferring 12.5 μL of the sample into a new well.

3.3.5 First Strand cDNA Synthesis

1. Add 1 μL of the primer 5′—AGA CGT GTG CTC TTC CG—3′ (10 μM stock, 10 pmol final concentration). Mix well by pipetting up and down approximately ten times.
2. Heat 70 °C for 2 min in a thermocycler, and transfer directly to a cold block.
3. To the RNA-primer mix add: 4.4 μL superscript Buffer (5× FS), 1 μL 100 mM DTT, 1 μL 10 mM dNTP Mix, 0.5 μL RNAse inhibitor, 0.9 μL SuperscriptIII enzyme.
4. Move the sample from ice to 50 °C in a thermocycler.
5. Incubate at 50 °C for 60 min, then allow the thermocycler to cool down to 4 °C before removing.
6. Place on ice or on cold block.
7. Add 3 μL ExoSap-it. Incubate 37 °C in a thermocycler for 12 min. This step will digest the oligo dT and primers from the sample. This is a possible stopping point—can store at −20 °C.

3.3.6 RNA Hydrolysis

1. Add 1 μL of 0.5 M EDTA.
2. Add 2.5 μL 1 M NaOH.
3. Incubate at 70 °C for 12 min in a thermocycler.
4. Add 2.5 μL 1 M HCl to neutralize NaOH.
5. Carry out cleanup in reduced volume of EtOH as in **steps 5–8** in Subheading 3.3.4, except that 12 μL of Silane beads should be resuspended in 90 μL RLT buffer, and the volume of 100% EtOH is 96 μL if small RNAs are to be maintained (0.8×) or 72 μL (0.6×) for larger sized RNAs.
6. Elute in 6.5 μL water, and transfer 5.5 μL into a new tube.

3.3.7 Second Ligation: Adapter Ligation to the cDNA

1. To the 5.5 μL of cDNA, add 0.5 μL of a 100 μM stock of the DNA adaptor 5′—/5Phos/AG ATC GGA AGA GCG TCG TGT AG/3ddC/—3′.
2. Incubate for 3 min at 75 °C and place on ice or cold block.
3. To the cDNA-adaptor mix add: 2 μL 10× NEB Buffer, 0.8 μL DMSO (100%), 0.2 μL ATP (100 mM), 10 μL PEG 8000 (50%), and 1.6 μL (48 U) T4 RNA Ligase 1, high concentration.
4. Incubate at 23 °C overnight, or at least 3 h.
5. Carry out cleanup in reduced volume of EtOH as in **steps 5–8** in Subheading 3.3.4, except that 5 μL of Silane beads should be resuspended in 60 μL RLT buffer, and the volume of 100% EtOH is 64 μL if small RNAs are to be maintained (0.8×) or 48 μL (0.6×) for larger-sized RNAs.
6. Elute in 23 μL water, and transfer 11.5 μL into each of two tubes. One tube could be used for the PCR enrichment and the other kept as frozen cDNA for an additional potential PCR reaction.

3.3.8 PCR Enrichment and Cleanup

1. To the tube with 11.5 μL cDNA intended for PCR, add 1 μL of a 25 μM each mixture of the primers and 12.5 μL of a 2× KAPA HiFi HotStart ReadyMix PCR Kit (KAPA Biosystems).
2. PCR program: 95 °C—2 min, followed by 4 cycles of: 98 °C—20 s, 65 °C—15 s, 72 °C—15 s, and 6 cycles of 98 °C—15 s, 72 °C—15 s. Lastly, 72 °C—2 min and hold at 10 °C.
3. Run 5 μL of the library on an agarose gel (Invitrogen E-Gel™ EX Agarose Gels, 2%, G402002 can be used). Libraries should appear as 200–300 bp smears, while a defined band at 140 bp usually indicates the presence of primer dimers (*see* **Note 7**).
4. SPRI cleanup—Using water, bring total volume of samples to 40 μL. Add 40 μL SPRI beads, mix well by pipetting ~10 times, let stand at room temperature for 2 min. Place on magnet until all beads have collected. Remove supernatant, wash twice in 100 μL 75% EtOH, (70% is useable here). For each wash, move back and forth on magnet 15–20 times, until beads are no longer clumpy. Remove supernatant carefully, and dry at room temperature on magnet until beads appear dry (2–3 min). Elute in 40 μL water, then place on magnet to collect beads. Transfer to a new tube.
5. Repeat SPRI cleanup: Add 40 μL SPRI beads, and repeat the clean up as before. Elute in 13 μL of water to give final library sample.

6. Measure library concentration by a Qubit fluorimeter, using the Qubit® dsDNA HS Assay Kit. An aliquot of the library can be diluted to the concentration required for Next-generation sequencing.

4 Notes

1. The RNA extraction protocol is written for samples originating from a confluent 15 cm plate of HEK293 cells. Scale volumes if needed. The protocol yields 15–20 μg of isolated RNA when isolating total RNA using TRI Reagent (Sigma) according to manufacturer's instructions.
2. If needed, cells can be stored at −80 °C at this stage. Alternatively, continue immediately to mitochondrial isolation.
3. The use of disposable 25-G needle enables quick processing of multiple samples, while keeping a relatively high yield of isolated RNA. However, homogenization of cells using a Dounce homogenizer usually increases RNA yield. A major drawback of the Dounce homogenizer is the need to clean it between samples, which increases handling time substantially. If using a Dounce homogenizer, resuspend each sample in 2 mL of MEB supplemented with 0.1% BSA and homogenize it with 15 strokes.
4. Repeating the homogenization step is an optional, but recommended, step that increases the final RNA yield. If conducting this step, keep the supernatant from **step 6** on ice until the next step.
5. In our experience, for the purpose of pseudouridine detection, sufficient mitochondrial enrichment is achieved even without benzonase treatment.
6. The protocol includes many "cleanup" steps. The purpose of these steps is to rinse the sample of reagents from prior reactions in order to continue to the next reaction with a clean sample eluted in water (unless otherwise specified). Cleanup includes binding the reaction mix to pre-cleaned Silane beads. Pre-cleaning of beads is detailed in **step 2** of Subheading 3.3.1. When applicable, cleaning of the beads can be conducted in parallel to the reaction it is meant to follow and thus save time for the user. Note that throughout the protocol the "pre-cleaning of Silane Beads" step involves different bead/buffer volumes, as specified in the relevant step of the protocol.
7. If library is not detectable at this stage, it is possible to repeat the second part of the PCR program for additional 4–5 cycles, and rerun on an E-gel. If a few rounds of PCR were required,

the rest of the cDNA kept in a second tube could be used for setting a new PCR with the calibrated number of cycles. However, requirement for a large number of PCR cycles may suggest that the library is of low complexity.

References

1. Contreras L, Drago I, Zampese E, Pozzan T (2010) Mitochondria: the calcium connection. Biochim Biophys Acta 1797:607–618
2. Burke PJ (2017) Mitochondria, bioenergetics and apoptosis in cancer. Trends Cancer Res 3:857–870
3. Ojala D, Montoya J, Attardi G (1981) tRNA punctuation model of RNA processing in human mitochondria. Nature 290:470–474
4. Mercer TR, Neph S, Dinger ME et al (2011) The human mitochondrial transcriptome. Cell 146:645–658
5. Machnicka MA, Milanowska K, Osman Oglou O et al (2013) MODOMICS: a database of RNA modification pathways—2013 update. Nucleic Acids Res 41:D262–D267
6. Arroyo JD, Jourdain AA, Calvo SE et al (2016) A genome-wide CRISPR death screen identifies genes essential for oxidative phosphorylation. Cell Metab 24:875–885
7. Auffinger P, Westhof E (1998) Effects of pseudouridylation on tRNA hydration and dynamics: a theoretical approach. In: Modification and editing of RNA. American Society of Microbiology, Washington, DC, pp 103–112
8. Durant PC, Davis DR (1997) The effect of pseudouridine and pH on the structure and dynamics of the anticodon stem-loop of tRNA (Lys, 3). Nucleic Acids Symp Ser (36):56–57
9. Motorin Y, Keith G, Simon C et al (1998) The yeast tRNA:pseudouridine synthase Pus1p displays a multisite substrate specificity. RNA 4:856–869
10. Fernandez-Vizarra E, Berardinelli A, Valente L et al (2007) Nonsense mutation in pseudouridylate synthase 1 (PUS1) in two brothers affected by myopathy, lactic acidosis and sideroblastic anaemia (MLASA). J Med Genet 44:173–180
11. Zeharia A, Fischel-Ghodsian N, Casas K et al (2005) Mitochondrial myopathy, sideroblastic anemia, and lactic acidosis: an autosomal recessive syndrome in Persian Jews caused by a mutation in the PUS1 gene. J Child Neurol 20:449–452
12. Zaganelli S, Rebelo-Guiomar P, Maundrell K et al (2017) The pseudouridine synthase RPUSD4 is an essential component of mitochondrial RNA granules. J Biol Chem 292:4519–4532
13. Antonicka H, Choquet K, Lin Z-Y et al (2017) A pseudouridine synthase module is essential for mitochondrial protein synthesis and cell viability. EMBO Rep 18:28–38
14. Calvo SE, Clauser KR, Mootha VK (2016) MitoCarta2.0: an updated inventory of mammalian mitochondrial proteins. Nucleic Acids Res 44:D1251–D1257
15. Safra M, Sas-Chen A, Nir R et al (2017) The m (1)A landscape on cytosolic and mitochondrial mRNA at single-base resolution. Nature. https://doi.org/10.1038/nature24456
16. Schwartz S, Bernstein DA, Mumbach MR et al (2014) Transcriptome-wide mapping reveals widespread dynamic-regulated pseudouridylation of ncRNA and mRNA. Cell 159:148–162
17. Safra M, Nir R, Farouq D et al (2017) TRUB1 is the predominant pseudouridine synthase acting on mammalian mRNA via a predictable and conserved code. Genome Res 27:393–406
18. Carlile TM, Rojas-Duran MF, Zinshteyn B et al (2014) Pseudouridine profiling reveals regulated mRNA pseudouridylation in yeast and human cells. Nature 515:143–146
19. Lovejoy AF, Riordan DP, Brown PO (2014) Transcriptome-wide mapping of pseudouridines: pseudouridine synthases modify specific mRNAs in S. cerevisiae. PLoS One 9:e110799
20. Li X, Zhu P, Ma S et al (2015) Chemical pull-down reveals dynamic pseudouridylation of the mammalian transcriptome. Nat Chem Biol 11:592–597
21. Grinberg M, Schwarz M, Zaltsman Y et al (2005) Mitochondrial carrier homolog 2 is a target of tBID in cells signaled to die by tumor necrosis factor alpha. Mol Cell Biol 25:4579–4590
22. Minczuk M, He J, Duch AM et al (2011) TEFM (c17orf42) is necessary for transcription of human mtDNA. Nucleic Acids Res 39:4284–4299
23. Quinodoz SA, Ollikainen N, Tabak B et al (2018) Higher-order inter-chromosomal hubs shape 3D genome organization in the nucleus. Cell 174:744–757.e24

24. Engreitz JM, Pandya-Jones A, McDonel P et al (2013) The Xist lncRNA exploits three-dimensional genome architecture to spread across the X chromosome. Science 341:1237973
25. Shishkin AA, Giannoukos G, Kucukural A et al (2015) Simultaneous generation of many RNA-seq libraries in a single reaction. Nat Methods 12:323–325
26. Van Nostrand EL, Pratt GA, Shishkin AA et al (2016) Robust transcriptome-wide discovery of RNA-binding protein binding sites with enhanced CLIP (eCLIP). Nat Methods 13:508–514

Chapter 10

High-Throughput Detection of mtDNA Mutations Leading to tRNA Processing Errors

Marita Annika Isokallio and James Bruce Stewart

Abstract

Some mutations in the tRNA genes of mitochondrial DNA (mtDNA) have been demonstrated to affect the processing of the mitochondrial transcriptome in human patients with mitochondrial disease. A recent analysis of mtDNA mutations in 527 human tumors revealed that approximately a quarter of the somatic mt-tRNA gene mutations lead to aberrant processing of the mitochondrial transcriptome in these tumors. Here, we describe a method, based on mtDNA mutations induced by the mtDNA mutator mouse, to map the sites that lead to transcript processing abnormalities. Mutations in the mtDNA are identified and quantified by amplicon-based mtDNA sequencing, and compared to the allelic ratios observed in matched RNASeq data. Strong deviation in the variant allele frequencies between the amplicon and RNASeq data suggests that such mutations lead to disruptions in mitochondrial transcript processing.

Key words Mitochondrial DNA, Transcriptome, Illumina sequencing, Mutation detection, tRNAs, RNA processing

1 Introduction

As we learn more of mitochondrial genomes and their architecture, it becomes nearly impossible to accurately generalize what a mitochondrial genome is [1]. Even within animals, apparent gene loss, gene acquisition, and variations in tRNA content and genetic code are well documented [2–4]. The mammalian mitochondrial DNA (mtDNA) itself encodes 13 protein-coding genes, including all core subunits of the mitochondrial respiratory chain complexes I, and III–IV. Another ~80 protein subunits of these complexes, and >1100 other proteins that carry out all other mitochondrial functions are transcribed from the nuclear DNA. These nuclear-encoded proteins are imported into mitochondria via a number of different mechanisms, depending on the sub-compartment of the mitochondria the protein is targeted to [5]. This dual-genome system has allowed the reduction of the coding content of the

Michal Minczuk and Joanna Rorbach (eds.), *Mitochondrial Gene Expression: Methods and Protocols*, Methods in Molecular Biology, vol. 2192, https://doi.org/10.1007/978-1-0716-0834-0_10,

mtDNA itself. Mammalian mtDNA contains the precise tRNA complement of 22 tRNAs and 2 rRNAs required to translate the mitochondrially encoded peptides with the vertebrate mitochondrial genetic code [6]. Animal mitochondria have even found ways to reduce the complement of RNAs that are normally found through the tree of life. For instance, the 5s rRNA subunit has been demonstrated to have been replaced by dual purposing tRNAs [7–9].

The mtDNA encoded tRNAs also play an important role in the "tRNA punctuation" model of mitochondrial RNA maturation. Early studies revealed that in mammalian mitochondria, transcription initiates from two promoters in the control region, and proceeds through the entire coding region in each direction, producing two large transcripts [10, 11]. The interspacing of the tRNA genes between the majority of the protein-coding and rRNA genes was noted early on [11], prompting the "tRNA punctuation model" of mitochondrial RNA maturation [10]. According to this model, tRNAs are recognized by a then-undefined mitochondrial RNase P and RNase Z activities, and then liberated mRNAs and rRNAs are identified and matured into their functional forms [10]. Human cell-line mitochondria were originally found to contain 18 distinct polyA-RNAs, all of which began at, or close to, an ATN of one of the protein-coding gene's open reading frames or one of the rRNA genes [10, 12]. In human [13] and mouse [14] mitochondria, sequence mapping has identified a conserved set of 11 mRNAs. These mRNAs encode the 13 protein open reading frames, with *Atp8/Atp6* and *Nd4L/Nd4* as bicistronic mRNAs, as one would predict by a strict application of the tRNA punctuation model. The remaining polyA-RNAs are interpreted as unprocessed transcript intermediates that appear to persist within the mitochondrial matrix. In *Drosophila*, differences in the Northern-blotting patterns revealed a different pool of RNAs suggesting five different transcriptional cassettes instead of the two seen in mammals [15]. However, these transcriptional initiation sites remain undefined. Interestingly, the same 11 mRNA remain conserved between the flies and mammals, including a processing event at the *Atp6–Cox3* gene boundary, which in mammals and flies lack an intervening tRNA [13, 14, 16], deviating from the tRNA punctuation model. RNASeq-based transcriptome analyses of human and fly mitochondria have confirmed this picture of the RNA species in the mitochondria [17, 18].

Recent work has clarified the enzyme complexes involved in the transcriptional processing. The mitochondrial RNase P is composed of at least four enzymatic subunits (*Mrpp1–3*, and *Hsd10*) [19–21], which have been shown to function without the ribozyme component found in the known, non-mitochondrial RNase Ps [19, 20, 22, 23]. The RNase Z activity is supplied by the *Elac2* gene product [24, 25], which has activity in both the nucleus and mitochondria [26]. These enzymes appear to act in concert, with the RNase P activity preceding the RNase Z activity [16, 21, 27]. The gene *Ptcd1* had previous been implicated in the processing of mitochondrial RNAs as well [28], but recent mouse knockout work implies that the previously observed processing defects may be the result of increased transcription, overwhelming the RNase P and RNase Z activities [29]. Instead, *Ptcd1* appears to act with other mitochondrial RNA granule proteins [30–32] to ensure the pseudouridylation of the *lrRNA*, and the stability of the *lrRNA* and non-polyadenylated *Nd6* mRNAs [29].

It was recognized early on in mitochondrial disease patients that mutations in the tRNAs can lead to alterations in the processing of the affected tRNA/mRNA boundaries [33–35]. More recently, naturally occurring variants in the RNase P complex have been shown to lead to quantifiable variations in the mitochondrial transcriptome [36]. In a previous study, we identified mtDNA mutations from whole-genome sequencing (WGS) data from The Cancer Genome Atlas (TCGA) and sought to confirm the presence of those mutations in polyA+ RNASeq data available for the same samples. Expectedly, for 616 confirmed mtDNA mutations, a strong linear correlation between the allelic ratios of the DNA and RNA datasets were observed, with the exception of 15 mutations. Surprisingly, 12 of these were in tRNA genes (26.7% of the tRNA mutations identified in the study), with the other 3 originating from the rRNAs and a protein-coding gene (<1% of these mutations detected) [27]. As tRNAs are not polyadenylated, size selection protocols for PolyA+ RNASeq should have excluded mature tRNAs. Inspection of the sequence reads revealed that these 12 specific tRNA mutations lead to the accumulation of RNA species bearing the unprocessed tRNA sequences within the mitochondrial RNA pool (Fig. 1a). Moreover, these mutations were predicted to lead to disruptions of the folding stability of the secondary structures of the tRNA genes, implying that their structure may be important to the recognition by the RNase P.

We recognized this as a powerful method to functionally screen the mtDNA for variants that may lead to such processing defects. Yet, that cancer study of the whole-genome DNA and RNA Illumina sequencing of 527 tumors only identified 45 mutations in the tRNA genes (2.3% of the tRNA-encoding bases according to the human mtDNA reference genome [37]). Thus, an accelerated model of mtDNA mutagenesis would be required: the mtDNA mutator mice, a mouse model with a knock-in allele for a proofreading-deficient mitochondrial DNA polymerase [38] which shows at least 40× the mtDNA mutation rate compared to wild-type mice of the same nuclear genetic background [39]. Female lineages of these mice have been shown to transmit, segregate, and clonally expand mtDNA mutations, especially in tRNA genes [40, 41]. Our preliminary work shows that the N2

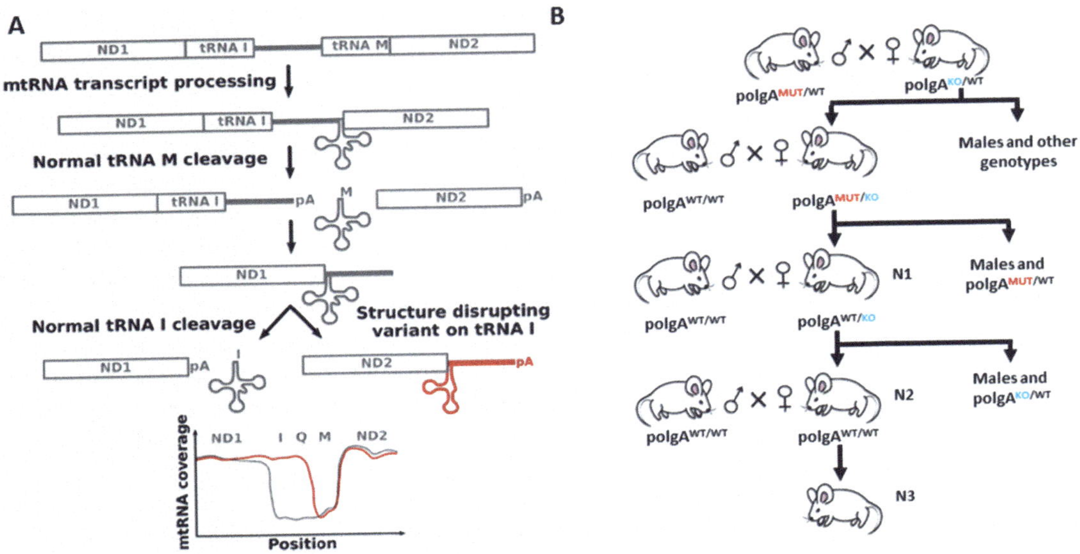

Fig. 1 High-throughput detection of mtDNA mutations leading to tRNA processing errors. (**a**) Schematic representation of mitochondrial tRNA processing in the presence of a mutation in *mtTI* that leads to aberrant RNA processing. Sequence coverage curves for the mutation-bearing RNASeq data (red line) are then compared to normal cells (gray line), as in [27]. (**b**) Schematic of mouse lineages and genotypes for the study. Preliminary data showed detection of these characteristic allelic mismatches in animals from the N2 and N3 generations. N2 animals will have more detectable mutations (mean = 1015 per animal) increasing the efficiency of the screening. Yet N3 animals (mean 423 SNPs per animal) will have higher relative allele frequencies. N3 progeny of female N2 animals with potential variants leading to allelic mismatches would provide verification of hits found in the N2

and N3 backcross generations provide the optimal signal. In these mice, certain point mutations have segregated to levels that allow statistical detection of mismatches between the variant allele frequency (AF) values.

Here, we describe a method to detect mtDNA mutations potentially inducing tRNA processing defects in lineages of the mtDNA mutator mice by detecting and characterizing the mtDNA and mtRNA variant AFs by an Illumina sequencing strategy. The use of large mtDNA amplicons in sequencing has been shown to highly enrich mtDNA, and efficiently decrease the detection of NUMTS [42], nuclear pseudogenes of mitochondrial origin which may confound mutation analysis [43, 44]. The mtDNA variants detected in this analysis are then matched to RNASeq data, and a mismatch between the AFs in the amplicon and RNASeq analyses is utilized to identify potentially compromised RNA processing intermediates.

2 Materials

2.1 Tissue Collection

1. Place two freshly collected ~50 mg pieces of liver into separate Eppendorf tubes and snap-freeze in liquid nitrogen. Store the tissues at −80 °C until use.

2.2 Amplicon Sequencing of Mouse mtDNA

2.2.1 Sample Collection

1. Scalpel, mortar, pestle.
2. Dry ice −80 °C.
3. Eppendorf tube.
4. Lysis buffer (20 mM Tris, 150 mM NaCl, 20 mM EDTA, 1% SDS, pH 8.75).
5. 0.02 mg/ml Proteinase K.
6. 0.02 mg/ml RNase A.

2.2.2 DNA Extraction

1. Chloroform:isoamyl alcohol in the presence of 1.2 M potassium acetate.
2. RNase A.
3. 96% ethanol.
4. 70% ethanol.
5. 5 mM Tris–HCl (pH 8.5).

2.2.3 Amplicon Production

1. PCR with Phusion® High-Fidelity DNA Polymerase (New England Biolabs).
2. 5× Phusion HF buffer.
3. 1.25 mM of dNTPs.

2.2.4 Amplicon Purification

1. Column-based PCR cleanup kit (Machery-Nagel NucleoSpin® Gel or PCR cleanup kit).
2. 5 mM Tris–HCl (pH 8.5) buffer.
3. Qubit™ 1× dsDNA HS Assay Kit (Thermo Fisher).
4. Qubit® 3.0 Fluorometer.

2.2.5 Amplicon Pooling

1. NEBNext Ultra II DNA Library preparation kit (New England Biolabs).
2. Illumina HiSeq2500 or HiSeq3000.

2.3 Total RNA Sequencing

2.3.1 Total RNA Extraction

1. Pre-clean mortar, pestle and pipettes with RNAZap.
2. RNase-Free 1.5 ml Eppendorf tube.
3. TRIzol.
4. Chloroform.
5. Isopropanol.

6. 75% ethanol.
7. Ethanol for rinsing purposes.
8. Nuclease-free water.

2.3.2 Removal of Contaminant DNA

1. TURBO DNA-free™ kit (Thermo Fisher).
2. Qubit™ RNA XR Assay Kit (Thermo Fisher).
3. Qubit® 3.0 Fluorometer (or similar).
4. Experion™ miniature electrophoresis system.
5. RNA StdSens Analysis kit (Bio-RAD).

2.3.3 rRNA Depletion

1. RiboZero rRNA Removal Kit (Human/Mouse/Rat) (Illumina).
2. NEBNext® Ultra Directional RNA Library Prep Kit (New England Biolabs).
3. Illumina HiSeq2500 or HiSeq3000.

2.4 Analysis of DNA Amplicon Sequencing Data

1. Sequence read trimming: Flexbar v.2.5.
2. DNA read aligner: BWA (mem) v.0.7.12-r1039.
3. Read filtering: samtools v.1.3.1 (or later).
4. Coverage calculation: bedtools v.2.22.1.
5. Variant calling: LoFreq* v2.1.2.
6. Variant filtering and annotation: SnpEff v.4.2.

2.5 Analysis of RNASeq Data

1. Sequence read trimming: Flexbar v.2.5.
2. RNA sequence aligner, STAR v2.4.1d.
3. Read filtering: samtools v.1.3.1 (or later).
4. Coverage calculation: bedtools v.2.22.1.
5. Variant calling: LoFreq* v2.1.2.
6. Variant filtering and annotation: SnpEff v.4.2.
7. Read visualization: IGV Genome browser.

3 Methods

3.1 Mouse Breeding

Three mtDNA mutator mouse variants have been published to date, all with the same *PolgA*-D257A mutation in the exonuclease domain, which leads to error-prone mtDNA replication, and the accumulation of mutations [38, 45, 46] (MGI:3046825, $Polg^{tm1.1Lrsn}$; MGI:3583920, $Polg^{tm1Prol}$; and MGI:5502688, $Polg^{tm1Jiha}$, respectively). The variant by the Prolla lab [45] is available for purchase from the Jackson Laboratories (Stock No: 017341).

Our preliminary analyses have shown the liver to be a good target for this work, due to its large size and active mitochondrial transcription. The entire liver is not used in the experiments described, allowing the use of the animal for many simultaneous experiments. However, alternative tissues could be investigated with appropriate optimization.

1. For our work, we initiated female lineages with female hemizygous mtDNA mutator mice, which resulted from a cross of a heterozygous polgA-knockout female [47] (MGI:3584444, $Polg^{tm1.2Lrsn}$) and a heterozygous $PolgA^{D257A}$ male, as in [39] to ensure all mtDNA mutations have occurred post-fertilization in the same individual (Fig. 1b). Depending on the breeding scheme of mtDNA mutator mice, complications may arise in continuous breeding of females that are heterozygous for a *PolgA*^{D257A} allele, which would transmit low levels of mtDNA to their offspring per each generation [39, 48]. The breeding scheme utilized here avoids this problem, and furthermore, it limits all mtDNA mutagenesis to the germline development in a single generation, reducing the problem of clonal expansion of specific mtDNA variants. The mtDNA mutator developed by the Larsson lab has a floxed *PolgA*^{D257A} allele, breeding a heterozygote $PolgA^{D257A}$ male to a germline-active cre-female, such as the β-actin *cre*-transgene, can produce the knockout allele described in [47].
2. Female $PolgA^{D257A}/PolgA^{KO}$ mice were selected and backcrossed to wildtype males. N1 female $WT/PolgA^{KO}$ mice were selected for backcrossing to generate the WT/WT N2 and N3 mice (Fig. 1b). The mtDNA mutations produced in the founder female will thus be transmitted, segregated, and allowed to clonally expand during these successive transmissions through the female germline bottleneck, as in [41]. Preliminary data show that each backcross reduces the mean number of variants that are subsequently detected (N1 mean = 7376, N2 mean = 1015, N3 = 423), while the AF for a given SNP detected in the mtDNA increases, making it easier to discern the transcript processing defects in the RNA-Seq data [49].

3.2 Amplicon Sequencing of Mouse mtDNA

1. For DNA extraction, cut the liver sample into fine pieces with a scalpel, and then grind in a mortar and pestle that was pre-cooled to −80 °C on dry ice.
2. Transfer the powdered tissue to a 1.5 ml Eppendorf tube and incubate overnight at 56 °C in 500 μl lysis buffer (20 mM Tris, 150 mM NaCl, 20 mM EDTA, 1% SDS, pH 8.75) with 0.02 mg/ml Proteinase K and 0.02 mg/ml RNase A added.

3. Extract DNA from the digested tissue with 500 μl chloroform: isoamyl alcohol in the presence of 1.2 M potassium acetate.
4. Briefly vortex the mixture and then spin down at top speed in a desktop centrifuge. Transfer the aqueous upper layer to a fresh tube, add ~150 ng of RNase A to the solution and incubate at 37 °C for approximately 1 h.
5. Add 2.1 times the volume of 96% ethanol to precipitate the DNA (*see* **Note 1**). Wash the pellet twice by addition of 500 μl of 70% ethanol and centrifugation at 16,000 rcf for 15 min. Dissolve the pellet in 20 μl of 5 mM Tris–HCl (pH 8.5). Confirm the DNA concentration with a spectrometer, and adjust the volume to a usable concentration.
6. Produce three amplicons by PCR with Phusion® High-Fidelity DNA Polymerase according to the manufacturer's instructions, using the supplied 5× Phusion HF buffer, in 20 μl reaction volumes. More than a single replicate of the amplification reaction may be needed per sample (*see* **Notes 2** and **3**).
7. Add primers to a final concentration of 10 μM, 1.25 mM of dNTPs, and 25 ng/μl total DNA extract. Optimized annealing temperatures and primer sequences for each amplicon are found in Table 1, and carry out amplicon cycling at;

$$\frac{98^{\circ}\text{C}}{30\,\text{s}}\left(\frac{98^{\circ}\text{C}}{5\,\text{s}}\ \frac{\text{annealing}}{2\ \text{min}}\ \frac{72^{\circ}\text{C}}{2\ \text{min}}\right)\times 20\,\text{cycles}\ \frac{72^{\circ}\text{C}}{10\ \text{min}}\ \frac{4\ \text{to}\ 8^{\circ}\text{C}}{\infty}.$$

8. Purify the amplicons using a column-based PCR cleanup kit.

Table 1
Amplicon Primers and annealing conditions

Amplicon number	Primer name [40]	Sequence (5′ → 3′) (M13 Tags underlined)	Start position	Annealing temperature (°C)
1	mp-6F	<u>TGTAAAACGACGGCCAGT</u>TTGA TGAGGATCTTACTCCC	9376	58
	mp-30R	<u>CAGGAAACAGCTATGACC</u>TCTA TGGAGGTTTGCATGTG	113	
2	mp-10F	<u>TGTAAAACGACGGCCAGT</u>GAAAC TTTATCAGACATCTGG	15773	51
	mp-13R	<u>CAGGAAACAGCTATGACC</u>GATAG TAGAGTTGAGTAGCG	4373	
3	mp-23F	<u>TGTAAAACGACGGCCAGT</u>CAAGCCC TCTTATTTCTAGG	3756	57
	mp-6R	<u>CAGGAAACAGCTATGACC</u>GTAGG TTGAGATTTTGGACG	10163	

9. Combine replicate PCR reactions of the same amplicon and adjust the volume up to 100 μl for each column, then follow the protocol as per the manufacturer's instructions.
10. Elute the column with 30 μl of the supplied 5 mM Tris–HCl (pH 8.5) buffer.
11. Perform a second elution with additional 30 μl and collect the flow through in the same collection tube.
12. Assess the concentration with a Qubit™ 1× dsDNA HS Assay Kit using a Qubit® 3.0 Fluorometer (or similar).
13. Pool the three amplicons at equimolar ratio, to a minimal combined concentration of 20 ng/μl in at least 10 μl final volume.
14. Fragment the library through either sonication or enzymatic fragmentations protocols, depending on your lab or sequencing center's protocols. Use 250 bp fragments to create the libraries using the NEBNext Ultra II DNA Library preparation kit as directed in the product protocol. Use sample barcoding protocols to allow the pooling of samples during sequencing.
15. Conduct sequencing on an Illumina HiSeq2500 or HiSeq3000 at 1 × 150 bp sequencing to obtain 1 Gb of sequencing per sample (*see* **Note 4**).

3.3 Total RNA Sequencing

1. Pre-clean mortar, pestle, and pipettes with RNAZap or an equivalent product to minimize the chance of exposing the sample to excess RNase.
2. For Total RNA extraction, mince the second 50 mg sample of tissue with a scalpel, and then ground in a mortar and pestle pre-cooled to −80 °C on dry ice.
3. Transfer the powdered tissue to an RNase-Free 1.5 ml Eppendorf tube. Extract the tissue using 1 ml TRIzol and incubate on ice for 5 min before adding 200 μl chloroform.
4. Briefly vortex the solution and incubate on ice for 2–3 min.
5. Transfer the aqueous phase to a clear, RNase-free tube and add 500 μl of isopropanol.
6. Incubate 20 min on ice, then pellet the RNA by centrifugation at 16,000 rcf for 30 min at 4 °C. Carefully draw the liquid off with a pipette without disturbing the RNA pellet. Wash the pellet with 1 ml 75% ethanol and centrifuge at 16,000 rcf for 5 min at 4 °C.
7. Draw the ethanol off of the pellet and wash the pellet with 500 μl of ethanol and centrifuge at 16,000 rcf for 5 min at 4 °C. After drawing off the ethanol, centrifuge pellet at 16,000 rcf for 1 min at 4 °C, then draw off any residual ethanol.

8. Incubate the RNA pellet at 55 °C for 2 min to evaporate any traces of ethanol. Dissolve the RNA pellet in 50 μl nuclease-free water with heating to 55 °C for 2 min to aid in the dissolving of the RNA, if necessary.
9. Remove contaminant DNA using the TURBO DNA-free™ kit with the Routine DNase treatment protocol supplied by the manufacturer.
10. Assess the Total RNA integrity using an Experion™ miniature electrophoresis system using the RNA StdSens Analysis kit or an equivalent method.
11. Finally, quantify the RNA using the Qubit™ RNA XR Assay Kit in a Qubit® 3.0 Fluorometer (or similar).
12. Deplete the rRNA from 1 μg of total RNA sample, using the RiboZero rRNA Removal Kit (Human/Mouse/Rat) as per the manufacturer's instructions (*see* **Note 5**).
13. Prepare directional RNA libraries with the NEBNext® Ultra Directional RNA Library Prep Kit, as per the manufacturer's instructions. Use sample barcoding protocols to allow the pooling of samples during sequencing.
14. Conduct sequencing on an Illumina HiSeq2500 or HiSeq3000 at 1 × 150 bp. Preliminary data suggests that 5 Gb of sequencing per sample results in 10–1000× coverage of the mitochondrial tRNA sequences [49].

3.4 Analysis of DNA Amplicon Sequencing Data

1. Obtain the Standard mouse mtDNA reference genome that is consistent with your mouse's mitochondrial haplogroup (e.g., The C57Bl/6J at GenBank Accession NC_005089.1; the C57Nl/6NCrl at GenBank accession JF286601, etc.).
2. Create a custom, second mtDNA reference by splitting the sequence in approximately the middle, and joining the first half of the sequence to the end. This will allow complete assembly across the break of the linearized reference sequences.
3. A step-by-step outline of the data analysis can be found at https://doi.org/10.17504/protocols.io.nfkdbkw but we have added an additional trimming step to this protocol, to remove the primer sequences from the data analysis and more stringent variant filtering better suitable for amplicon data.
4. Perform trimming of the sequencing reads with Flexbar v.2.5 [50] for quality and adapter sequences (parameters -q 28 -m 50 -ao 10 -at 1 -ae ANY). Use an additional trimming step to remove the M13-tagged reads by adding the forward and reverse primer sequences from Table 1 to a fasta file and use that for additional filtering (parameters -bo 15 -bt 2 -bu -be ANY). This will remove M13 primer-tagged reads allowing exclusion of the amplicon ends (including the primer sequences) from the downstream sequence analysis and correction of the coverage at overlapping amplicon regions.

5. Align the trimmed reads to the mitochondrial reference genome with BWA version 0.7.12-r1039, invoking mem (-T 19 -B 3 -L 5,4) [51] (*see* **Note 6**).
6. Keep only uniquely aligned reads with samtools (–q 1) [52] and calculate the per-position coverage with bedtools v.2.22.1 (genomecov –d) [53].
7. Call the variants using LoFreq∗ v2.1.2 [54], a variant caller which does not assume a diploid genome, making it suitable for mitochondrial heteroplasmy analysis. Set indel qualities (indelqual –dindel), and call the variants in LoFreq∗ (--parallel-threads 20 -N -B -q 30 -Q 30 --call-indels --no-default-filter) and filter them with the filter parameters (--snvqual-thres 70 --sb-incl-indels -B 60 --no-defaults).
8. Filter and annotate the variants using SnpEff [55, 56] using the vertebrate mitochondrial codon table. Set the filtering conditions to require 15 alternative base supporting reads to call the SNP ($DP*AF \geq 15$) and with a minimum of 3 supporting reads on each strand ($DP4[2] \geq 3$ and $DP4[3] \geq 3$).
9. Keep all variants except the 200 positions closest to the first and to the last reference genome positions. Repeat **steps 4** to **8** using the custom reference genome made in Subheading 3.4, **step 2**. Keep variants detected at the 400 middle positions of this genome i.e., 200 first and last positions in the original reference genome and correct the position numbering to correspond to the original reference genome positions. Combine the two resulting files in order to obtain variant results for the entire mtDNA genome. To reduce the false positive calls inherent to amplicon-based methods, use $AF \geq 0.5$–1.0% for final filtering of the data.

3.5 Analysis of RNASeq Data

1. Perform the analysis on the RNA reads, using the standard mouse mtDNA reference genome. Correction to the linearized genome as described for the DNA analysis above is not required, because the *mtTF* variants will not be detected with our rRNA depletion strategy. If a polyA-RNASeq strategy is attempted, alignment to the custom reference from Subheading 3.4, **step 2** should avoid potential assembly issues for the *mtTF* gene variant detection.
2. Perform a similar analysis as the described steps in Subheading 3.4, except use an RNA sequence aligner, STAR v2.4.1d [57] instead of BWA. Align the reads with the default parameters, except for genome indexing (--genomeSAindexNbases 6).
3. Match the detected RNASeq variants to those found in the amplicon dataset, and compare the variations in the DNA and RNA. Assume that variants found in the RNASeq data but not in the amplicon data are artifacts and sequencing errors for

further analysis. In [27] we could easily identify the mismatched alleles, as the mutations present in the tumors tended to have clonally expanded significantly, and were often present in more than half of the mtDNAs in the tumor. Given that the AF of some variants will still be quite small, calculate the allelic imbalance (AI) between the datasets as;

$$\mathrm{AI} = \log 2\left(\frac{\text{RNASeq AF}}{\text{Amplicon AF}}\right)$$

4. To visualize the results, plot these AI values versus the genome positions of the variants.
5. To identify the interesting RNA variants, inspect the RNA reads with a genome browser e.g., IGV Genome browser [58] to confirm that the interesting RNA variants originate from continuous, unprocessed RNA sequence intermediates. Where possible, confirm variants with AI by using another animal of the same female lineage, or better, in the N3 progeny of the mouse bearing the variant of interest.

4 Notes

1. Normally, precipitation is immediate in these conditions, but prolonged incubation or incubation at −20 °C or −80 °C could be done.
2. We found that 20 μl reactions were more efficient than larger volumes, so multiple 20 μl reactions were set up to obtain sufficient ng of amplified product DNA.
3. Phusion polymerase was used due to our familiarity with the enzyme. Any high-fidelity polymerase with the ability to amplify large fragments could be substituted in the protocol. Amplification conditions would need to be re-optimized accordingly.
4. In our work, we have performed sequencing only on HiSeq2500 or 3000 models and chemistry, and these provided sufficient sequence quality for low level heteroplasmy detection. MiSeq, other HiSeq, or non-Illumina sequencing would need to be optimized and/or tested by the user. We used 1 × 150-bp read lengths, as we found in other experiments that the second read of a 2 × 150-bp sequencing rather decreased than increased the quality of the results. With 1 Gb of 1 × 150 bp reads, you normally obtain >40,000× coverage across the mtDNA genome. If all reads would be of good quality and align to the mtDNA, 1 Gb would provide >61,000× average coverage.

5. In our pilot study, we chose to optimize non-ribosomal coverage by using the RiboMinus RNA depletion strategy. This lead to reduced ability to detect SNPs in the RNASeq data from the *mtTF, mtTV, and mtTL1* tRNAs, which abut the mt-rRNAs. As the previous cancer study was carried out using polyA+ RNASeq protocols [28], and small oligoA tails are found on the rRNAs of mouse mitochondria [14], polyA+ RNASeq could provide an alternative strategy for detection of SNPs on those missing tRNAs.

6. Our preliminary analysis revealed that with amplicon enrichment, ~99% of the sequenced reads originated from the mtDNA, allowing alignment directly to only the mtDNA reference genome instead of the entire mouse genome [50]. For the mouse, this is helpful, as a large number of highly identical NUMTs [59] are found in the nuclear reference genome: for instance a 4.65 kb insertion in chromosome 1 (GRCm38.p4 C57BL/6J, NC_000067.6, positions 24611535 to 24616184), aligning to positions 6394–11042 of the mitochondrial reference genome NC_005089.1 with 99.98% identity. In our analysis using unique mapping, aligning the reads against the entire mouse genome leads to no alignment at all over 28.6% of the mitochondrial genome, from *mtCO1* to *mtNd4* [50]. With this high mtDNA-specific enrichment, miscalls due to variant NUMT sequence contamination is not a problem.

References

1. Burger G, Gray MW, Lang BF (2003) Mitochondrial genomes: anything goes. Trends Genet 19(12):709–716. S0168952503003044 [pii]
2. Lavrov DV, Pett W (2016) Animal mitochondrial DNA as we do not know it: mt-genome organization and evolution in nonbilaterian lineages. Genome Biol Evol 8(9):2896–2913. https://doi.org/10.1093/gbe/evw195
3. Bernt M, Bleidorn C, Braband A, Dambach J, Donath A, Fritzsch G, Golombek A, Hadrys H, Juhling F, Meusemann K, Middendorf M, Misof B, Perseke M, Podsiadlowski L, Reumont BV, Schierwater B, Schlegel M, Schrodl M, Simon S, Stadler PF, Stoger I, Struck TH (2013) A comprehensive analysis of bilaterian mitochondrial genomes and phylogeny. Mol Phylogenet Evol. https://doi.org/10.1016/j.ympev.2013.05.002
4. Bernt M, Braband A, Schierwater B, Stadler PF (2013) Genetic aspects of mitochondrial genome evolution. Mol Phylogenet Evol 69 (2):328–338. https://doi.org/10.1016/j.ympev.2012.10.020
5. Wiedemann N, Pfanner N (2017) Mitochondrial machineries for protein import and assembly. Annu Rev Biochem 86:685–714. https://doi.org/10.1146/annurev-biochem-060815-014352
6. Boore JL (1999) Animal mitochondrial genomes. Nucleic Acids Res 27(8):1767–1780
7. Desai N, Brown A, Amunts A, Ramakrishnan V (2017) The structure of the yeast mitochondrial ribosome. Science 355(6324):528–531. https://doi.org/10.1126/science.aal2415
8. Rorbach J, Gao F, Powell CA, D'Souza A, Lightowlers RN, Minczuk M, Chrzanowska-Lightowlers ZM (2016) Human mitochondrial ribosomes can switch their structural RNA composition. Proc Natl Acad Sci U S A 113(43):12198–12201. https://doi.org/10.1073/pnas.1609338113
9. Greber BJ, Bieri P, Leibundgut M, Leitner A, Aebersold R, Boehringer D, Ban N (2015) Ribosome. The complete structure of the 55S

mammalian mitochondrial ribosome. Science 348(6232):303–308. https://doi.org/10.1126/science.aaa3872

10. Ojala D, Montoya J, Attardi G (1981) tRNA punctuation model of RNA processing in human mitochondria. Nature 290 (5806):470–474
11. Ojala D, Merkel C, Gelfand R, Attardi G (1980) The tRNA genes punctuate the reading of genetic information in human mitochondrial DNA. Cell 22(2 Pt 2):393–403
12. Montoya J, Ojala D, Attardi G (1981) Distinctive features of the 5′-terminal sequences of the human mitochondrial mRNAs. Nature 290 (5806):465–470
13. Temperley RJ, Wydro M, Lightowlers RN, Chrzanowska-Lightowlers ZM (2010) Human mitochondrial mRNAs—like members of all families, similar but different. Biochim Biophys Acta 1797(6–7):1081–1085. https://doi.org/10.1016/j.bbabio.2010.02.036
14. Ruzzenente B, Metodiev MD, Wredenberg A, Bratic A, Park CB, Cámara Y, Milenkovic D, Zickermann V, Wibom R, Hultenby K, Erdjument Bromage H, Tempst P, Brandt U, Stewart JB, Gustafsson CM, Larsson N-G (2012) LRPPRC is necessary for polyadenylation and coordination of translation of mitochondrial mRNAs. EMBO J 31(2):443–456. https://doi.org/10.1038/emboj.2011.392
15. Berthier F, Renaud M, Alziari S, Durand R (1986) RNA mapping on Drosophila mitochondrial DNA: precursors and template strands. Nucleic Acids Res 14(11):4519–4533
16. Stewart JB, Beckenbach AT (2009) Characterization of mature mitochondrial transcripts in Drosophila, and the implications for the tRNA punctuation model in arthropods. Gene 445 (1–2):49–57
17. Mercer TR, Neph S, Dinger ME, Crawford J, Smith MA, Shearwood AM, Haugen E, Bracken CP, Rackham O, Stamatoyannopoulos JA, Filipovska A, Mattick JS (2011) The human mitochondrial transcriptome. Cell 146 (4):645–658. https://doi.org/10.1016/j.cell.2011.06.051
18. Torres TT, Dolezal M, Schlotterer C, Ottenwalder B (2009) Expression profiling of Drosophila mitochondrial genes via deep mRNA sequencing. Nucleic Acids Res 37 (22):7509–7518. https://doi.org/10.1093/nar/gkp856
19. Reinhard L, Sridhara S, Hallberg BM (2015) Structure of the nuclease subunit of human mitochondrial RNase P. Nucleic Acids Res. https://doi.org/10.1093/nar/gkv481
20. Deutschmann AJ, Amberger A, Zavadil C, Steinbeisser H, Mayr JA, Feichtinger RG, Oerum S, Yue WW, Zschocke J (2014) Mutation or knock-down of 17beta-hydroxysteroid dehydrogenase type 10 cause loss of MRPP1 and impaired processing of mitochondrial heavy strand transcripts. Hum Mol Genet 23 (13):3618–3628. https://doi.org/10.1093/hmg/ddu072
21. Rackham O, Busch JD, Matic S, Siira SJ, Kuznetsova I, Atanassov I, Ermer JA, Shearwood AM, Richman TR, Stewart JB, Mourier A, Milenkovic D, Larsson NG, Filipovska A (2016) Hierarchical RNA processing is required for mitochondrial ribosome assembly. Cell Rep 16(7):1874–1890. https://doi.org/10.1016/j.celrep.2016.07.031
22. Holzmann J, Rossmanith W (2009) tRNA recognition, processing, and disease: hypotheses around an unorthodox type of RNase P in human mitochondria. Mitochondrion 9 (4):284–288. https://doi.org/10.1016/j.mito.2009.03.008
23. Holzmann J, Frank P, Loffler E, Bennett KL, Gerner C, Rossmanith W (2008) RNase P without RNA: identification and functional reconstitution of the human mitochondrial tRNA processing enzyme. Cell 135 (3):462–474. https://doi.org/10.1016/j.cell.2008.09.013
24. Takaku H, Minagawa A, Takagi M, Nashimoto M (2003) A candidate prostate cancer susceptibility gene encodes tRNA 3′ processing endoribonuclease. Nucleic Acids Res 31 (9):2272–2278
25. Brzezniak LK, Bijata M, Szczesny RJ, Stepien PP (2011) Involvement of human ELAC2 gene product in 3′ end processing of mitochondrial tRNAs. RNA Biol 8(4). 15393 [pii]
26. Siira SJ, Rossetti G, Richman TR, Perks K, Ermer JA, Kuznetsova I, Hughes L, Shearwood AJ, Viola HM, Hool LC, Rackham O, Filipovska A (2018) Concerted regulation of mitochondrial and nuclear non-coding RNAs by a dual-targeted RNase Z. EMBO Rep. https://doi.org/10.15252/embr.201846198
27. Stewart JB, Alaei-Mahabadi B, Sabarinathan R, Samuelsson T, Gorodkin J, Gustafsson CM, Larsson E (2015) Simultaneous DNA and RNA mapping of somatic mitochondrial mutations across diverse human cancers. PLoS Genet 11(6):e1005333. https://doi.org/10.1371/journal.pgen.1005333
28. Sanchez MI, Mercer TR, Davies SM, Shearwood AM, Nygard KK, Richman TR, Mattick JS, Rackham O, Filipovska A (2011) RNA processing in human mitochondria. Cell Cycle 10

(17):2904–2916. https://doi.org/10.4161/cc.10.17.17060

29. Perks KL, Rossetti G, Kuznetsova I, Hughes LA, Ermer JA, Ferreira N, Busch JD, Rudler DL, Spahr H, Schondorf T, Shearwood AJ, Viola HM, Siira SJ, Hool LC, Milenkovic D, Larsson NG, Rackham O, Filipovska A (2018) PTCD1 is required for 16S rRNA maturation complex stability and mitochondrial ribosome assembly. Cell Rep 23(1):127–142. https://doi.org/10.1016/j.celrep.2018.03.033
30. Jourdain AA, Koppen M, Wydro M, Rodley CD, Lightowlers RN, Chrzanowska-Lightowlers ZM, Martinou JC (2013) GRSF1 regulates RNA processing in mitochondrial RNA granules. Cell Metab 17(3):399–410. https://doi.org/10.1016/j.cmet.2013.02.005
31. Antonicka H, Sasarman F, Nishimura T, Paupe V, Shoubridge EA (2013) The mitochondrial RNA-binding protein GRSF1 localizes to RNA granules and is required for posttranscriptional mitochondrial gene expression. Cell Metab 17(3):386–398. https://doi.org/10.1016/j.cmet.2013.02.006
32. Tu YT, Barrientos A (2015) The human mitochondrial DEAD-Box protein DDX28 resides in RNA granules and functions in mitoribosome assembly. Cell Rep. https://doi.org/10.1016/j.celrep.2015.01.033
33. Bindoff LA, Howell N, Poulton J, McCullough DA, Morten KJ, Lightowlers RN, Turnbull DM, Weber K (1993) Abnormal RNA processing associated with a novel tRNA mutation in mitochondrial DNA. A potential disease mechanism. J Biol Chem 268 (26):19559–19564
34. Maniura-Weber K, Helm M, Engemann K, Eckertz S, Mollers M, Schauen M, Hayrapetyan A, von Kleist-Retzow JC, Lightowlers RN, Bindoff LA, Wiesner RJ (2006) Molecular dysfunction associated with the human mitochondrial 3302A>G mutation in the MTTL1 (mt-tRNALeu(UUR)) gene. Nucleic Acids Res 34(22):6404–6415
35. Mollers M, Maniura-Weber K, Kiseljakovic E, Bust M, Hayrapetyan A, Jaksch M, Helm M, Wiesner RJ, von Kleist-Retzow JC (2005) A new mechanism for mtDNA pathogenesis: impairment of post-transcriptional maturation leads to severe depletion of mitochondrial tRNASer(UCN) caused by T7512C and G7497A point mutations. Nucleic Acids Res 33(17):5647–5658
36. Hodgkinson A, Idaghdour Y, Gbeha E, Grenier JC, Hip-Ki E, Bruat V, Goulet JP, de Malliard T, Awadalla P (2014) High-resolution genomic analysis of human mitochondrial RNA sequence variation. Science 344 (6182):413–415. https://doi.org/10.1126/science.1251110
37. Andrews RM, Kubacka I, Chinnery PF, Lightowlers RN, Turnbull DM, Howell N (1999) Reanalysis and revision of the Cambridge reference sequence for human mitochondrial DNA. Nat Genet 23(2):147
38. Trifunovic A, Wredenberg A, Falkenberg M, Spelbrink JN, Rovio AT, Bruder CE, Bohlooly YM, Gidlof S, Oldfors A, Wibom R, Tornell J, Jacobs HT, Larsson NG (2004) Premature ageing in mice expressing defective mitochondrial DNA polymerase. Nature 429 (6990):417–423
39. Ross JM, Stewart JB, Hagstrom E, Brene S, Mourier A, Coppotelli G, Freyer C, Lagouge M, Hoffer BJ, Olson L, Larsson NG (2013) Germline mitochondrial DNA mutations aggravate ageing and can impair brain development. Nature 501:412–415. https://doi.org/10.1038/nature12474
40. Stewart JB, Freyer C, Elson JL, Wredenberg A, Cansu Z, Trifunovic A, Larsson N-G (2008) Strong purifying selection in transmission of mammalian mitochondrial DNA. PLoS Biol 6 (1):e10
41. Kauppila JH, Baines HL, Bratic A, Simard ML, Freyer C, Mourier A, Stamp C, Filograna R, Larsson NG, Greaves LC, Stewart JB (2016) A phenotype-driven approach to generate mouse models with pathogenic mtDNA mutations causing mitochondrial disease. Cell Rep 16 (11):2980–2990. https://doi.org/10.1016/j.celrep.2016.08.037
42. Li M, Schroeder R, Ko A, Stoneking M (2012) Fidelity of capture-enrichment for mtDNA genome sequencing: influence of NUMTs. Nucleic Acids Res 40(18):e137. https://doi.org/10.1093/nar/gks499
43. Samuels DC, Han L, Li J, Quanghu S, Clark TA, Shyr Y, Guo Y (2013) Finding the lost treasures in exome sequencing data. Trends Genet 29(10):593–599. https://doi.org/10.1016/j.tig.2013.07.006
44. Dayama G, Emery SB, Kidd JM, Mills RE (2014) The genomic landscape of polymorphic human nuclear mitochondrial insertions. Nucleic Acids Res 42(20):12640–12649. https://doi.org/10.1093/nar/gku1038
45. Kujoth GC, Hiona A, Pugh TD, Someya S, Panzer K, Wohlgemuth SE, Hofer T, Seo AY, Sullivan R, Jobling WA, Morrow JD, Van Remmen H, Sedivy JM, Yamasoba T, Tanokura M, Weindruch R, Leeuwenburgh C, Prolla TA (2005) Mitochondrial DNA mutations, oxidative stress,

and apoptosis in mammalian aging. Science 309(5733):481–484

46. Mito T, Kikkawa Y, Shimizu A, Hashizume O, Katada S, Imanishi H, Ota A, Kato Y, Nakada K, Hayashi J (2013) Mitochondrial DNA mutations in mutator mice confer respiration defects and B-cell lymphoma development. PLoS One 8(2):e55789. https://doi.org/10.1371/journal.pone.0055789
47. Hance N, Ekstrand MI, Trifunovic A (2005) Mitochondrial DNA polymerase gamma is essential for mammalian embryogenesis. Hum Mol Genet 14(13):1775–1783
48. Kauppila TES, Kauppila JHK, Larsson NG (2017) Mammalian mitochondria and aging: an update. Cell Metab 25(1):57–71. https://doi.org/10.1016/j.cmet.2016.09.017
49. Isokallio MA (2017) The source and fate of mitochondrial DNA mutations using high-sensitivity next-generation sequencing technologies. PhD Thesis, Universität zur Köln, Köln, Deutchland
50. Dodt M, Roehr JT, Ahmed R, Dieterich C (2012) FLEXBAR-flexible barcode and adapter processing for next-generation sequencing platforms. Biology 1(3):895–905. https://doi.org/10.3390/biology1030895
51. Li H (2013) Aligning sequence reads, clone sequences and assembly contigs with BWA-MEM. arXiv 1303.3997
52. Li H, Handsaker B, Wysoker A, Fennell T, Ruan J, Homer N, Marth G, Abecasis G, Durbin R (2009) The Sequence Alignment/Map format and SAMtools. Bioinformatics 25 (16):2078–2079. https://doi.org/10.1093/bioinformatics/btp352
53. Quinlan AR, Hall IM (2010) BEDTools: a flexible suite of utilities for comparing genomic features. Bioinformatics 26(6):841–842. https://doi.org/10.1093/bioinformatics/btq033
54. Wilm A, Aw PP, Bertrand D, Yeo GH, Ong SH, Wong CH, Khor CC, Petric R, Hibberd ML, Nagarajan N (2012) LoFreq: a sequence-quality aware, ultra-sensitive variant caller for uncovering cell-population heterogeneity from high-throughput sequencing datasets. Nucleic Acids Res 40(22):11189–11201. https://doi.org/10.1093/nar/gks918
55. Cingolani P, Platts A, Wang le L, Coon M, Nguyen T, Wang L, Land SJ, Lu X, Ruden DM (2012) A program for annotating and predicting the effects of single nucleotide polymorphisms, SnpEff: SNPs in the genome of Drosophila melanogaster strain w1118; iso-2; iso-3. Fly 6(2):80–92. https://doi.org/10.4161/fly.19695
56. Cingolani P, Patel VM, Coon M, Nguyen T, Land SJ, Ruden DM, Lu X (2012) Using Drosophila melanogaster as a model for genotoxic chemical mutational studies with a new program, SnpSift. Front Genet 3:35. https://doi.org/10.3389/fgene.2012.00035
57. Dobin A, Davis CA, Schlesinger F, Drenkow J, Zaleski C, Jha S, Batut P, Chaisson M, Gingeras TR (2013) STAR: ultrafast universal RNA-seq aligner. Bioinformatics 29(1):15–21. https://doi.org/10.1093/bioinformatics/bts635
58. Thorvaldsdottir H, Robinson JT, Mesirov JP (2013) Integrative Genomics Viewer (IGV): high-performance genomics data visualization and exploration. Brief Bioinform 14 (2):178–192. https://doi.org/10.1093/bib/bbs017
59. Hazkani-Covo E, Zeller RM, Martin W (2010) Molecular poltergeists: mitochondrial DNA copies (numts) in sequenced nuclear genomes. PLoS Genet 6(2):e1000834. https://doi.org/10.1371/journal.pgen.1000834

Chapter 11

High-Throughput Measurement of Mitochondrial RNA Turnover in Human Cultured Cells

Anna V. Kotrys, Lukasz S. Borowski, and Roman J. Szczesny

Abstract

RNA turnover is an essential part of the gene expression pathway, and there are several experimental approaches for its determination. High-throughput measurement of global RNA turnover rates can provide valuable information about conditions or proteins that impact gene expression. Here, we present a protocol for mitochondrial RNA turnover analysis which involves metabolic labeling of RNA coupled with quantitative high-throughput fluorescent microscopy. This approach gives an excellent opportunity to discover new factors involved in mitochondrial gene regulation when combined with loss-of-function screening strategy.

Key words Mitochondrial RNA, Bromouridine (BrU), RNA turnover, Metabolic labeling

1 Introduction

The steady state level of RNA is a result of two opposite processes—formation and destruction, which encompass RNA synthesis, post-transcriptional processing and decay. These processes respond to internal and external stimuli to fine tune the levels of functional RNA molecules. Their regulation involves different mechanisms, which rely on protein–RNA interactions and RNA folding. Mitochondrial RNA (mtRNA) turnover is still not fully understood. We know the key components of mitochondrial transcription machinery [1–3], RNA processing factors [4–7] and main RNA-degrading enzymes [8, 9]. However, regulatory mechanisms for these factors are largely unknown. A typical analysis of RNA turnover includes measurement of transcription rates as well as determination of RNA decay. In the case of mitochondria, measurement of transcriptional rates most often involves isolation of these organelles and assessing incorporation of labeled ribonucleotides [10, 11]. Although this *in organello* method gives an excellent opportunity to study the direct effect of a given stimuli on the mitochondrial transcription and

Michal Minczuk and Joanna Rorbach (eds.), *Mitochondrial Gene Expression: Methods and Protocols*,
Methods in Molecular Biology, vol. 2192, https://doi.org/10.1007/978-1-0716-0834-0_11,

analysis of individual RNAs, it suffers from a limited number of conditions that can be tested at once. On the contrary, metabolic labeling of transcripts in cultured cells allows studies in the whole cellular context and provides an opportunity to analyze many conditions simultaneously (if combined with appropriate technical strategy), although it has limited ability to track individual transcripts. Here, we describe a protocol for global mtRNA turnover measurement without isolation of mitochondria (Fig. 1). Total cellular RNA is labeled with bromouridine (BrU) in cultured cells (Fig. 1a), detected in fixed cells using anti-BrU immunostaining (Fig. 1b) and quantified with the help of fluorescent microscopy (Fig. 1c, d). Immunodetection of BrU-labeled transcripts is combined with staining of nuclei and mitochondria. Thus,

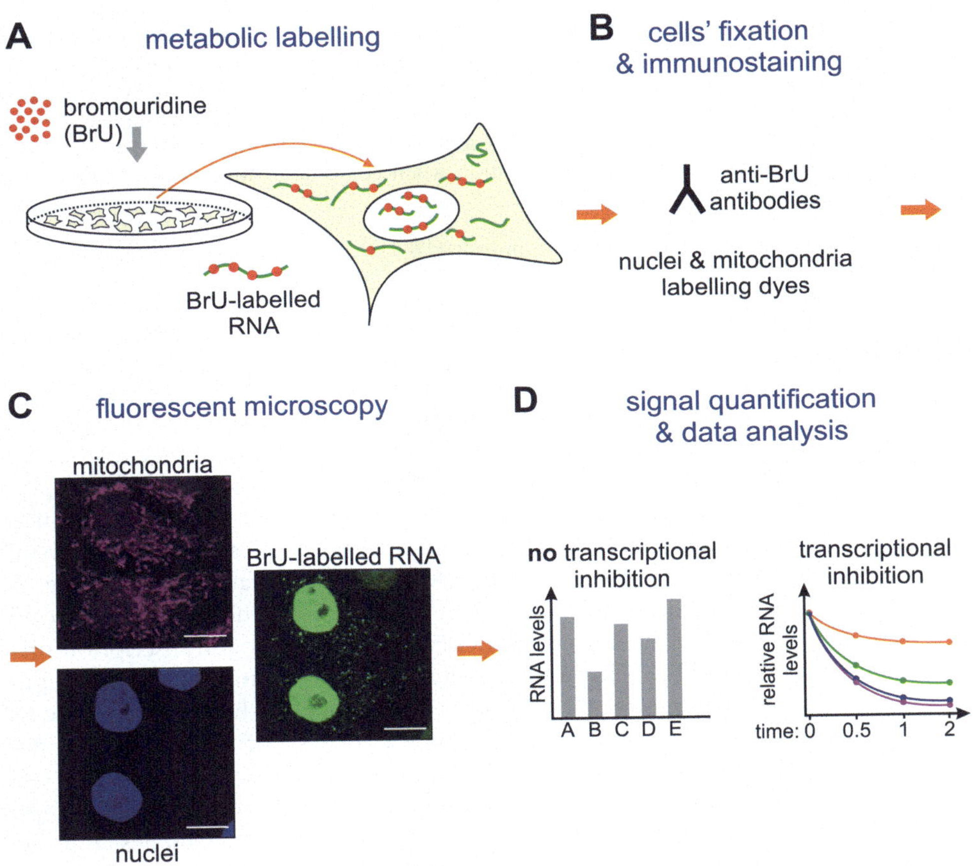

Fig. 1 Schematic representation of the procedure. (**a**) Bromouridine is added to the cell culture and is incorporated to nascent nuclear and mitochondrial encoded transcripts. (**b**) Cells are fixed following staining of BrU-labeled RNAs with anti-BrU antibodies. Nuclei and mitochondria are stained with specific labeling dyes. (**c**) Fluorescent microscopy is carried out to envision BrU-labeled transcripts. (**d**) Signal quantification enables analysis of relative RNA levels in studied samples. If the analysis includes transcription inhibition step, a decay rate of BrU-labeled can be determined (graph on the right)

mitochondrial transcripts can be distinguished from nuclear encoded ones, with the resolution limit of applied microscopy technique. A variant of this approach includes a step of transcriptional shut-off after BrU labeling. This strategy enables the determination of RNA stability providing a possibility to identify factors which are involved in mtRNA decay (Fig. 1d, the graph on the right). Moreover, modification of this method allows investigation of proteins involved in mtDNA transcription [12]. Importantly, this approach can be optimized for the high-throughput procedure enabling the application of screening strategies, such as siRNA screening. The procedure consists of the following steps: (1) transcriptional labeling of RNA with BrU, (2) inhibition (or not) of transcription, (3) immunodetection of BrU-labeled RNAs combined with staining of mitochondria and nuclei, (4) acquisition of fluorescent microscopy images and quantification. The levels of BrU-labeled mtRNAs are compared in different conditions, revealing ones which impact transcriptional capacity and/or change transcripts' stability. A few steps which require optimization are discussed and example results are presented.

2 Materials

2.1 Labeling of RNA with BrU and Inhibition of Transcription

1. Desired mammalian cell line (for example HeLa).
2. Cell culture vessels: 384-well microplates (Greiner Bio-One) (*see* **Notes 1** and **2**).
3. Cell culture medium suitable for applied cells (here DMEM, Gibco).
4. Cell culture supplements (if applicable): 10% FBS, Penicillin/Streptomycin mixture (final concentration of 100 U and 0.1 mg/mL, respectively) (*see* **Note 3**).
5. Cell culture incubator set to 37 °C with a humidified 5% CO_2 atmosphere.
6. Multidrop Combi Reagent Dispenser (Thermo Fisher Scientific) (*see* **Note 1**).
7. 100 mM 5-Bromouridine solution (Sigma) dissolved in sterile water (*see* **Note 4**). Store at −20 °C.
8. 0.5 mg/mL Actinomycin D (ActD) solution (Sigma) prepared in sterile water (*see* **Note 4**). Store at −20 °C.

2.2 Cells Fixation and Immunostaining of BrU-Labeled Transcripts

1. Phosphate Buffered Saline (PBS): 137 mM NaCl, 2.7 mM KCl, 10 mM phosphate buffer solution, pH 7.4 (Sigma).
2. 2× Fixing solution: 10% (v/v) formaldehyde, 0.5% (w/v) Triton X-100, 4 ng/mL Hoechst 33342 dye (Invitrogen).

3. 2× Blocking solution: 6% (w/v) Bovine Serum Albumin (BSA) in PBS (*see* **Note 5**).
4. Primary antibodies: anti-BrU/BrdU (Abcam) (*see* **Note 6**).
5. Secondary antibodies: anti-rat conjugated with Alexa Fluor 555 (Thermo Fisher Scientific) (*see* **Note 7**).
6. Multidrop Combi Reagent Dispenser (Thermo Fisher Scientific).
7. 405 LS Microplate Washer (Bio Tek) (*see* **Note 8**).

2.3 Fluorescent Microscopy: Data Acquisition

1. ScanR fluorescence microscopy system, Olympus (*see* **Note 9**).
2. MT20 lighting system based on a 150 W xenon burner.
3. Objective: UPlanSApo 20.0×, NA 0.75 (Olympus).
4. Hamamatsu Orca-R2 (C10600) CCD camera.

2.4 Image Data Analysis

1. ScanR 2.7.2 analysis software (Olympus) (*see* **Note 10**).

2.5 siRNA Transfection in 384-Well Format

1. Cell culture vessels: 384-well microplates (Greiner Bio-One) (*see* **Note 2**).
2. Opti-MEM I Reduced Serum Medium (Gibco).
3. Lipofectamine RNAiMAX Transfection Reagent (Invitrogen).
4. siRNAs: Control non-targeting siRNA D-001810-10-20 (Dharmacon), PNPase targeting siRNA L-019454-01-0020 (Dharmacon).
5. Multichannel pipette.
6. Multidrop Combi Reagent Dispenser (Thermo Fisher Scientific).

3 Methods

3.1 Labeling of RNA with BrU

1. Seed cells on 384-well plates. Dispose 20 μL of the medium at room temperature to the wells, following addition of 20 μL cell suspension at desired concentration. Use Multidrop Combi Reagent Dispenser or equivalent apparatus to assure equal seeding amounts and conditions (*see* **Notes 11–13**).
2. Incubate plates at room temperature for 60 min before placing plates to the incubator (*see* **Note 14**).
3. Grow cells at 37 °C with a humidified 5% CO_2 atmosphere.
4. After desired time add BrU to the cell culture medium to a final concentration of 2.5 mM (*see* **Notes 15** and **16**).
5. Return plates into the incubator and incubate for 60 or 120 min (*see* **Note 17**).

6. Add ActD to the cell culture medium to the final concentration of 5 μg/mL (*see* **Notes 18** and **19**).
7. Return plates into the incubator and incubate for desired time (*see* **Note 20**).
8. Wash cells twice with 100 μL PBS. Leave 25 μL PBS in the wells after each washing step (*see* **Note 21**).

3.2 Cells Fixation and Immunostaining of BrU-Labeled Transcripts

1. Fix cells by addition of 25 μL of 2× fixing solution to each well.
2. Incubate plates for 30 min at room temperature.
3. Wash cells four times with 100 μL PBS. Leave 25 μL PBS in the wells after each washing step (*see* **Note 21**).
4. Add 25 μL of 2× blocking solution to each well.
5. Incubate plates for 30 min at room temperature.
6. Aspirate 40 μL of blocking solution so that 10 μL of 1× blocking solution remains in each well.
7. Prepare 2× concentrated solution of primary antibodies by diluting antibodies 1:300 with 1× blocking solution (*see* **Note 22**).
8. Add 10 μL of 2× concentrated primary antibodies to each well (final dilution of antibodies 1:600).
9. Incubate at 4 °C overnight.
10. Wash cells four times with 100 μL PBS. Leave 10 μL PBS in the wells after the last washing (*see* **Note 21**).
11. Prepare 2× concentrated solution of secondary antibodies by diluting antibodies 1:400 with 2× blocking solution (*see* **Note 23**).
12. Add 10 μL of 2× concentrated secondary antibodies to each well (final dilution of antibodies 1:800).
13. Incubate plates for 60 min at room temperature. Protect from light.
14. Wash cells four times with 100 μL PBS. Leave 50 μL PBS in the wells after the last washing (*see* **Note 21**). Fixed cells are kept in PBS for imaging.
15. Seal the plates with an adhesive sealing tape.
16. Store the plates at 4 °C until imaging (*see* **Note 24**).

3.3 Fluorescence Microscopy: Data Acquisition

1. Remove the plates from 4 °C 1 h before imaging and keep in a dark place at room temperature to adjust the temperature of the plates. After incubation wipe the bottom to remove water vapor.
2. Turn on the microscope and the burner at least 10 min before imaging (the time can vary depending on the applied imaging system). Allow the burner to stabilize light emission and the microscope to calibrate the motorized stage.

3. Mount the plate in the motorized stage.
4. Check the auto-focus settings. Verify if the system can properly focus on cells growing in wells at the edges of the plate (*see* **Note 25**).
5. Set the appropriate fluorescent channels to be imaged: at least Nuclei and BrU. Collect the z-stacks for the BrU channel (*see* **Note 26**).
6. Set the appropriate acquisition time for each channel (*see* **Note 27**).
7. Set the number of images to be collected per well (*see* **Note 28**).
8. Perform high-throughput imaging using automated microscopy station (*see* **Notes 22** and **29**).

3.4 Image Data Analysis

1. Create virtual channels for each channel to be analyzed and subtract the background (*see* **Note 30**).
2. Create the main-object mask from the virtual channel of the nuclei. Use module "Edge." Do not detect the objects on the borders of the image.
3. Create the sub-object mask from the virtual channel of BrU. Use "spot-detector" module. Manually adjust setting to identify the highest number of spots with the intensity of fluorescence above the background level (*see* **Note 31**).
4. Define the main-object mask for sub-objects to be measured outside the nuclei. Use distance = 1 and width = 50 (*see* **Note 32**).
5. Define the parameters to be measured for each type of objects. For main-objects measure: area, circularity factor, fluorescence total intensity of nuclei, foci count. For sub-objects measure: area and total intensity of BrU foci fluorescence.
6. Define the derived parameters: total and mean intensity of BrU foci. Total intensity of BrU foci is a sum of the parameter "total intensity of BrU foci fluorescence." Mean intensity of BrU foci is a sum of the parameter "total intensity of BrU foci fluorescence" divided by the parameter "foci area."
7. Run and save the analysis.
8. Create the dot plot from parameters for main objects: a circularity factor and an area. Set the gate to exclude from the analysis cells with abnormally shaped nuclei. The nuclei should all have a comparable size and an approximately round shape (a circularity factor close to 1.0).
9. Export the following data for gated population: nuclei count, foci count, total intensity of BrU foci, mean intensity of BrU foci.

10. Analyze the exported data with the appropriate statistical analysis software (for example R, GraphPad Prism or Microsoft Excel).

3.5 siRNA Transfection in 384-Well Format: Method Validation and Anticipated Results

1. Dilute siRNA to 140 nM with Opti-MEM medium.
2. Pipette 5 μL of siRNA solution to the wells of 384-well plate (*see* **Note 33**).
3. Dilute RNAiMAX transfection reagent with Opti-MEM medium 1:100 and add 10 μL of prepared solution to each well containing siRNA (*see* **Note 34**).
4. Incubate plates for 40 min at room temperature.
5. While incubation of siRNA with transfection reagent is in progress harvest cells and prepare cell suspension at desired concentration (*see* **Note 4**). Seed cells by placing 20 μL of cell suspension to the wells of 384-well plates with prepared siRNA transfection mix.
6. Incubate plates at room temperature for 60 min before putting plates to the incubator (*see* **Note 14**).
7. Culture cells for desired time (routinely 72 h), label with BrU, subject to staining procedure and imaging. Anticipated results are presented on Fig. 2. Please note that in the presented case it

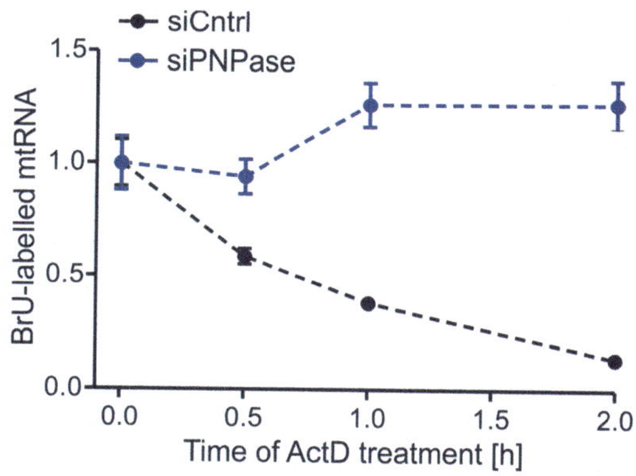

Fig. 2 Silencing of PNPase, a mitochondrial RNA degradosome component, stabilizes mitochondrial RNA. HeLa cells were transfected with siRNA targeting PNPase [9] or control non-targeting siRNA. Cells were cultured for 72 h following BrU labeling. BrU was added to the cell culture for 1 h then cells were treated (or not) with ActD (5 μg/mL) for the indicated time. Next, cells were fixed and BrU-labeled transcripts were detected with anti-BrU antibodies. Fluorescent microscopy images were obtained and relative BrU-labeled mtRNAs levels were quantified. Dashed lines show trend of BrU-labeled mtRNA decay. In the case of PNPase silencing, stabilization of mitochondrial transcripts is observed. This observation is in line with the anticipated result, showing that the lack of main mitochondrial RNA degradation machinery component results in inhibition of mtRNA degradation ($n = 4$, ±SEM)

was feasible to track decline of BrU-labeled RNAs in a few time points after addition of ActD as only one gene was silenced. This can be difficult to achieve if many genes are examined.

4 Notes

1. The protocol presented here describes a high-throughput procedure using 384-well plates and automated dispensing and washing stations. Nevertheless, it is possible to scale down described experiment and perform all steps with the use of manual electronic or multichannel pipettes and standard culture vessels and slides.
2. We recommend to apply poly-L-lysine coated plates. In particular, if you plan to perform the protocol with cells that do not adhere well (e.g., 293, also known as HEK293) consider using coated plates. If you wish to perform poly-L-lysine coating by yourself in low-throughput experimental format see coating protocol described previously [13].
3. Use of the antibiotics in the cell culture may be necessary as many steps of manipulations may lead to a contamination.
4. Prepare the solution in sterile water, store at −20 °C in aliquots of 0.5–1 mL. Before using, make sure that the reagents are thawed completely and no precipitants are present in the solution.
5. Filter the solution with a 0.22 μm filter before use to get rid of any remaining undissolved BSA. BSA solution can be prepared in advance and frozen at −20 °C.
6. There are several commercially available anti-BrU/BrdU antibodies. These antibodies detect both 5-Bromouridine (BrU) and 5-Bromodeoxyuridine (BrdU) which are incorporated into RNA or DNA, respectively. You may search for antibodies raised in different organisms or possessing specific isotype to fit your multiple staining experiment. Remember to test a new set of primary and secondary antibodies as described in **Note 21**.
7. Choice of the secondary antibodies depends strictly on the primary antibodies used. Make sure that your secondary antibodies recognize host species or specific isotype of the primary antibodies used.
8. Use of the automated wash station 405 LS Microplate Washer is not necessary although it is highly recommended for performing high-throughput experiments. Equivalent washing apparatus can be used.

9. Collection of images can be performed with any automated microscopy system.
10. Another software may be used for performing quantification. For small subsets of images, analysis can be performed with Image J (Fiji) [14], for larger subsets of data the CellProfiler [15] will be the alternative tool.
11. Determine the number of cells that you will seed for labeling. Density of the cell culture depends on the experiment, typically is around 70–90% on the day of labeling. If you plan to perform labeling 24 h after seeding we recommend starting at around 2400 HeLa or 143B human osteosarcoma cells per well and around 3000 293 cells per well. When performing siRNA transfection, consider that applied siRNA may be toxic for the cells, at least to some extent, and thus a higher number of the cells may be needed for seeding. Start at around 800 HeLa cells per well for labeling after 72 h of culture, increase cell number to around 1000–1200 per well if you observe siRNA toxicity.
12. If you observe cell aggregation, consider using cell strainer to separate the cells and to assure even growth in the well.
13. Seed cells and add reagents with an automated dispenser or multichannel pipette to assure equal seeding.
14. Incubating plates at room temperature helps to obtain even cell distribution within a well. Placing plates into the incubator directly after seeding may result in undesired cell migration due to temperature gradient in the wells.
15. Time of the culture prior to BrU labeling depends on the experimental design.
16. Consider that the medium evaporates during cell culture. Estimate volume of the medium remaining in the well before adding reagents to maintain their proper concentration. Note that BrU concentration may need to be adjusted for a specific cell line.
17. BrU labeling time might differ depending on the cell line and experimental design. We recommend to examine different BrU labeling times to make sure that the signal can be well distinguished from the background (*see* also **Note 23**). *See* Fig. 3 to compare different BrU labeling times for HeLa cells.
18. For sole examination of transcription rates, it is sufficient to perform immunostaining directly after BrU labeling, therefore, the addition of transcription inhibitors is not necessary. Treatment with transcription inhibitors enables investigation of transcripts stability.

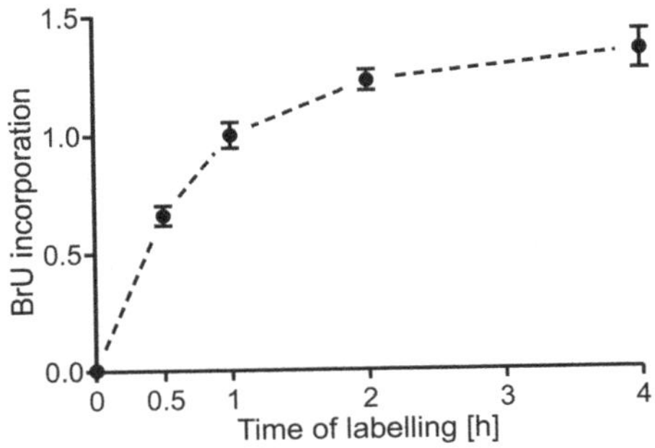

Fig. 3 Time-dependent increase of BrU labeling of mitochondrial RNA. HeLa cells were incubated with BrU for the indicated time. Cells were then fixed and BrU-labeled RNAs were detected with the use of anti-BrU antibodies. Quantification was performed to asses relative BrU incorporation, results were normalized to 1 h labeling time ($n = 6$, ±SEM)

19. ActD concentration and treatment time may vary between the cell types. To adapt the procedure to a high-throughput format, it is beneficial to reduce the number of steps during the process. In this example, we omit washing off BrU. Therefore, it is important that the condition which you apply (type of inhibitor, its concentration) ensures relatively quick and efficient inhibition of the transcription. Otherwise, decay rate data will be affected by the persistent labeling. Generally, you should choose the concentration of ActD and treatment time allowing for a complete transcription inhibition (i.e., with BrU signal increase not being observed) after ActD treatment. To optimize ActD treatment conditions perform a preliminary experiment by treating cells with various ActD concentrations at different time points prior to addition of BrU to the culture and subsequent immunofluorescent staining of BrU. To establish an optimal dose, you could consider ActD concentration ranging from 1 to 10 μg/mL. You should use conditions at which mitochondrial RNA labeling is blocked within 5 min of inhibitor treatment. *See* Fig. 4 as an example.
20. ActD treatment time may vary depending on the cell type, conditions, and experiment design. It is possible to perform a time-course of ActD treatment although in the high-throughput format it would be usually single, selected time point. The choice of the optimal time point depends on the extent of the effect/phenotype which you expect. If possible, perform a preliminary experiment using conditions (positive controls) which cause changes of the similar intensity as the one which you may expect in your final experiment. You may consider the following treatment times 30, 60, and 120 min.

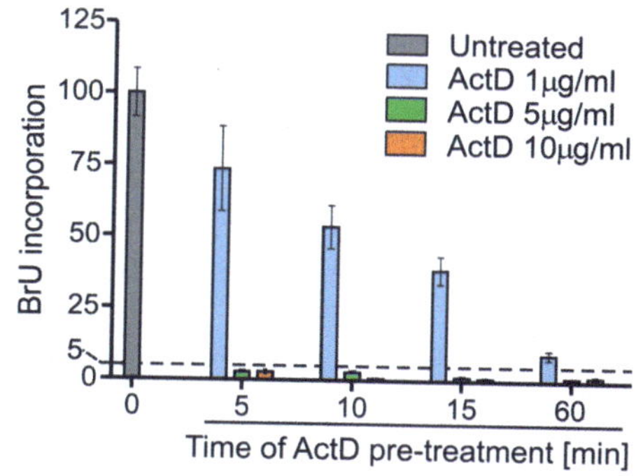

Fig. 4 Optimization of transcription inhibition. HeLa cells were preincubated with 1, 5 and 10 μg/mL of ActD for the indicated time (or untreated). Subsequently, BrU was added for 1 h, cells were fixed, and subjected to staining of BrU-labeled transcripts. Images were collected with the use of fluorescence microscopy. Signal intensity corresponding to non-nuclear RNA was quantified, showing inhibition of BrU incorporation upon ActD treatment ($n = 4$, ±SEM)

21. Perform wash steps with the use of 405 LS Microplate Washer (Bio Tek) or equivalent apparatus to assure equal washing conditions.
22. If you plan to use different antibodies, perform additional optimization step. Test various dilutions of primary and secondary antibodies (usually a final antibody dilution ranges from 1 to 5 μg/mL). If you plan to perform immunostaining with several primary antibodies test if you do not observe cross-reactivity of secondary antibodies. For this, perform staining with single primary antibody and add all secondary antibodies, except the one which is designated for applied primary antibody. You should not observe any signal in these conditions.
23. To determine the background level of anti-BrU staining, include a control where you do not add BrU to the medium. Perform staining with primary and secondary antibodies and examine signal intensities obtained.
24. Perform imaging preferably within 1–2 weeks after plates preparation. After prolonged storage time, you may observe a diffused fluorescent signal and/or that cells detach from the plate surface. Inspect plates under the microscope prior to running the scan to assure that cells are still attached. You may consider the addition of any antimicrobial preservative and/or antifade reagent to prevent microbial growth and increase fluorescent signal.
25. We strongly recommend using a microscope with Z-Drift Compensation System which continually monitors the distance between the objective lens and the sample surface, thus maintaining accurate focus and helping to overcome imperfections in the bottom surface of the plate.

26. Collecting z-stacks increases the number of BrU foci imaged.
27. Check histograms of fluorescence intensity for each channel in control wells. Check the wells with the highest expected intensity and the lowest one. Adjust exposure time to obtain the best dynamic range, avoiding detector saturation.
28. With 20× objective and Orca-R2 CCD camera we image area of 433 μm × 330 μm, at the confluency of 80%, ~200 HeLa cells can be detected with these settings.
29. To assure mitochondrial localization of the signal obtained from BrU-labeled transcripts, additional control immunostaining can be performed with antibodies against mitochondrial RNA granules components or to utilize specific mitochondrial dyes (e.g., MitoTracker, Thermo Fisher Scientific) to examine colocalization with BrU signal (Fig. 5). Alternatively, BrU labeling and staining can be performed in cells lacking mtDNA (rho0). In this case, no signal outside nucleus should be observed. Please note that rho0 culture medium is supplemented with uridine which can outcompete BrU. Wash off uridine supplemented medium before labeling.

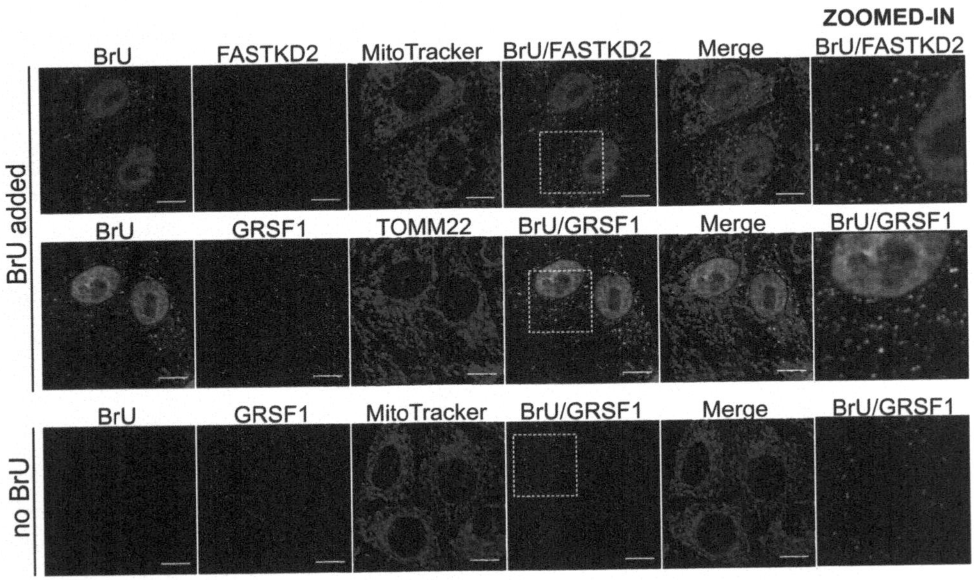

Fig. 5 Intracellular localization of BrU foci. Immunofluorescence was performed to examine the intracellular localization of BrU spots. BrU was added or not to the cell culture prior to staining of BrU-labeled transcripts with anti-BrU antibodies. FASTKD2 and GRSF1, well-known components of mitochondrial RNA granules, were detected with anti-FASTKD2 and anti-GRSF1 antibodies, respectively. Mitochondria were stained with MitoTracker or anti-TOMM22 antibodies. BrU/FASTKD2 as well as BrU/GRSF1 overlays show colocalization of BrU foci (green) with mitochondrial RNA granules components (red). Zoomed-in images are shown on the right. Merge images show colocalization of BrU foci (green), RNA granules components (red) with mitochondria (blue). Lack of BrU addition (no BrU) results in no signal observed in BrU channel. The same acquisition settings were applied for the BrU channel in BrU-labeled and unlabeled cells. Scale bar, 10 μm

30. To subtract the background from images of nuclei typically we use the filter with 50–100 pixel size (rolling ball algorithm). In BrU images we are focused on small foci and that is why we use a filter with 2–4 pixel size to subtract the background from these images.
31. It is useful to compare the results of spot detection between the wells with the highest expected fluorescence intensity and the lowest one (e.g., BrU unlabeled sample but subjected to BrdU staining).
32. For the exact definition of cell area staining with HCS Cell-Mask stain can be performed. Images from this channel should be used to create another sub-object mask. Foci detected inside nuclei must always be excluded from the analysis because they are mostly artifacts generated after background subtraction.
33. The way of adding siRNA solution to the wells depends on the number of siRNAs to be dispensed. For a large number of siRNA use of an automated pipetting workstation may be necessary. Otherwise, manual single or multichannel pipette is an option.
34. Transfection solution might be distributed with the use of reagent dispenser, automated pipetting workstation or any other pipetting device. Use of reagent dispenser, like Multi-drop Combi Reagent Dispenser (Thermo Fisher Scientific) is the method of choice.

Acknowledgments

Studies were supported by the National Science Centre, Poland [UMO-2014/12/W/NZ1/00463 to R.J.S.]. Experiments were carried out with the use of CePT infrastructure financed by the European Union: the European Regional Development Fund (Innovative economy 2007–13, Agreement POIG.02.02.00-14-024/08-00).

References

1. Litonin D, Sologub M, Shi Y, Savkina M, Anikin M, Falkenberg M, Gustafsson CM, Temiakov D (2010) Human mitochondrial transcription revisited: only TFAM and TFB2M are required for transcription of the mitochondrial genes in vitro. J Biol Chem 285:18129–18133
2. Minczuk M, He J, Duch AM, Ettema TJ, Chlebowski A, Dzionek K, Nijtmans LGJ, Huynen MA, Holt IJ (2011) TEFM (c17orf42) is necessary for transcription of human mtDNA. Nucleic Acids Res 39:4284–4299
3. Hillen HS, Temiakov D, Cramer P (2018) Structural basis of mitochondrial transcription. Nat Struct Mol Biol 25:754–765
4. Tomecki R, Dmochowska A, Gewartowski K, Dziembowski A, Stepien PP (2004) Identification of a novel human nuclear-encoded mitochondrial poly(A) polymerase. Nucleic Acids Res 32:6001–6014

5. Holzmann J, Frank P, Löffler E, Bennett KL, Gerner C, Rossmanith W (2008) RNase P without RNA: identification and functional reconstitution of the human mitochondrial tRNA processing enzyme. Cell 135:462–474
6. Brzezniak LK, Bijata M, Szczesny RJ, Stepien PP (2011) Involvement of human ELAC2 gene product in 3′ end processing of mitochondrial tRNAs. RNA Biol 8:616–626
7. Rorbach J, Minczuk M (2012) The post-transcriptional life of mammalian mitochondrial RNA. Biochem J 444:357–373
8. Szczesny RJ, Borowski LS, Brzezniak LK, Dmochowska A, Gewartowski K, Bartnik E, Stepien PP (2010) Human mitochondrial RNA turnover caught in flagranti: involvement of hSuv3p helicase in RNA surveillance. Nucleic Acids Res 38:279–298
9. Borowski LS, Dziembowski A, Hejnowicz MS, Stepien PP, Szczesny RJ (2013) Human mitochondrial RNA decay mediated by PNPase-hSuv3 complex takes place in distinct foci. Nucleic Acids Res 41:1223–1240
10. Enríquez JA, Fernández-Silva P, Pérez-Martos A, López-Pérez MJ, Montoya J (1996) The synthesis of mRNA in isolated mitochondria can be maintained for several hours and is inhibited by high levels of ATP. Eur J Biochem 237:601–610
11. Park CB, Asin-Cayuela J, Cámara Y, Shi Y, Pellegrini M, Gaspari M, Wibom R, Hultenby K, Erdjument-Bromage H, Tempst P, Falkenberg M, Gustafsson CM, Larsson N-G (2007) MTERF3 is a negative regulator of mammalian mtDNA transcription. Cell 130:273–285
12. Kotrys AV, Cysewski D, Czarnomska SD, Pietras Z, Borowski LS, Dziembowski A, Szczesny RJ (2019) Quantitative proteomics revealed C6orf203/MTRES1 as a factor preventing stress-induced transcription deficiency in human mitochondria. Nucleic Acids Res 47:7502–7517
13. Szczesny RJ, Kowalska K, Klosowska-Kosicka-K, Chlebowski A, Owczarek EP, Warkocki Z, Kulinski TM, Adamska D, Affek K, Jedroszkowiak A, Kotrys AV, Tomecki R, Krawczyk PS, Borowski LS, Dziembowski A (2018) Versatile approach for functional analysis of human proteins and efficient stable cell line generation using FLP-mediated recombination system. PLoS One 13:e0194887
14. Schindelin J, Arganda-Carreras I, Frise E, Kaynig V, Longair M, Pietzsch T, Preibisch S, Rueden C, Saalfeld S, Schmid B, Tinevez J-Y, White DJ, Hartenstein V, Eliceiri K, Tomancak P, Cardona A (2012) Fiji: an open-source platform for biological-image analysis. Nat Methods 9:676–682
15. Jones TR, Kang IH, Wheeler DB, Lindquist RA, Papallo A, Sabatini DM, Golland P, Carpenter AE (2008) CellProfiler Analyst: data exploration and analysis software for complex image-based screens. BMC Bioinformatics 9:482

Chapter 12

RNA Crosslinking to Analyze the Mitochondrial RNA-Binding Proteome

Selma L. van Esveld and Johannes N. Spelbrink

Abstract

Even though the mammalian mitochondrial genome (mtDNA) is very small and only codes for 13 proteins, all being subunits of the oxidative phosphorylation system, it requires several hundred nuclear encoded proteins for its maintenance and expression. These include replication and transcription factors, approximately 80 mitoribosomal proteins and many proteins involved in the posttranscriptional modification, processing, and stability of mitochondrial RNAs. In recent years, many of these factors have been identified and functionally characterized, but the complete mtRNA-interacting proteome is not firmly established. Shotgun proteomics has been used successfully to define whole-cell polyadenylated RNA (poly(A)-RNA) interacting proteomes using the nucleotide analogue 4-thiouridine (4SU) combined with UV crosslinking, poly(A)-RNA isolation and mass spectrometry to identify all poly(A)-RNA bound proteins. Although in this case also a considerable number of mitochondrial proteins were identified, the method was not specifically directed at the mitochondrial poly(A)-RNA bound proteome. Here we describe a method for enrichment of the mitochondrial poly(A)-RNA bound proteome based on 4SU labeling and UV crosslinking. The method can be applied either for isolated mitochondria prior to UV crosslinking or for whole-cell crosslinking followed by mitochondrial isolation.

Key words Mitochondrial RNA, 4-Thiouridine, Crosslinking, Mass spectrometry, mtDNA

1 Introduction

Human mitochondrial DNA (mtDNA) is a small circular double-stranded DNA that contains 13 protein-coding genes, 2 genes for the rRNAs of the large and small mitoribosomal subunits, and 22 genes for all tRNAs necessary for mitochondrial translation [1]. Maintenance of mtDNA, transcription, RNA processing, and translation are completely reliant on nuclear encoded proteins that are translated on cytosolic ribosomes and imported into the mitochondrial matrix. Perhaps as much as a quarter of the whole mitochondrial proteome is thus involved in the expression of the 13 mtDNA-encoded proteins of the oxidative phosphorylation system. These are foremost proteins involved in mitochondrial

Michal Minczuk and Joanna Rorbach (eds.), *Mitochondrial Gene Expression: Methods and Protocols*,
Methods in Molecular Biology, vol. 2192, https://doi.org/10.1007/978-1-0716-0834-0_12,

RNA metabolism. The mitoribosome already constitutes some 80 proteins in addition to its RNA components. Mitochondrial transcripts are initially polycistronic and need to be processed to yield individual RNA species, as originally proposed in the tRNA punctuation model [2]; rRNAs and tRNAs are posttranscriptionally modified; mRNAs are polyadenylated and need to be stabilized, while used; incomplete or otherwise damaged RNAs eventually need to be degraded. All these steps require various proteins and enzymes, many of which reside in so-called mitochondrial RNA granules (MRGs) [3].

A method to identify RNA-interacting proteins uses protein–RNA UV crosslinking, followed by poly(A)-RNA isolation and identification of crosslinked proteins via mass spectrometry. The efficiency of crosslinking can be enhanced by the use of nucleoside analogs such as 4-thiouridine (4SU). Here we describe how we use 4SU cell-labeling and either mitochondrial or whole-cell crosslinking followed by mitochondrial isolation, and subsequent isolation of poly(A)-RNA with crosslinked proteins, in order to specifically identify mitochondrial poly(A)-RNA-bound proteins. The methods we use are based on previously published protocols for whole-cell crosslinking [4] with the notable exception that we use further mitochondrial enrichment prior to poly(A)-RNA isolation. Subsequent mass spectrometry identification is only outlined in brief, as it is in part facility and instrumentation dependent. A comparison of enrichment for mitochondrial proteins of previously published whole-cell crosslinking [5, 6] and mitochondrially targeted crosslinking methods as described in this chapter is shown in Fig. 1, and is described in more detail in van Esveld et al. [7].

2 Materials

Order materials and chemicals RNase-free whenever possible, otherwise autoclave materials or treat in another way to remove possible RNase contamination. Prepare all solutions using autoclaved ultrapure water unless indicated otherwise.

1. HEK293 cell line (ATCC CRL-1573).
2. 37 °C incubator at 5% CO_2.
3. Biorad imager with a 302 nm UV lamp in the drawer.
4. Nanodrop™ spectrophotometer (Thermo Scientific™).
5. 96-well plate reader, capable to measure absorbance at 595 nm.
6. Cooled Eppendorf centrifuge.
7. Cooled centrifuge for 50 mL Falcon tubes.
8. Ultracentrifuge, e.g., Beckman Optima Max-XP with MLS 50 swing-out rotor.

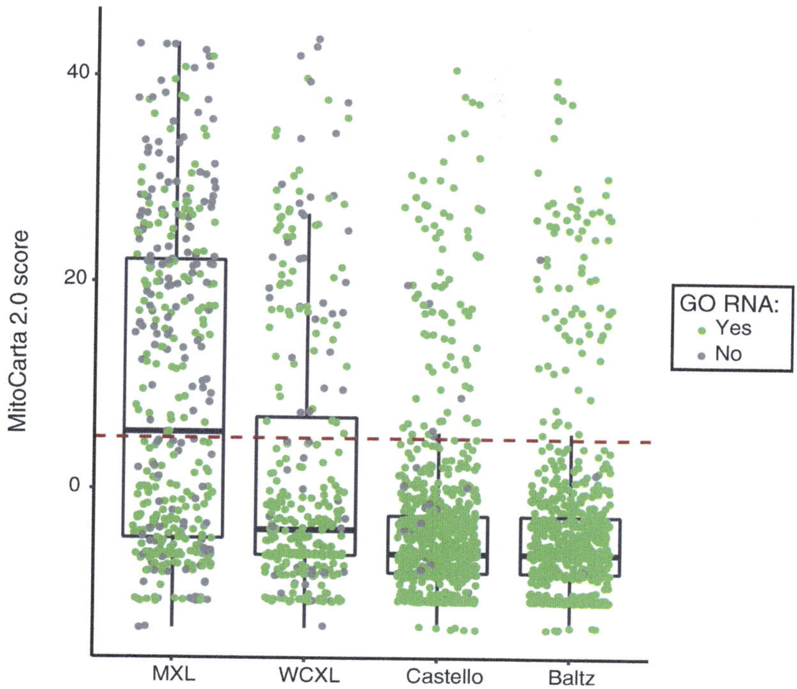

Fig. 1 Comparison of mitochondrial localization prediction scores (MitoCarta2.0, [11]) of enriched proteins in MXL, WCXL, and published whole-cell mRNA interactomes. Enriched proteins that were identified with mass spectrometry by us or others [5, 6], "Baltz" and "Castello" respectively (note that the order is inverted in the graph), with a log2(intensity fold-change crosslinking over no-crosslinking) larger or equal to log2(3) are shown. Each dot in the graph represent an enriched protein, green color indicates that the protein is annotated with the molecular function RNA-binding GO-term (GO:0003723, [12–14]). All proteins above the dotted red line are predicted to be mitochondrial proteins. For more details *see* van Esveld [7]

9. SW60 tubes (for ultracentrifuge).
10. Magnetic Separation Rack.
11. Rotary agitator.
12. 50 mL falcon tubes.
13. 1.5 and 2 mL Eppendorf tubes.
14. Pipette tips and pipettors.
15. Glass-Teflon Dounce homogenizer for 55 mL.
16. 1× PBS
17. Amicon 3K filters (Merck Millipore).
18. RNase Cocktail™ Enzyme Mix (ThermoFisher Scientific).
19. Magnetic mRNA Isolation Kit (New England Biolabs) containing (*see* **Note 1**):
    (a) Oligo d(T)25 Magnetic Beads (5 mg/mL).
    (b) Lysis/Binding Buffer.

(c) Wash Buffer I.

(d) Wash Buffer II.

(e) Low Salt Buffer.

(f) Elution Buffer.

20. 5× Bradford solution: Protein Assay Dye Reagent Concentrate (Biorad).

21. Bradford standards: Quick Start Bovine Serum Albumin Standard Set (Biorad) containing protein standards at seven prediluted concentrations (0.125, 0.25, 0.5, 0.75, 1.0, 1.5, and 2.0 mg/mL).

22. Ultrapure water.

23. Medium: supplement Dulbecco's modified Eagle's medium (DMEM) with 10% fetal calf serum (FCS), stored at 4 °C. Warm up to 37 °C before use.

24. 4SU stock solution: dissolve 100 mM 4-Thiouridine in 1× PBS, filter sterilize and store at −20 °C (*see* **Note 2**).

25. 10× homogenization buffer: 400 mM TRIS hydrochloride, pH 7.8, 250 mM sodium chloride, 50 mM magnesium chloride, autoclave, and store at 4 °C.

26. PMSF stock solution: 100 mM phenylmethanesulfonyl fluoride in 100% isopropanol, store at 4 °C (*see* **Note 3**).

27. Lysis buffer: 50 mM TRIS hydrochloride, pH 7.4, 150 mM sodium chloride, 1 mM Ethylenediaminetetraacetic acid (EDTA), 1% Triton™ X-100, stored at 4 °C. Add PMSF to a final concentration of 2.5 mM (40× dilution of PMSF stock) shortly before use.

28. 4× SDS-sample buffer: 250 mM TRIS hydrochloride, pH 6.8, 8% sodium dodecyl sulfate, 40% glycerol, 0.05% Serva Blue, 4% β-mercaptoethanol. Store at −20 °C before addition of β-mercaptoethanol and after addition at room temperature.

29. 10× RNase buffer: 100 mM TRIS hydrochloride, pH 7.4, 1.5 M sodium chloride, 0.5% NP40, 5 mM DL-dithiothreitol (DTT). Autoclave buffer before the addition of DTT, then add DTT, filter sterilize completed buffer and store at 4 °C.

30. 3K Filter buffer: 10 mM TRIS hydrochloride, pH 7.5, 50 mM sodium chloride, autoclave and store at 4 °C.

31. 1.0 M Sucrose in 10 mM HEPES, pH 7.4, 10 mM EDTA, filter sterilize and store at 4 °C.

32. 1.5 M Sucrose in 10 mM HEPES pH 7.4, 10 mM EDTA, filter sterilize and store at 4 °C.

3 Methods

Carry out all procedures on ice or at 4 °C with cold buffers unless otherwise specified. When performing an experiment, always include a non-crosslinking control and a crosslinking sample to assess enrichment of a protein in the crosslinking sample compared to the control sample. Subheadings 3.2 and 3.4 therefore are only performed when crosslinking is required for that condition.

3.1 Cell Culture

Culture HEK293 cells in DMEM at 37 °C in a humidified incubator at 5% CO_2 and split 1:3 the day before harvest toward thirty 150 mm petri dishes per condition (*see* **Note 4**). For the crosslinking conditions, add 4SU stock solution to the medium to a final concentration of 100 μM 18 h before harvesting the cells (*see* **Note 5**). Ideally the plates should be ~70% confluent on the day of harvest (*see* **Note 4**).

3.2 Whole-Cell UV Crosslinking

Remove medium from cell culture plates and place each plate for ~1 min above a 302 nm UV-light to crosslink nucleic acids to proteins (*see* **Note 6**). Continue with Subheading 3.3 from **step 2** onward.

3.3 Cell Harvest and Mitochondrial Isolation

1. Remove medium from plates.
2. Harvest each plate in 10 mL PBS, pipet up and down to detach all cells and combine cells of one condition in 50 mL tubes.
3. Pellet cells at 500 × *g* for 3 min and discard supernatant.
4. Combine each condition in one tube with 25 mL PBS, sequentially rinse tubes with an additional 25 mL PBS and combine to get 50 mL sample.
5. Pellet cells at 500 × *g* for 3 min and discard supernatant.
6. Make 25 mL 0.1× homogenization buffer per condition by mixing 250 μL 10× homogenization buffer, 0.625 mL PMSF stock solution, and 24.125 mL autoclaved MQ.
7. Resuspend cell pellets per condition in 25 mL 0.1× homogenization buffer and incubate on ice for 6 min to allow the cells to swell.
8. Transfer cells to the Dounce homogenizer and disrupt with 20 strokes.
9. Transfer disrupted cells to a new 50 mL tube and add 3.125 mL 10× homogenization buffer.
10. Pellet cell debris at 1200 × *g* for 3 min and transfer mitochondria containing supernatant to a new tube.
11. Repeat **step 10** once.

12. Pellet mitochondria at 13,000 × *g* for 10 min and discard supernatant.
13. When performing a mitochondrial crosslinking experiment, continue as specified below: (a) Resuspend mitochondrial pellet in 300 μL PBS, measure volume and fill up with PBS to 500 μL.
    (b) Add 2 mL 1.5 M sucrose buffer to a SW60 tube.
    (c) Add 2 mL 1.0 M sucrose buffer on top of the 1.5 M sucrose buffer.
    (d) Add mitochondrial suspension on top of the 1.0 M sucrose buffer.
    (e) Weight tubes and create pairs of tubes with equal weight using PBS. These tubes are inserted in the MLS 50 swing-out rotor in the ultracentrifuge opposite each other.
    (f) Spin at 60,000 × *g* for 20 min with medium acceleration and no break on deceleration.
    (g) Discard around 1 mL of the top layer and carefully collect around 500 μL of the mitochondrial layer that formed between the two sucrose layers in an Eppendorf tube.
    (h) Add 1 mL of PBS to dilute the sucrose and pellet mitochondria at 13,000 × *g* for 5 min.
    (i) Discard supernatant, resuspend in 1 mL PBS and pellet mitochondria at 13,000 × *g* for 5 min.
    (j) Discard supernatant and resuspend in 700 μL PBS, measure volume and fill up with PBS to 2 mL.
    (k) Take 50 μL suspension apart for protein content measurements and SDS-PAGE analysis of input, and continue with the remainder with Subheading 3.4.
14. When the mitochondrial isolation followed whole-cell crosslinking as described under Subheading 3.2, continue with the mitochondrial pellet as specified below:
    (a) Resuspend pellet in 700 μL PBS, transfer to an Eppendorf tube and measure volume. Adjust volume with PBS to a final volume of 2 mL.
    (b) Take 50 μL suspension apart for protein content measurements and SDS-PAGE analysis of input.

3.4 Mitochondrial UV Crosslinking

1. Add mitochondrial suspension to wells of a 6-well plate, with a maximum of 1 mL suspension per well to allow proper exposure to the UV-light.
2. Place 6-well plate on a 302 nm UV lamp for 6 min to crosslink nucleic acids to proteins, shake plate to mix sample after 3 min.
3. Transfer crosslinked sample to an Eppendorf tube.

3.5 Protein Concentration Measurements and Input SDS-PAGE Sample Preparation

1. Pellet mitochondria of the 50 μL sample collected under Subheading 3.3, **step 13k** or **14b** at 13,000 × *g* for 5 min and discard supernatant.
2. Resuspend pellet in 50 μL lysis buffer and vortex to lyse the mitochondria.
3. Spin cell debris down at 14,000 × *g* for 5 min and split sample:
   (a) Transfer 45 μL supernatant to a new tube. Add 15 μL 4× SDS-sample buffer, mix and boil for 5 min at 95 °C to denature the proteins. Make protein concentrations of samples equal across conditions with 1× SDS-sample buffer (diluted with MQ from the 4× buffer) using the Bradford outcome. Store as input SDS-PAGE sample at −20 °C.
   (b) Use remaining supernatant for Bradford measurements to determine protein concentration in samples.
      - Make 1× Bradford solution by dilution of the 5× Bradford concentrate with MQ. Filter the 1× solution using Whatman #1 filter to get rid of particles.
      - Protein standard is measured in duplo and is linear in the range of 0.5–5 μg/well of a 96-well plate. Add 8 μL MQ and 2 μL standard to each well. Use 10 μL MQ as a blanc sample. Do not use the 0.125 μg/μL standard as it will fall outside the linear range.
      - Sample is measured in duplicate. Add 9 μL MQ to wells of a 96-well plate and add 1 μL of lysate. As a blanc use 9 μL MQ with 1 μL lysis buffer.
      - Add to both the standard and the sample wells 200 μL 1× Bradford solution, mix and incubate 5 min at room temperature.
      - Measure extinction at 595 nm in a 96-well plate reader, construct a standard curve and use this to determine the protein concentration in the 2 mL mitochondrial lysate prepared in Subheading 3.3, **step 13j** or **14a**.

3.6 Oligo(dT) Bead Purification

1. Pellet mitochondria at 13,000 × *g* for 5 min and discard supernatant.
2. Resuspend pellet in 700 μL Lysis/Binding buffer. Measure volume, adjust with Lysis/Binding buffer to a final volume of 1 mL and incubate 5 min to lyse the sample with occasional tapping of the tube to mix the solution (*see* **Note 7**).
3. Adjust sample volumes with Lysis/Binding buffer to create 3 mg/mL lysates using the Bradford outcome. When required the RNA concentration can be measured using nanodrop.

4. The pull-down protocol is performed with 100 μL beads suspension for mitochondrial crosslinking experiments, while it is performed with 400 μL beads suspension for whole-cell crosslinking experiments (*see* **Note 8**). Volume of washing and elution steps differs as well. Below volumes for mitochondrial crosslinking are stated, with the volumes for whole-cell crosslinking between brackets.
   (a) Resuspend oligo(dT)-magnetic beads and take 100 μL (400 μL) per condition to a 2 mL tube (*see* **Note 9**).
   (b) Add 200 μL (800 μL) Lysis/Binding buffer to the beads, vortex briefly and mix with agitation for 2 min.
   (c) Collect magnetic beads using the magnetic separator and discard supernatant.
   (d) Add 1 mL (1 mL) mitochondrial lysate to the beads and incubate for 45 min on a rotation device.
   (e) Collect magnetic beads using the magnetic separator and take supernatant to a new tube (*see* **Note 10**). When required the RNA concentration can be measured using nanodrop.
   (f) Wash beads twice with 500 μL (1.8 mL) Wash buffer 1.
   (g) Wash beads twice with 500 μL (1.8 mL) Wash buffer 2.
   (h) Wash beads once with 500 μL (1.8 mL) Wash buffer 3.
   (i) Add 100 μL (400 μL) Elution buffer, vortex to suspend the beads and incubate at 50 °C for 2 min.
   (j) Collect magnetic beads using the magnetic separator and transfer eluate to a new tube. When required the RNA concentration can be measured using nanodrop.
5. When performing a whole-cell crosslinking experiment, continue with the steps below (*see* **Note 8**):
   (a) Prepare beads for re-use:
      - Wash beads once with 400 μL Elution buffer.
      - Wash beads once with 200 μL Lysis/Binding buffer.
   (b) Repeat **steps 4d–5a** twice with the supernatant of **step 4e** as 1 mL lysate input to allow capture of all mRNA species present in the lysate.
   (c) Combine the three whole-cell crosslinking eluates. When required the RNA concentration can be measured using nanodrop.

3.7 Sample Processing to Obtain Protein Sample

Adjust volumes in protocol below to the volume of sample obtained in Subheading 3.6.

1. Treat eluted samples with RNase A and T1 to degrade the RNA attached to its interacting proteins.

   (a) Add 11.1 μL 10× RNase buffer and 2 μL RNase Cocktail™ Enzyme Mix per 100 μL eluate, mix and incubate at 37 °C for 1 h.

2. Concentrate obtained protein sample using Amicon 3K filters. In all steps place the tubes with the cap strap toward the center of the centrifuge.

   (a) Take one 3K filter per condition. These filters can contain a maximum volume of 500 μL, so it might be necessary to add sample in multiple centrifugation rounds.

      - When volume is larger than 500 μL, add 500 μL sample to the filter, spin at 14,000 × *g*, room temperature for 15 min, and discard flow through. Repeat this, but add a maximum of 400 μL sample to the 3K filter (as about 100 μL remains inside the filter). Continue adding sample and spinning until less than 400 μL sample is left.
      - Add remaining sample to the filter and top off with 3K filter buffer when necessary and spin at 14,000 × *g*, room temperature for 30 min.

   (b) Add 500 μL 3K filter buffer to each filter and spin at 14,000 × *g*, room temperature for 30 min.

   (c) Transfer filter to a new tube, this time place filter upside down (leave tube open!).

   (d) Spin at 1000 × *g* for 2 min to collect sample.

   (e) Transfer sample to Eppendorf tube, measure the volume and adjust with 3K filter buffer to a final volume of 45 μL. Sample can be stored at −20 °C indefinitely.

The obtained protein sample is ready for Bradford analysis to determine protein yield (*see* **Note 11**). It can also be used for SDS-PAGE and western blot analysis (together with the input SDS-PAGE samples) when mixed with SDS-sample buffer to a final 1× SDS-sample buffer concentration and boiled for 5 min at 95 °C. Besides the obtained protein sample can be used for mass spectrometry measurements. This requires additional processing steps, which depend on the mass spectrometry instrument available in the lab (*see* **Note 12**).

4 Notes

1. For the whole-cell crosslinking polyadenylated RNA pull down the kit contains too small volumes of the buffers. Therefore, additional buffers with the same composition as mentioned in the kit were made. The buffers were autoclaved before the

addition of lithium dodecyl sulfate (LiDS) and/or DTT and after addition of these compounds finished by passing the solution through a 0.45 μm filter.

2. Store 4SU stock solution in aliquots to avoid repeated freezing and thawing. Solution is stable at −20 °C for several months.
3. PMSF stock solution can also be made with 100% ethanol as solvent.
4. It is important to split the cells the day before harvest and to have plates which are not too confluent at the moment of harvest to obtain a sample with active mitochondria. Also, be sure that there is no mycoplasma infection by routinely checking cells for this contamination.
5. Before addition of 4SU to the medium, check if most cells are attached to the plate. Eighteen hour treatment with 4SU might otherwise result in many floating cells and/or small, round looking attached cells. Also, when cells are attached when adding 4SU, the cells might look a bit disturbed after treatment compared to the control cells that are not treated with 4SU.
6. Only perform the UV crosslinking steps when they are required for that condition. If not required, skip these sections. Make sure the UV-light is already on for at least 5 min before incubation with the first sample to ensure that emitted light is equal for all samples. We use a 302 nm UV-light, but when available a UV lamp of 365 nm in case of 4SU treatment or of 254 nm without 4SU would give a more efficient crosslinking [4].
7. Lysates can be frozen at −80 °C for up to 1 week before starting oligo(dT) beads pull down.
8. Mitochondrial crosslinking samples contain less contamination of cytosolic RNA species compared to whole-cell crosslinking samples due to sucrose gradient purification and crosslinking after isolation of mitochondria. Therefore, total amount of RNA within mitochondrial crosslinking samples is smaller, allowing a smaller amount of beads to capture all polyadenylated RNA species present.
9. Make sure the oligo(dT)-magnetic beads are resuspended properly before dividing the solution over Eppendorf tubes to have equal amount of beads for each condition. Proper resuspension can for example be achieved by incubating the bead suspension on a rotor 5 min before pipetting or by tapping until bead pellet disappears.
10. The beads collected by the magnetic rack will form a nice compact pellet when no UV crosslinking is performed. A halo will be visible when crosslinking is performed. This is also described for published oligo(dT) capture approaches [4].

11. Bradford analysis of the processed protein sample can be performed according to the above described Bradford protocol with 1 μL out of the 45 μL sample. The 1 μL blanc sample needs to be prepared like the protein samples, so mix 1200 μL elution buffer with 133.32 μL RNase buffer and concentrate this according to the described protocol to a sample of 45 μL. This is important since the 3K filters concentrate the components of the elution, RNase and 3K filter buffers and influence the background signal of the Bradford assay. Our eluted protein yields were typically in the range of 20–100 μg of protein.
12. The protein sample contains NP-40 detergent, this should be removed during mass spectrometry sample preparation to prevent interference with peptide measurements. We have done this using the FASP digestion protocol [8] as described in Castello et al. [4], which also concentrates, reduces, alkylates, and digests the samples. The only deviations from this protocol are the use of chloroacetamide for 20 min instead of iodoacetamide for 5 min for alkylation and 0.25 μg of trypsin instead of 0.5 μg. After elution from the filter and a second elution with salt, the combined sample is acidified with TFA to a final concentration of 1%. The sample was desalted using "Stop And Go Extraction (STAGE) tips" [9] and the peptide sample was further purified by Pierce Detergent Removal Spin Columns (Thermo Scientific) before injection of 28% of the sample in triplicate on a nanoLC 1000 (Thermo Scientific) chromatography coupled online to Q Exactive hybrid quadrupole-Orbitrap mass spectrometer (Thermo Scientific). Raw mass spectrometry data is converted into proteins with peptide counts and label-free-quantification intensities (LFQ) using MaxQuant software (version 1.5.0.25, [10]) and further analysis in R (version 3.2.3). For more details *see* van Esveld [7].

Acknowledgement

This work was supported by the Radboud Institute for Molecular Life Sciences; Radboudumc (R0002792) and by the "Prinses Beatrix Spierfonds" and the "Stichting Spieren voor Spieren" (W. OR15-05 to J.N.S.).

References

1. Anderson S, Bankier AT, Barrell BG, de Bruijn MH, Coulson AR, Drouin J, Eperon IC, Nierlich DP, Roe BA, Sanger F, Schreier PH, Smith AJ, Staden R, Young IG (1981) Sequence and organization of the human mitochondrial genome. Nature 290(5806):457–465. https://doi.org/10.1038/290457a0
2. Ojala D, Montoya J, Attardi G (1981) tRNA punctuation model of RNA processing in human mitochondria. Nature 290

(5806):470–474. https://doi.org/10.1038/290470a0

3. Pearce SF, Rebelo-Guiomar P, D'Souza AR, Powell CA, Van Haute L, Minczuk M (2017) Regulation of mammalian mitochondrial gene expression: recent advances. Trends Biochem Sci 42(8):625–639. https://doi.org/10.1016/j.tibs.2017.02.003
4. Castello A, Horos R, Strein C, Fischer B, Eichelbaum K, Steinmetz LM, Krijgsveld J, Hentze MW (2013) System-wide identification of RNA-binding proteins by interactome capture. Nat Protoc 8(3):491–500. https://doi.org/10.1038/nprot.2013.020
5. Baltz Alexander G, Munschauer M, Schwanhäusser B, Vasile A, Murakawa Y, Schueler M, Youngs N, Penfold-Brown D, Drew K, Milek M, Wyler E, Bonneau R, Selbach M, Dieterich C, Landthaler M (2012) The mRNA-bound proteome and its global occupancy profile on protein-coding transcripts. Mol Cell 46(5):674–690. https://doi.org/10.1016/j.molcel.2012.05.021
6. Castello A, Fischer B, Eichelbaum K, Horos R, Beckmann Benedikt M, Strein C, Davey Norman E, Humphreys David T, Preiss T, Steinmetz Lars M, Krijgsveld J, Hentze Matthias W (2012) Insights into RNA biology from an atlas of mammalian mRNA-binding proteins. Cell 149(6):1393–1406. https://doi.org/10.1016/j.cell.2012.04.031
7. van Esveld SL, Cansız-Arda Ş, Hensen F, van der Lee R, Huynen MA, Spelbrink JN (2019) A combined mass spectrometry and data integration approach to predict the mitochondrial poly(A) RNA interacting proteome. Front Cell Dev Biol 7(283). https://doi.org/10.3389/fcell.2019.00283
8. Wisniewski JR, Zougman A, Nagaraj N, Mann M (2009) Universal sample preparation method for proteome analysis. Nat Methods 6(5):359–362. https://doi.org/10.1038/nmeth.1322
9. Rappsilber J, Ishihama Y, Mann M (2003) Stop and go extraction tips for matrix-assisted laser desorption/ionization, nanoelectrospray, and LC/MS sample pretreatment in proteomics. Anal Chem 75(3):663–670
10. Cox J, Mann M (2008) MaxQuant enables high peptide identification rates, individualized p.p.b.-range mass accuracies and proteome-wide protein quantification. Nat Biotechnol 26(12):1367–1372. https://doi.org/10.1038/nbt.1511
11. Calvo SE, Clauser KR, Mootha VK (2015) MitoCarta2.0: an updated inventory of mammalian mitochondrial proteins. Nucleic Acids Res. https://doi.org/10.1093/nar/gkv1003
12. The Gene Ontology Consortium (2017) Expansion of the Gene Ontology knowledgebase and resources. Nucleic Acids Res 45(D1):D331–D338. https://doi.org/10.1093/nar/gkw1108
13. Ashburner M, Ball CA, Blake JA, Botstein D, Butler H, Cherry JM, Davis AP, Dolinski K, Dwight SS, Eppig JT, Harris MA, Hill DP, Issel-Tarver L, Kasarskis A, Lewis S, Matese JC, Richardson JE, Ringwald M, Rubin GM, Sherlock G (2000) Gene ontology: tool for the unification of biology. The Gene Ontology Consortium. Nat Genet 25(1):25–29. https://doi.org/10.1038/75556
14. Carbon S, Ireland A, Mungall CJ, Shu S, Marshall B, Lewis S (2009) AmiGO: online access to ontology and annotation data. Bioinformatics (Oxford, England) 25(2):288–289. https://doi.org/10.1093/bioinformatics/btn615

Chapter 13

Visualizing Mitochondrial Ribosomal RNA and Mitochondrial Protein Synthesis in Human Cell Lines

Matthew Zorkau, Yasmin Proctor-Kent, Rolando Berlinguer-Palmini, Andrew Hamilton, Zofia M. Chrzanowska-Lightowlers, and Robert N. Lightowlers

Abstract

Human mitochondria contain their own DNA (mtDNA) that encodes 13 proteins all of which are core subunits of oxidative phosphorylation (OXPHOS) complexes. To form functional complexes, these 13 components need to be correctly assembled with approximately 70 nuclear-encoded subunits that are imported following synthesis in the cytosol. How this complicated coordinated translation and assembly is choreographed is still not clear. Methods are being developed to determine whether all members of a particular complex are translated in close proximity, whether protein synthesis is clustered in submitochondrial factories, whether these align with incoming polypeptides, and if there is evidence for co-translational translation that is regulated and limited by the interaction of the incoming proteins with synthesis of their mtDNA-encoded partners. Two methods are described in this chapter to visualize the distribution of mitochondrial ribosomal RNAs in conjunction with newly synthesized mitochondrial proteins. The first combines RNA *F*luorescent *In S*itu *H*ybridization (FISH) and super-resolution immunocytochemistry to pinpoint mitochondrial ribosomal RNA. The second localizes nascent translation within the mitochondrial network through non-canonical amino acid labeling, click chemistry and fluorescent microscopy.

Key words Mitochondria, Mitochondrial RNA, Mitoribosome, Translation, Click chemistry, Single-molecule RNA FISH, Fluorescence microscopy, Stimulated emission depletion microscopy, Super-resolution microscopy

1 Introduction

1.1 Background

Mitochondrial protein synthesis requires mitochondrially encoded mRNAs (mt-mRNAs) to be delivered to their translation machinery, the mitoribosome. The newly generated hydrophobic polypeptides must be correctly inserted into the inner mitochondrial membrane (IMM) such that they can interact with their partner

Matthew Zorkau and Yasmin Proctor-Kent contributed equally to this work.

Michal Minczuk and Joanna Rorbach (eds.), *Mitochondrial Gene Expression: Methods and Protocols*, Methods in Molecular Biology, vol. 2192, https://doi.org/10.1007/978-1-0716-0834-0_13,

proteins to form four of the five complexes required for oxidative phosphorylation (OXPHOS). It is not yet clear whether all transcripts encoding members of specific complexes are colocalized prior to translation allowing for discrete synthesis sites for each complex, or if mitoribosomes commence translation and arrest after sufficient peptide has emerged, to allow sufficient time to interact with chaperone/partner proteins to promote co-translational assembly. Distribution of the mt-mRNAs and the translation machinery may be random but the current method of analyzing de novo synthesis by [^{35}S]-Met/Cys radiolabel incorporation [1], although effective to measure newly synthesized proteins, is not a suitable approach to localize nascent protein synthesis in intact cells. We have, therefore, been modifying a click chemistry/fluorescence microscopy protocol to visualize localization of nascent mitochondrial proteins in situ. In tandem, we have been refining Fluorescence In Situ Hybridization (FISH), to establish the distribution of the large (39S; mt-LSU; 16S or *RNR2* mt-rRNA containing) and small (28S; mt-SSU; 12S or *RNR1* mt-rRNA containing) mitochondrial ribosomal subunits with the sites of active translation. Single molecule labelling of RNA via DNA probes allows visualization and quantification of both mt-rRNA and mt-mRNA and could determine the position of mitoribosomes and their association with specific mt-mRNAs. This method generates highly specific signals with very low false positives [2, 3] and has been used in embryos to quantify and display distribution of *RNR1* and *RNR2* [4], however not in adherent cells or in combination with super-resolution microscopy. Using this technique, the distribution of these mt-rRNAs within the mitochondrial network can indicate the proportion of assembled mitoribosomes. In combination with FISH for mt-mRNAs, it may also distinguish between active assembled and quiescent or partially assembled mitoribosomes. The combination of these approaches should permit a better understanding of the spatial organization of 28S and 39S subunits, and the assembled/active mitoribosomes.

1.2 Super-Resolution Mitochondrial RNA Fluorescent In Situ Hybridization and Immunocytochemistry to Visualize Partial or Intact Mitochondrial Ribosomes

Fluorescence microscopy is limited by the fixed size of a single point of light that can be resolved by a conventional confocal light microscope. This limitation is ~180 nm× >500 nm in the focal plane and optic axis [5]. Since mitochondrial networks are often similar in size or larger, they can be resolved in this way. To gain submitochondrial definition, however, super-resolution such as STimulated Emission Depletion (STED) microscopy is required [6]. This allows resolution of structures beyond the diffraction limit of conventional optical microscopy [7, 8]. In simple terms this enhancement is achieved by eliminating all the fluorescence from dye molecules at the periphery of the excitation focus. This is done with stimulated emission from a laser that directs intense light to these peripheral regions causing most of the excited molecules to return to their ground state. Thus, only fluorescence emitted at the center of the STED beam is detected, allowing resolution at sub-diffraction limited objects. Intramitochondrial protein structures have been reported using this technique [9] and we have increased the definition of mt-rRNA distribution from amorphous signals with conventional confocal microscopy to resolved puncta (Fig. 1). By combining RNA FISH, which uses multiple DNA oligonucleotides to bind specific RNA targets, with immunocytochemistry this method allows quantification of both the RNA targets and spatial information on the location of translated products (Fig. 2).

Here we present a robust method to visualize and localize mitochondrial ribosomal RNAs (*RNR1* and *RNR2*). Colocalization measurements of *RNR1* and *RNR2* indicate the percentage of subunits that are likely to be present as mitoribosomal monomers and are potentially active for mitochondrial protein synthesis. We have based our method on a similar protocol described by others

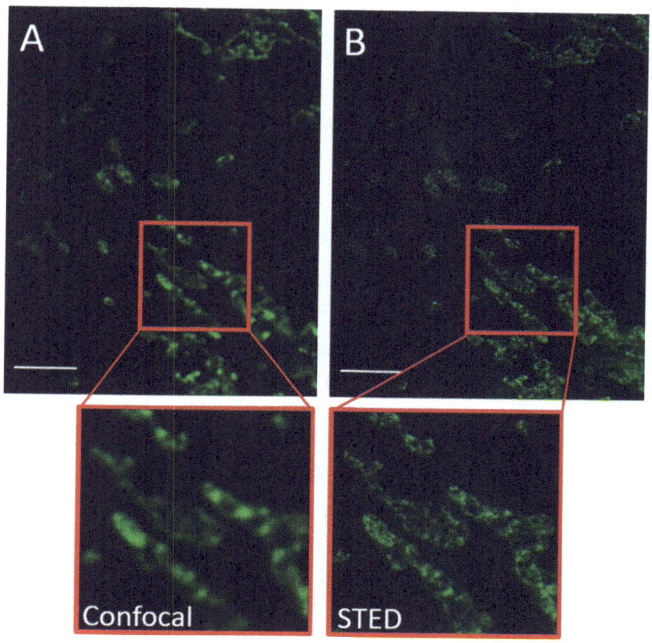

Fig. 1 Confocal and STED images of RNA FISH in fixed U2OS cells. (**a**) Depicts labelling of *RNR1* with RNA FISH oligonucleotides conjugated to Quasar 570 fluorophores using confocal microscopy. (**b**) Depicts the corresponding image taken using STED imaging. Scale bars are 5 μm. Boxes below are enlargements of the red boxed areas from the upper images, revealing the improvement in resolution achieved by STED microscopy. The images presented are single not deconvolved images. All images were taken on Leica TCS SP8 described in Subheading 2.1

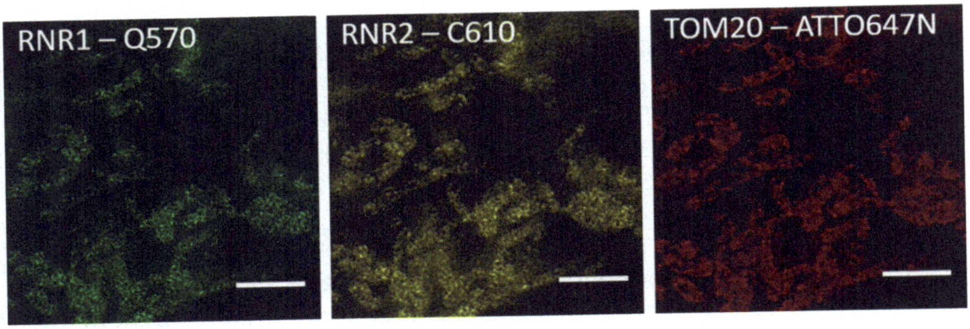

Fig. 2 STED images of RNA FISH-coupled with immunofluorescent labelling of mitochondrial components. Fixed U2OS cells were prepared as per the described protocol. *RNR1* is labeled by RNA FISH with oligonucleotides conjugated to Quasar 570 fluorophores (left panel) and *RNR2* oligonucleotides are conjugated to CAL Fluor 610 fluorophores (center panel). Polyclonal antibodies against Tom20 are decorated with Atto 647N conjugated secondary antibodies. The images were captured on a Leica TCS SP8 microscope and deconvolved in Huygens Professional Deconvolution software as described in Subheading 3.1.4, **step 6**. Scale bar 2 μm

[10], however, we describe optimized sample preparation for specifically targeting mitochondrial RNAs and mitochondrial proteins such that they can be imaged by STED microscopy. Super-resolution STED imaging resolved indistinct signals into more specific puncta giving a more accurate representation of RNA localization within the mitochondria, in combination with protein markers.

1.3 Click Chemistry Approach to Visualize Nascent Mitochondrial Protein Synthesis by Fluorescence Microscopy

Mitochondrial translation is typically investigated by the incorporation of [^{35}S]-Met/Cys radiolabel into nascent mitochondrial proteins, which are then separated by SDS-PAGE or BN-PAGE and visualized by phosphorimaging [1]. In contrast, microscopy can provide spatial information at a cell and ultrastructural level. This approach has been used to investigate nascent synthesis of mtDNA and mtRNA molecules, and has provided excellent insights into the dynamic regulation and localization of nucleic acids within the mitochondrial network [10, 11]. We aim to combine labelling of nascent proteins with spatial distribution to expand our understanding of mitochondrial gene expression.

Until recently, visualizing mtDNA-encoded proteins has been limited to establishing the distribution of their steady state levels through fluorescent immunocytochemistry [12]. Developments of new fluorophores, as well as the introduction of imaging mass cytometry has increased the capacity so that many antibodies targeting multiple individual targets can be applied simultaneously [13]. Nevertheless, this is still limited to steady state and not nascent synthesis. Using a fluorescent alternative to radiolabeled methionine provides the potential for visualizing the spatial distribution of active translation machinery within the mitochondrial network. Click chemistry is now routinely used to measure cytosolic protein synthesis [14] and provides a fast, sensitive, nontoxic and nonradioactive alternative to conventional radiolabelling approaches.

Following inhibition of cytosolic translation, cells are bathed with the non-canonical amino acids L-azidohomoalanine (AHA) or L-homopropargylglycine (HPG) allowing incorporation of these methionine analogues into growing peptide chains of mtDNA-encoded proteins. AHA and HPG have been chemically modified to contain an azido or alkyne group, respectively. Copper-catalyzed azide/alkyne cycloaddition (CuAAC) click chemistry reactions attach the corresponding molecule to the azido or alkyne group. Importantly, CuAAC approaches build upon the capacity of radioactive methods by providing two outputs: comparable analysis of cell lysates by SDS-PAGE or mass spectrometry as can be achieved with radiolabelling [15], but additionally it permits visualization by microscopy of nascent proteins in intact cells via a fluorescent moiety [16], which is not possible with the radiolabel approach.

Here we describe a method that advances on previous methods [17] harnessing these modified methionine analogues to gain a better understanding of protein synthesis within the human mitochondrial network. HPG-containing mitochondrial proteins are labeled with Alexa Fluor-conjugated-azide molecules to allow visualization of mitochondrial translation by fluorescence microscopy [18].

This method will provide a novel tool to analyze mitochondrial translation in intact cells under different conditions such as genetically modified cell lines (knock-out or siRNA depleted of specific factors) or those derived from patient cells with mitochondrial disease (with either nuclear or mtDNA mutations). Further development of this technology provides the potential to visualize nascent mtDNA, mtRNA and mitochondrial protein synthesis in concert, improving the capacity to investigate dynamic regulation of mitochondrial gene expression within the network.

2 Materials

2.1 Super-Resolution Mitochondrial RNA Fluorescent In Situ Hybridization and Immunocytochemistry to Visualize Partial or Intact Mitochondrial Ribosomes

All reagents should be prepared using diethyl pyrocarbonate treated (DEPC-treated) water to be RNase free. Standard cell culture and other consumables are as used in general molecular biology labs but should all be of analytical grade. The Leica TCS SP8 confocal laser scanning and gated STED microscope (Leica Microsystems, Wetzlar, Germany) was used to image all sample preparations. Other commercial or custom STED microscopes may be used.

2.1.1 Probe Design

We recommend using the tools at http://www.biosearchtech.com/stellarisdesigner/ to design and order RNA FISH probes. Based on the selected input sequence, this software custom designs whole probe sets of 20–45 short DNA oligonucleotides, each labeled with a fluorophore. Following consultation with the Bioimaging Unit at Newcastle University, Quasar 570, CAL Fluor 610 and Quasar 670 were determined as the most STED-compatible fluorophores available from this company. We have obtained good quality STED images with all three of these fluorophores. Atto 647N is a commonly used STED fluorophore in immunofluorescence experiments. As Atto 647N and Quasar 670 share a similar excitation and emission spectra, CAL Fluor 610 should be used as a replacement.

2.1.2 General Supplies and Solutions

1. High performance 0.17 mm coverslips (Carl Zeiss, Germany) (*see* **Note 1**).
2. Microscope slides (76 mm × 26 mm, 1–1.2 mm thick).
3. Fine point forceps, sterilized by baking.
4. A humidified chamber (*see* **Note 2**).
5. DEPC-treated water: prepared by addition of 0.1% DEPC to ultrapure water before leaving overnight and then autoclaving.
6. 1 × PBS: 137 mM NaCl, 2.7 mM KCl, 10 mM Na_2HPO_4, 1.76 mM KH_2PO_4, pH 7.4.
7. 1× PBS: mix 5 mL 10× PBS, 45 mL DEPC-treated water.
8. Fixation solution: 50 mL 4% paraformaldehyde solution, 400 μL 25% glutaraldehyde solution. Store at 4 °C, stable for months.
9. 70% Ethanol: 35 mL absolute ethanol, 15 mL DEPC-treated water. Store at room temperature.
10. Prolong Glass Antifade Mountant (ThermoFisher Scientific).
11. Clear nail polish.

2.1.3 RNA FISH

1. Hybridization buffer: 1 mL 20× nuclease-free SSC, 1 mL formamide, 1 g dextran sulfate (Mw > 500,000), 7 mL DEPC-treated water. Prepare by slow addition of dextran sulfate to the DEPC-treated water, mix by rotation; this can take up to 30 min. Once dissolved, add the formamide and 20× SSC then make up to 10 mL with DEPC-treated water. Store as 500 μL aliquots at −20 °C.
2. Wash Buffer: 5 mL 20× nuclease-free SSC, 5 mL formamide, 40 mL DEPC-treated water. Store at room temperature.
3. TE buffer: 10 mM Tris–HCl, 1 mM EDTA, pH 8.0.

4. Probe stock solutions: resuspend dried oligonucleotides in 50 μL of TE buffer to generate 100 μM stock. Dilute 12.5 μL of this stock in 87.5 μL TE buffer for working concentration of 12.5 μM.

2.1.4 Immunofluorescence Labelling

1. Blocking and permeabilization buffer: 200 μL 200 mM vanadyl ribonucleoside complexes (*see* **Note 3**), 600 μL 10% Triton X-100, 2 mL 10% BSA, 10 mL 2× PBS, 7.2 mL DEPC-treated water.
2. Primary antibody: anti-Tom20, FL-145, rabbit polyclonal 1:500.
3. Fluorescent secondary antibody: anti-rabbit Atto 647N, goat polyclonal 1:200. If DAPI is to be used, we recommend the ThermoFisher product at a final concentration of 0.5 μg/mL.

2.2 Click Chemistry Approach to Visualize Nascent Mitochondrial Protein Synthesis by Fluorescence Microscopy

2.2.1 Pulse Labeling of Cultured Cells

1. Cell in culture to be labeled (*see* **Note 4**).
2. Tissue culture 6-well plates.
3. Sterilized 22 × 22 mm glass coverslips and fine point forceps, sterilized by baking.
4. Labeling medium: Methionine-free DMEM supplemented with 10% dialyzed fetal bovine serum (10,000 molecular weight cut off), 1% Minimum Essential Medium (MEM) nonessential amino acids solution, 200 μM L-cysteine, 10 mM HEPES and 50 μg/mL uridine. Filter sterilize prior to use.
5. High glucose DMEM: supplemented with 10% FBS, 1% MEM nonessential amino acids solution, 10 mM HEPES and 50 μg/mL uridine. Filter sterilize prior to use.
6. 50 mM L-Homopropargylglycine (HPG, Jena Bioscience): in a 1:1 solution of molecular grade DMSO and ddH_2O, store at −20 °C.
7. 50 mg/mL molecular biology grade chloramphenicol (CAP) in 100% ethanol, store at −20 °C.
8. 10 mg/mL molecular biology grade cycloheximide (CHI) in 100% ethanol, store at 4 °C.

2.2.2 Pre-permeabilizing and Fixing Intact Cells

1. Mitochondria-protective buffer (MPB): 10 mM HEPES/KOH, pH 7.5, 10 mM NaCl, 5 mM $MgCl_2$, 300 mM sucrose in ddH_2O, store at 4 °C.
2. Digitonin: 0.5% (w:v) in MPB, make 70 μL aliquots, store at −20 °C.
3. Formaldehyde: 3.7% in MPB diluted 1:10 from 37% stock solution, store in the dark at 4 °C.

2.2.3 Blocking Procedures

1. Bovine serum albumin (BSA): 5% (w:v) in PBS, store at 4 °C for up to 2 weeks.

2.2.4 Detection of HPG-Labeled Mitochondrial Proteins

1. Phosphate buffered saline (PBS): 137 mM NaCl, 2.7 mM KCl, 10 mM Na_2HPO_4, 1.76 mM KH_2PO_4, pH 7.4, store at room temperature.
2. Copper sulfate: 20 mM in ddH_2O, store at 4 °C.
3. [2-(4-((bis((1-(tert-butyl)-1*H*-1,2,3-triazol-4-yl)methyl) amino)methyl)-1*H*-1,2,3-triazol-1-yl)acetic acid] (BTTAA, Jena Bioscience): 20 mM in ddH_2O, store at −20 °C.
4. 100% molecular biology grade dimethyl sulfoxide (DMSO), store at room temperature.
5. Picolyl-azide-Alexa Fluor 594 (Picolyl AF594, Jena Bioscience): 10 mM in ddH_2O, store at −20 °C.
6. Sodium ascorbate: 200 or 2 mM in PBS on the day of the experiment.
7. 2× click reaction mixture. 10 μM Picolyl AF594, 600 μM $CuSO_4$, 1.2 mM BTTAA, 5% molecular grade DMSO in PBS on the day of the experiment.
8. Humidified chamber. An airtight plastic box (at least 20 × 20 cm) has its base covered with damp paper towel and is then lined with aluminum foil. The surface is labeled to identify each sample. The plastic box is then sealed with its lid (*see* **Note 2**).
9. Paper towels.
10. Aluminum foil.
11. Fine point forceps, sterilized by baking.

2.2.5 Immunofluorescence Labelling

1. 10× Tris Buffered Saline (TBS): 0.2 M Tris base, 1.38 M NaCl, pH to 7.6, adjust to 1 L ddH_2O, store at room temperature.
2. 1× TBS with Tween-20 (TBS-T): 1× TBS in ddH_2O, 0.1% Tween-20, store at room temperature.
3. Bovine serum albumin (BSA): 5% (w:v) in TBS-T, store at 4 °C for up to 2 weeks.
4. Primary antibody: unconjugated rabbit polyclonal IgG anti-Tom20.
5. Secondary antibody: goat anti-rabbit IgG (H + L), Alexa Fluor 488, store undiluted in the dark at 4 °C.
6. Hoechst 33342 DNA dye.

2.2.6 Mounting Coverslips onto Microscope Slides

1. ProLong Glass Antifade Mountant, store at 4 °C and bring to room temperature just before use.
2. Glass microscope slides (1.0–1.2 mm thickness) and forceps.

3. Clear nail polish.

2.2.7 Analyzing Samples with Fluorescence Microscopy

1. An epifluorescence inverted microscope (we recommend use of a confocal microscope for optimal resolution) with ×63 oil immersion lens.
2. Huygens software for deconvolution of images and colocalization analysis.
3. ImageJ software with FIJI plugin for image analysis including calculation of mean fluorescence and colocalization.

3 Methods

1. Place a coverslip into a chamber of a 6-well plate or 35 mm dish using baked forceps.
2. Seed 100 μL of diluted adherent cultured cells onto the coverslip in a droplet and incubate for 2–4 h (Fig. 3 *see* **Notes 5** and **6**).

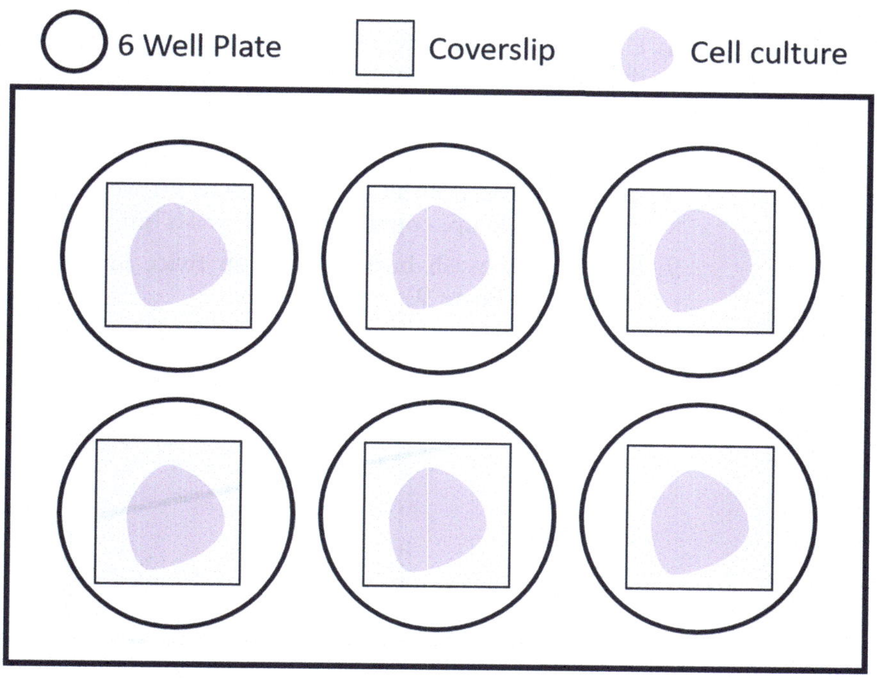

Fig. 3 How to seed cells in preparation for RNA FISH. Coverslips were placed into individual wells of a 6-well plate using sterile forceps and a 100 μL droplet of cell suspension (*see* **Note 6**) was pipetted onto the center of the coverslip. Cells were incubated at 37 °C for 2–4 h before the addition of 2 mL cell culture medium to each well. Cells were allowed to proliferate overnight or until the desired confluency was reached

3.1 Super-Resolution Mitochondrial RNA Fluorescent In Situ Hybridization and Immunocytochemistry to Visualize Partial or Intact Mitochondrial Ribosomes

3.1.1 Cell Culture and Fixation, RNA FISH and Immunofluorescence

3. After allowing the cells to adhere for 2–4 h, add 2 mL pre-warmed media to the well and leave the cells to grow overnight to achieve 20–30% confluency.
4. Remove the culture medium and wash twice with 1 mL warm 1× PBS to prevent cell shock (*see* **Note 7**).
5. Remove PBS and fix for 10 min with 1 mL fixative.
6. Remove fixative and wash twice with 1 mL 1× PBS.
7. Add 1 mL 70% ethanol for 1 h at room temperature or overnight at 4 °C (*see* **Note 8**).

3.1.2 RNA FISH Labelling of *mt*-RNR1 and *mt*-RNR2

1. Remove ethanol solution and wash twice with 1× PBS.
2. Add 1 mL of wash buffer for 5 min to equilibrate cells.
3. During this time prepare a humidified chamber (*see* **Note 2**).
4. To each experiment add 0.5 μL of 12.5 μM probe stock to 50 μL of hybridization buffer (final probe concentration of 125 nM).
5. Place a 50 μL droplet onto parafilm (labeled with experiment designation) within the humidified chamber.
6. Using forceps, gently lower the coverslip, cell side down, into the probe-hybridization buffer droplet and ensure that no bubbles are formed (Fig. 4).
7. Seal the humidified chamber and incubate at 37 °C overnight.
8. Using forceps, transfer the coverslip to a 6-well plate or 35 mm dish, cell side up, containing 1 mL wash buffer.
9. Remove the wash buffer and wash twice in wash buffer for 30 min (*see* **Note 9**).

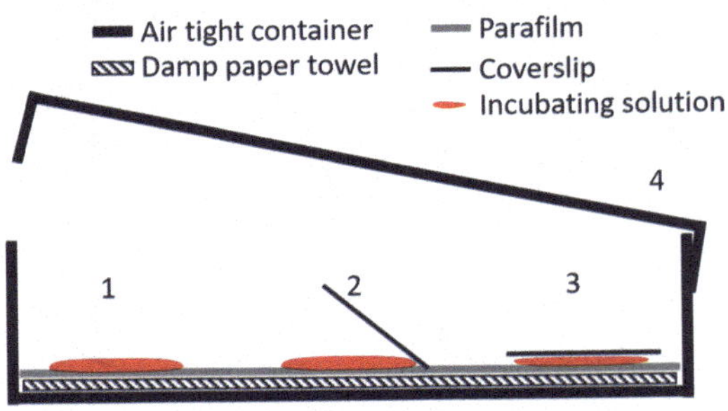

Fig. 4 Preparation of the Humidified Chamber. A damp paper towel was placed in the bottom of a lidded, airtight, plastic box and covered with parafilm (1). A 100 μL droplet of incubating solution (RNA FISH probes or antibody dilution) was placed onto the parafilm (2). A coverslip was angled to the edge of the liquid droplet and then gently lowered onto the droplet, avoiding the formation of air bubbles (3). The lid was then closed to retain a humidified environment (4)

10. Remove the wash buffer and keep the coverslips in 1× PBS until mounted.
11. Add a small drop of ProLong Glass Antifade Mountant to a microscope slide.
12. Using forceps, carefully lower the coverslip, cell side down, onto the mountant droplet avoiding the formation of air bubbles. Let the mountant set overnight for confocal imaging, or for 3–4 days for STED imaging (*see* **Note 10**).
13. If desired, seal the coverslips with nail polish to avoid any coverslip movement during handling or cleaning (*see* **Note 11**).

3.1.3 Sequential Immunofluorescence and RNA FISH

In order to couple RNA FISH to immunofluorescence some additional steps, including blocking and antibody incubations, need to be carried out before the RNA FISH hybridization. Here we describe the labelling of Tom20, an outer membrane mitochondrial marker, in fixed cells followed by RNA FISH labelling of the mitochondrial ribosomal RNAs.

1. Grow and fix adherent mammalian cells on coverslips as described in Subheading 3.1. Do not carry out ethanol permeabilization.
2. Incubate coverslip in 1 mL blocking and permeabilization buffer for 1 h at room temperature on a platform rocker. During this time prepare the humidified chamber and antibody dilution.
3. Dilute the primary antibody to double the recommended concentration in blocking/permeabilization buffer (*see* **Note 12**). Vortex briefly and centrifuge for 1 min at 13,000 × *g*.
4. Place 100 μL of antibody dilution onto labeled parafilm within the humidified chamber.
5. Using forceps, gently lower the coverslip, cell side down, onto the antibody dilution droplet avoiding the formation of bubbles.
6. Seal the humidified chamber and incubate at 4 °C overnight.
7. Using forceps, transfer the coverslip to a 6-well plate or 35 mm dish, cell side up, containing 1 mL 1× PBS.
8. Wash cells three times in 1× PBS for a minimum of 5 min on lab rocker. During this time prepare the humidified chamber and antibody dilution.
9. Dilute labeled secondary antibody to double the recommended final concentration in blocking/permeabilization buffer (*see* **Note 12**). Vortex briefly and centrifuge for 1 min at 13,000 × *g*.

10. Place 100 μL of antibody dilution into the humidified chamber.
11. Using forceps, gently lower the coverslip, cell side down, onto the antibody dilution droplet avoiding the formation of bubbles.
12. Seal the humidified chamber and incubate for 1 h at room temperature in the dark. N.B. all the following steps should be carried out in the dark where possible.
13. Transfer the coverslip to a 6-well plate or 35 mm dish, cell side up, containing 1 mL 1× PBS.
14. Wash cells in 1× PBS three times (each wash is a minimum of 5 min) on a lab rocker.
15. Remove PBS and add 1 mL of fixative for 10 min at room temperature.
16. Remove the fixative and wash cells three times in 1× PBS (each wash is a minimum of 5 min) on lab rocker.
17. Equilibrate cells in RNA FISH wash buffer for a minimum of 5 min and carry out RNA FISH protocol as described in Subheading 3.1.2 from **step 3**.

3.1.4 Imaging

1. Place your slide onto the microscope using immersion oil as appropriate. For STED, images were acquired with a 100× NA 1.4 oil objective on a Leica SP8 gated STED microscope fitted with a Leica HyD hybrid detector.
2. Focus your signal using the rhodamine channel, the *RNR1* and *RNR2* signals should be extremely bright, which allows this visualization (*see* **Note 13**).
3. In most cases, the Quasar 570 labeled probes are excited with two white light (WL) lasers at 520 and 548 nm and depleted with a 660 nm STED laser. The acquisition window of the Leica HyD hybrid detector was limited to 560–574 nm when imaging Quasar 570 and CAL Fluor610 concurrently. CAL Fluor610 labeled probes are excited by the WL laser at 590 nm and depleted with a 660 nm STED laser. Atto 647N labeled probes are excited by the WL laser at 647 nm and depleted with a 775 nm STED laser.
4. For each sample preparation, imaging parameters such as WL laser power, STED laser power and gating will need to be optimized (*see* **Note 14**).
5. In general, images were acquired as stacks at 4–10 μm intervals in order to allow better quality deconvolution of the images. However, stack acquisition results in greater photobleaching of the sample.

6. Deconvolution (e.g., Fig. 2) of images was carried out using the Huygens Professional Deconvolution software (version 14.10; Scientific Volume Imaging).
7. When samples are not being imaged, store them in the dark at 4 °C. The signal may fade over time. Best results are obtained when images are taken within 2 weeks of staining.

3.1.5 Analysis

1. To analyze fluorescence intensity across a variety of cellular conditions, we have used FIJI Software (https://fiji.sc/). The first step is to define a region of interest using the threshold setting and then measure the mean intensity. To compare fluorescence intensities, samples must be prepared at the same time and visualized using the same imaging parameters.
2. To analyze colocalization of *RNR1*, *RNR2* and antibody decorated proteins, we used Huygens Professional colocalization software. This software allows a range of colocalization methods to be applied to the image.

3.2 Click Chemistry Approach to Visualize Nascent Mitochondrial Protein Synthesis by Fluorescence Microscopy

3.2.1 Pulse Labelling in Cultured Cells

1. 1–2 days before starting the experiment: plate cells at 30–40% confluence with regular DMEM onto coverslips that had been placed into 6-well plates (9.6 cm^2) with sterilized forceps. Each well is used for a separate experiment condition or cell line. The experiment should be conducted when the cells are in the log phase of cell growth and 60–80% confluent.

   Negative controls should include:

   (a) A well with regular methionine-containing DMEM (no HPG added).

   (b) A well with HPG + 50 μg/mL cycloheximide (for cytosolic) and 50 μg/mL CAP (for mitochondrial) to block total protein synthesis.

   (c) A well with HPG but lacking any inhibitors, to visualize cytosolic protein synthesis as a point of comparison.

   The mitochondria-specific signal will be obtained in the well containing HPG and 50 μg/mL cycloheximide.
2. Methionine starvation and inhibition of protein synthesis: aspirate away regular DMEM and replace with 500 μL methionine-free DMEM with or without inhibitors. Incubate cells for 1 min at 37 °C, under 5% CO_2 in a humidified incubator (*see* **Note 15**).
3. HPG pulse labelling: aspirate away medium and replace with 500 μL methionine-free DMEM with or without inhibitors and 500 μM HPG for 2 h, then incubate cells at 37 °C and under 5% CO_2 in a humidified incubator (*see* **Note 16**).

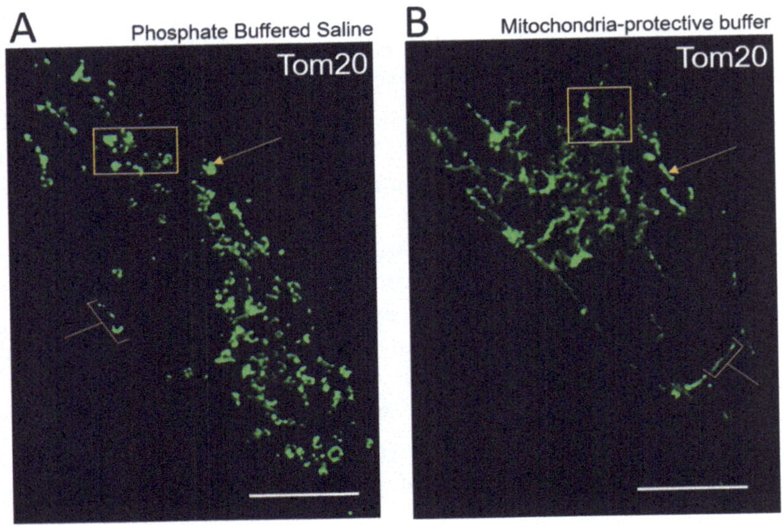

Fig. 5 Preserving the integrity of the mitochondrial network during digitonin pre-permeabilization. Cells were retrieved from culture and washed once, treated with digitonin (0.005%) for 2 min on ice, washed once more and fixed for 10 min at room temperature. The buffer used for washing and for dilution of digitonin and fixative was either phosphate buffer saline (**a**) or mitochondria-protective buffer (**b**, *see* Subheading 2.2.2). The fixative used for (**a**) was 3.7% formaldehyde solution made from paraformaldehyde powder while for (**b**) it was 3.7% formaldehyde diluted 1/10 from a 37% formaldehyde solution. Yellow annotations highlight fragmentation and swelling of mitochondria (**a**) and intact mitochondria (**b**). Scale bar is 5 μm

3.2.2 Pre-permeabilizing and Fixing Intact Cells

1. Quenching HPG labelling pulse: retrieve cells from the incubator, aspirate away medium and wash once with ice cold mitochondria-protective buffer (*see* **Note 17**).
2. Pre-permeabilization (*see* **Note 18**): add 500 μL digitonin diluted in ice cold mitochondria-protective buffer to 0.005% to each well, with the plate kept on ice for 2 min (*see* **Note 19**, Fig. 5).
3. Fixation: aspirate away digitonin and wash once with ice cold PBS before adding 500 μL ice cold 3.7% formaldehyde in mitochondria-protective buffer. Keep plates at room temperature in the dark for 10 min before washing once with ice cold mitochondria-protective buffer and moving to blocking if required (*see* **Note 20**).

3.2.3 Blocking Procedures

1. Blocking nonspecific binding of antigens and antibodies: add 500 μL ice cold 5% (w:v) BSA to cells for 1 h, incubating at room temperature with agitation for 1 h.

3.2.4 Detection of HPG-Labeled Mitochondrial Proteins

1. Creating a humidified container: use a sealable plastic container that can hold a suitable number of samples. Dampen a single layer of paper towel with water, ensuring the paper covers the entire surface of the dish. Pour excess liquid out of the dish. Cover the paper towel with a single layer of aluminum foil. Place labels in the container corresponding to the correct sample (each glass coverslip).
2. Preparing components for click reaction to label HPG-containing mitochondrial proteins (*see* **Note 21**): add components to a microfuge tube and briefly vortex (*see* **Note 22**).
3. Addition of click components to cells: using forceps, remove glass coverslip, dry to remove excess liquid by dabbing edge onto paper towels and place coverslip with cells facing up in the humidified chamber (*see* **Note 23**). Add 50 μL of the 2× click reaction mixture to each coverslip, then seal the chamber that should also be protected from light. Allow 40 min for components to enter cells (*see* **Note 24**). All steps from this point on should minimize the cells exposure to light.
4. Initiating the click chemistry reaction to label HPG-containing mitochondrial proteins: add 50 μL of 2× sodium ascorbate solution to each coverslip and then seal the chamber. Incubate for a further 30 min to complete the reaction.
5. Washing: using forceps, place coverslips back into 6-well plates and to remove unattached Picolyl AF594, wash three times with PBS for 5 min each. For all washing and incubation steps the 6-well plate should be covered in aluminum foil to protect cells from light exposure prior to imaging.

3.2.5 Immuno-fluorescence Labelling

1. Primary antibody incubation: dilute rabbit polyclonal IgG anti-Tom20 1:1000 in TBS-T with 1% (w:v) BSA to label the mitochondrial network. Add 500 μL to cells for 1 h in the dark with agitation.
2. Wash three times for 5 min each with TBS-T to remove unattached antibody.
3. Secondary antibody incubation: dilute goat anti-Rabbit IgG (H + L), Alexa Fluor 488 1:200 to fluorescently label primary anti-Tom20 antibody. Add 500 μL to cells for 1 h in the dark, with agitation.
4. Wash three times for 5 min each with TBS-T to remove unattached antibody.
5. Nuclear staining: dilute 1 mg/mL stock solution of Hoechst 33342 DNA dye 1:1000 in PBS to give a final concentration of 1 μg/mL. Add 500 μL to cells for 10 min in the dark before washing once with PBS and replacing with 1 mL of PBS.

3.2.6 Mounting Coverslips onto Microscope Slides

1. Add one droplet of ProLong Glass Antifade Mountant to each microscope slide (*see* **Note 25**).
2. Wash cells once with PBS and remove excess liquid from coverslip by dabbing the edge onto paper towel. Carefully lower the coverslips with cells facing down onto the mounting medium, taking care to avoid air bubble formation.
3. Allow to set for 18–24 h at room temperature in the dark before imaging with a fluorescence microscope. For long-term storage, seal the edges of the coverslip with clear nail polish and store at 4 °C or −20 °C.

3.2.7 Analyzing Samples by Fluorescence Microscopy

1. To capture images use an epifluorescence inverted microscope (confocal or standard emission depletion microscopes are recommended for optimal resolution) with ×63 oil immersion lens (Fig. 6).
   (a) Images must be taken using identical filter settings and laser power/exposure time for all samples.
   (b) We recommend using a confocal microscope to create a Z-stack series, allowing the entire sample volume to be visualized and rendered. Analyzing 3D reconstructed images of the Z series allows quantification of signal within the entire sample volume.
2. Use Huygens software for deconvolution of images, using identical settings for all samples within a given experiment.
3. Use image analysis software to measure mitochondrial translation levels and distribution. This is completed by calculating the mean fluorescence of HPG signal (we have used ImageJ with the FIJI plugin) and determining colocalization within the mitochondrial network (we have used Huygens), respectively. Identical settings are to be used when comparing samples for a given experiment.
   (a) *Mean fluorescence*: this is used to quantify translation levels and compare this parameter between samples, e.g., between different cell lines, different experimental conditions or between control and patient-derived cell lines. Cell areas are selected manually as a "region of interest" and pixel/intensity threshold settings between images are kept identical. The mean gray value of the region of interest is calculated with the measurement tool to quantify fluorescence. At least eight separate cells are measured from each experiment for each sample, with the average over three separate experiments calculated. Standard error of the mean is calculated and data is tabulated with Microsoft Excel.

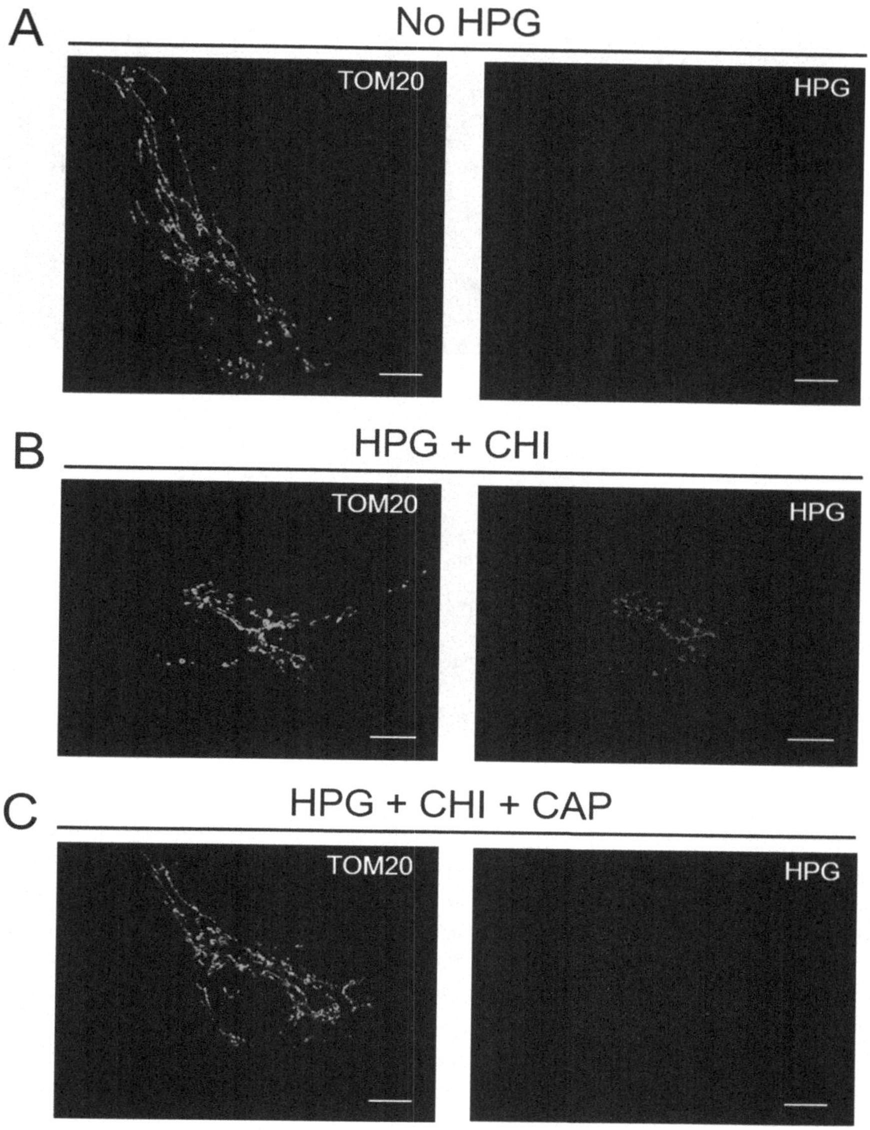

Fig. 6 Visualizing nascent mitochondrial protein synthesis. Cells were incubated in supplemented but methionine-free DMEM for 20 min before addition of HPG and inhibitors in fresh methionine-free media for 2 h. Pre-permeabilization (0.005% digitonin) preceded fixation with 3.7% formaldehyde and further permeabilization with 0.01% Triton X-100. A copper-catalyzed reaction was used to label HPG with Picolyl AF594 before counterstaining with antibodies to Tom20 to label the mitochondrial network. (**b**) Demonstrates nascent mitochondrial protein synthesis while (**a**) and (**c**) are used as negative controls. (**a**) Indicates nonspecific staining of Picolyl AF594 and (**c**) demonstrates the background staining caused by labelling of unincorporated HPG. *HPG* homopropargylglycine, *Tom20* translocase of the outer mitochondrial membrane 20, *CHI* cycloheximide, *CAP* chloramphenicol. Scale bar is 10 μm

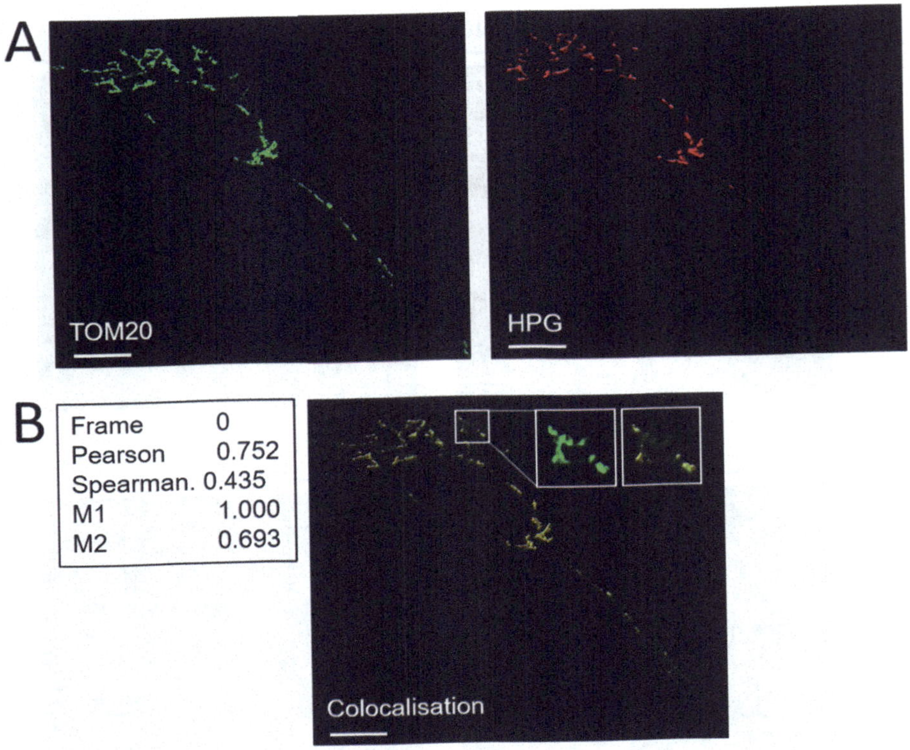

Fig. 7 Colocalization of HPG with the mitochondrial network. Cells were incubated in supplemented but methionine-free DMEM for 20 min before addition of HPG and cycloheximide in fresh methionine-free media for 2 h. Pre-permeabilization with 0.005% digitonin preceded fixation with 3.7% formaldehyde and further permeabilization with 0.01% Triton X-100. A copper-catalyzed reaction was used to label HPG with Picolyl AF594 (**a**, left panel) before counterstaining with Tom20 (Alexa Fluor 488) to label the mitochondrial network (**a**, right panel). Regions of colocalization are visualized as yellow (**b**). The expanded boxes (white) highlight that only a subset of the HPG colocalizes (yellow) with Tom20 (green). Different quantification programs were used to evaluate this and derived data presented in the box (**b**)

(b) *Colocalization*: between Picolyl AF594 and AF488 this is used to establish that the HPG (nascent mitochondrial protein synthesis, Picolyl AF594) signal is specific to the mitochondrial network (AF488). It also provides spatial information on whether the nascent synthesis signal is uniform or distributive throughout the network (*see* Fig. 7).

4 Notes

1. High performance coverslips are used to ensure an even thickness of the coverslip. Further, objectives may be optimized for different coverslips. The Leica objectives used to image the preparations presented here are optimized for 0.17 mm thick coverslips.

2. A humidified chamber is used for RNA FISH and immunofluorescence hybridizations to minimize evaporation of small volumes of reagents. The chamber is prepared using a lidded air tight plastic box with damp paper towels on the base and lined with parafilm. The parafilm should be labeled to designate each separate experiment (Fig. 4).
3. Vanadyl ribonucleoside complexes solution (1 mL, 200 mM) were prepared from powder, reconstituting in DEPC-treated water according to manufacturer's data sheet. The solution should be heated to 65 °C for 10 min with intermittent mixing until the power is dissolved. Aliquots (200 μL) were stored at −20 °C until needed. If, when thawed, the powder comes out of solution, reheat to 65 °C until dissolved before using.
4. The cell type used to demonstrate this technique was control primary fibroblasts. The rationale for this was twofold: these cells have distinct and elaborate mitochondrial networks, and patient cells with mitochondrial defects are often obtained as fibroblasts. This technique will be of value to compare mitochondrial translation between healthy and diseased patient cell lines, which is of great interest.
5. The labelling and imaging described here was carried out predominantly on human osteosarcoma (U2OS) cells as they generate a very defined mitochondrial network. Labelling has been successful in multiple other mammalian cell types including HEK293K and HeLa cells, although the former have less uniform morphology.
6. We have found that cells at a lower confluency are better for mitochondrial imaging as the cells have a greater area in which to expand thus allowing for better visualization of the mitochondrial network, with less interference from out of focus light. We, therefore, suggest seeding cells from an exponentially growing population, at approximately 10–15% confluency (for U2OS cells) to achieve approximately 20–30% coverage the following day.
7. We have found that cells "shocked" before fixation can result in fragmented mitochondrial networks. Even mild "shock" can have an impact and so it is important to use warm or room temperature PBS before fixation and ensure that the cells do not dry out on the coverslips.
8. The cells were permeabilized for 1 h at room temperature but we have had success with overnight permeabilization at 4 °C. If the sample is to be permeabilized overnight, seal the edges of the plate with parafilm to minimize evaporation. If cells/coverslips have dried out, *do not* proceed to labelling steps.

9. During the second wash step, 1 μL 1:100 DAPI can be added if nuclear staining is desired (*see* Subheading 2.1.4, **item 3**).
10. The mountant needs to harden for 3–4 days for STED imaging such that the refractive index is uniform across the slide. Avoid moving the coverslip once the cells are in contact with the mountant as this can crush cells and generate distorted images with smeared signals from the fluorescent probes.
11. Nail polish is routinely used to seal microscope samples by carefully applying the nail polish around the coverslip edges. Clear nail polish should be used to avoid any additional fluorescence in colored or glittered alternatives.
12. In order to counter the effects of photobleaching caused through STED imaging, higher antibodies concentrations are recommended, we successfully used double the standard concentrations. We do not see a different distribution when using a lower antibody concentration, but the effects of bleaching following STED imaging are greater. For decorating Tom20, the final antibody concentration was ~2 μg/mL and the final concentration of Atto 647N labeled secondary antibody was ~10 μg/mL.
13. The *RNR1* and *RNR2* signals are extremely bright as a high concentration of probe is recommended. This is used to combat the effects of photobleaching by STED microscopy and removes the need for DAPI in order to focus easily on the cells. We do not see a different distribution when using a lower probe concentration, but the effects of bleaching following STED imaging are greater.
14. Laser power should be adjusted for each sample preparation as the fluorescence can vary between preparations. Gated STED is a type of STED microscopy that can remove any light within the depletion laser that is not completely depleted. This is done by filtering photo detection by arrival time to the detector. This setting may also vary between preparations.
15. We have found that 1 min pre-incubation in methionine-free media with inhibitors is sufficient to allow the HPG labelling to be effective. We have found increased incubation periods to be unnecessary, and potentially could alter protein expression levels, affecting potential physiological validity of any data.
16. HPG pulse time can be varied, and a chase can also be performed, whereby inhibitors and HPG are washed out at completion of the pulse and replaced with 500 μL complete methionine-containing DMEM medium. This allows analysis of the distribution of nascent proteins throughout the time course.

17. It is important to use mitochondria-protective buffer for all steps following the end of the HPG pulse until fixation has been completed. The sucrose and isotonic nature of the buffer preserves morphology of mitochondrial network during the washing, pre-permeabilizing and fixation steps. Use of PBS for these steps causes mitochondria swelling and fragmentation, resulting in a disintegrated mitochondrial reticulum.
18. This step is important for removing unincorporated HPG molecules, which otherwise cause a diffuse background signal across the cell that obscures detection of the specifically incorporated mitochondrial HPG. At low concentrations (0.015% and below), it is thought that digitonin selectively permeabilizes the cholesterol-rich plasma membranes of cells while leaving intracellular organelles intact. This procedure has been performed to allow entry of molecules into cells for the purposes of other assays [19], but here it allows free efflux of HPG molecules from cells. Pre-permeabilization conditions (length, concentration, etc.) should be optimized for each cell type to achieve the optimal balance between complete removal of unincorporated HPG and preserved integrity of the mitochondrial network.
19. BSA blocking is only necessary if HPG labelling is to be followed by immunofluorescent labelling of mitochondrial markers, such as Tom20, as in our example.
20. Copper is the catalyst for these reactions, while DMSO protects against degradation of biomolecules. Picolyl azides possess an internal copper chelating moiety that (1) accelerates the CuAAC reaction by maintaining the Cu(I) oxidation state and (2) protects proteins and nucleic acids from oxidative damage. For any given copper concentration there is an increase in the efficiency of labelling, which is an important factor when measuring a low signal such as nascent mitochondrial protein synthesis. Therefore, picolyl azides are the fluorophores of choice. Biotinylated picolyl azides are also available, and are suggested for SDS-PAGE and mass spectrometry applications.
21. There are two options when preparing the reaction solution, a high or low copper version. Although the low copper reaction results in a weaker signal, in our experience it is the preferred option for preserving structural integrity of mitochondria. It has also been shown to be essential for compatibility with RNA FISH labeling due to preservation of RNA molecules [18]. In the low copper reaction BTTAA is included, as it is a very effective ligand for CuAAC when used in conjunction with picolyl azides [20].

(a) 2× Low copper reaction buffer solution: 600 μM $CuSO_4$, 10% (v:v) DMSO, 1.2 mM BTTAA and 20 μM Picolyl AF594 in room temperature PBS. 1 mM sodium ascorbate added during the click reaction.

(b) 2× High copper reaction buffer solution: 2 mM $CuSO_4$, 10% (v:v) DMSO and 20 μM Picolyl AF594 in room temperature PBS. Briefly vortex. 100 mM sodium ascorbate added during the click reaction.

22. Use of the humidified chamber allows the volume to be reduced to 20% of that normally used in the well of a 6-well plate, thus greatly increasing the number of experiments possible with the same volume of click chemistry reagents.

23. We have found that this pre-incubation before triggering the click reaction with sodium ascorbate results in more uniform labelling across the cell population.

24. ProLong Glass Antifade Mountant is recommended for its antifade protective properties. In our experience, it provides the brightest signal and lowest background, which is important for achieving high-definition fluorescent images. Coverslips can also be allowed to cure onto microscope slides for 4 days at 4 °C instead of overnight at room temperature.

25. Colocalization analysis consists of at least two distinct sets of methods which can be used in tandem to address separate biological questions. These parameters are termed co-occurrence and correlation [21] (*see* Fig. 7). Co-occurrence describes the extent of spatial overlap between two fluorophores. Such co-occurrence measurements can be utilized to determine what proportion of HPG is present within the mitochondrial network. Manders M1 and M2 are recommended. Correlation determines the degree to which the abundance of two spatially overlapping fluorophores are related to each other. For instance, it can be used to examine the relationship between the intensity of the signals. For these analyzes, Pearson and Spearman are recommended.

Acknowledgements

We thank Dr. Kurt Hoogewijs for advice and suggestions. This work was supported by The Wellcome Trust [203105/Z/16/Z] R.N.L. and Z.C.L. and the REMIX (REgulation of MItochondrial gene eXpression) grant of the Marie Curie Network. The Marie Skłodowska-Curie Action ITN is offered by the European Commission as part of the Horizon 2020 programme for funding research, technological development, and innovation.

References

1. Chomyn A (1996) In vivo labeling and analysis of human mitochondrial translation products. Methods Enzymol 264:197–211
2. Raj A et al (2008) Imaging individual mRNA molecules using multiple singly labeled probes. Nat Methods 5(10):877–879
3. Femino AM et al (1998) Visualization of single RNA transcripts in situ. Science 280 (5363):585–590
4. Zheng Z et al (2016) Unequal distribution of 16S mtrRNA at the 2-cell stage regulates cell lineage allocations in mouse embryos. Reproduction 151(4):351–367
5. Patterson GH (2009) Fluorescence microscopy below the diffraction limit. Semin Cell Dev Biol 20(8):886–893
6. Hell SW, Wichmann J (1994) Breaking the diffraction resolution limit by stimulated emission: stimulated-emission-depletion fluorescence microscopy. Opt Lett 19(11):780–782
7. Galbraith CG, Galbraith JA (2011) Super-resolution microscopy at a glance. J Cell Sci 124(Pt 10):1607–1611
8. Hell SW, Dyba M, Jakobs S (2004) Concepts for nanoscale resolution in fluorescence microscopy. Curr Opin Neurobiol 14 (5):599–609
9. Jakobs S, Wurm CA (2014) Super-resolution microscopy of mitochondria. Curr Opin Chem Biol 20:9–15
10. Lentz SI et al (2010) Mitochondrial DNA (mtDNA) biogenesis: visualization and duel incorporation of BrdU and EdU into newly synthesized mtDNA in vitro. J Histochem Cytochem 58(2):207–218
11. Mitra K, Lippincott-Schwartz J (2010) Analysis of mitochondrial dynamics and functions using imaging approaches. Curr Protoc Cell Biol Chapter 4:Unit 4.25.1–21
12. Grunewald A et al (2014) Quantitative quadruple-label immunofluorescence of mitochondrial and cytoplasmic proteins in single neurons from human midbrain tissue. J Neurosci Methods 232:143–149
13. Spitzer MH, Nolan GP (2016) Mass cytometry: single cells, many features. Cell 165 (4):780–791
14. Beatty KE (2011) Chemical strategies for tagging and imaging the proteome. Mol Biosyst 7 (8):2360–2367
15. Landgraf P et al (2015) BONCAT: metabolic labeling, click chemistry, and affinity purification of newly synthesized proteomes. Methods Mol Biol 1266:199–215
16. Tom Dieck S et al (2012) Metabolic labeling with noncanonical amino acids and visualization by chemoselective fluorescent tagging. Curr Protoc Cell Biol Chapter 7:Unit 7.11
17. Zhang Y et al (2016) The mitochondrial outer membrane protein MDI promotes local protein synthesis and mtDNA replication. EMBO J 35(10):1045–1057
18. Estell C et al (2017) In situ imaging of mitochondrial translation shows weak correlation with nucleoid DNA intensity and no suppression during mitosis. J Cell Sci 130 (24):4193–4199
19. Adam SA (2016) Nuclear protein transport in digitonin permeabilized cells. Methods Mol Biol 1411:479–487
20. Besanceney-Webler C et al (2011) Increasing the efficacy of bioorthogonal click reactions for bioconjugation: a comparative study. Angew Chem Int Ed Engl 50(35):8051–8056
21. Aaron JS, Taylor AB, Chew TL (2018) Image co-localization - co-occurrence versus correlation. J Cell Sci 131(3). https://doi.org/10.1242/jcs.211847

Chapter 14

Mitoribosome Profiling from Human Cell Culture: A High Resolution View of Mitochondrial Translation

Sarah F. Pearce, Miriam Cipullo, Betty Chung, Ian Brierley, and Joanna Rorbach

Abstract

Ribosome profiling (Ribo-Seq) is a technique that allows genome-wide, quantitative analysis of translation. In recent years, it has found multiple applications in studies of translation in diverse organisms, tracking protein synthesis with single codon resolution. Traditional protocols applied for generating Ribo-Seq libraries from mammalian cell cultures are not suitable to study mitochondrial translation due to differences between eukaryotic cytosolic and mitochondrial ribosomes. Here, we present an adapted protocol enriching for mitoribosome footprints. In addition, we describe the preparation of small RNA sequencing libraries from the resultant mitochondrial ribosomal protected fragments (mtRPFs).

Key words Mitoribosome, Ribosome profiling, Mitochondria, MitoRibo-Seq

1 Introduction

Genome-wide gene expression profiles generated using microarray or RNA sequencing approaches attempt to quantify all mRNA species within a cell. However, frequent discordance between mRNA and protein levels highlights the complexity of translational and post-translational regulation and the need for techniques that directly monitor protein synthesis.

Ribosome profiling, or *Ribo-Seq*, is a technique developed by Ingolia et al. based upon the principle that each translating ribosome protects a well-defined *footprint* of an mRNA undergoing translation, shielding this region from nuclease activity [1, 2]. The *footprints* (ribosome-protected fragments, RPFs) are isolated and subjected to deep sequencing analysis, providing single-nucleotide resolution of translating ribosomes [3]. The density of protected footprints for a given transcript reports on its rate of translation. Studies using ribosome profiling have provided new insights into

Michal Minczuk and Joanna Rorbach (eds.), *Mitochondrial Gene Expression: Methods and Protocols*, Methods in Molecular Biology, vol. 2192, https://doi.org/10.1007/978-1-0716-0834-0_14,

the fundamental mechanisms of protein synthesis in numerous species [4].

Due to structural differences and divergent modes of translation, Ribo-Seq protocols currently employed for the studies of cytosolic ribosomes (cytoribosomes) cannot be effectively applied to mitochondrial ribosomes (mitoribosomes). Mitoribosomes are less abundant than cytoribosomes, their sedimentation coefficients differ, and mitoribosomal subunits dissociate easily during purification, complicating molecular analyses. Notably, mtRPFs are longer than those of cytosolic ribosomes (~33–35 nt reads vs. ~30 nt) [5, 6].

Recently, several groups have reported adaptations of ribosome profiling protocols to ensure the enriched capture of mitochondrial ribosome footprints in yeast and mammalian cells [5–8]. Here, we describe a mitoribosome profiling protocol that utilizes sucrose gradient fractionation to isolate mitochondrial monosomes and associated mtRPFs (Fig. 1). In addition, we describe the steps required to produce small RNA-like sequencing libraries from the resultant mtRPFs for deep sequencing.

2 Materials (*See* Note 1)

2.1 Cell Lysis

1. Cell lysis buffer: 50 mM Tris–HCl, pH 7.4, 150 mM NaCl, 1 mM EDTA, 1% Triton X-100, 20 mM MgOAc, 1 mM dithiothreitol, TURBO DNase I (2000 U/ml, Thermo Fisher Scientific).
2. 1× Phosphate buffered saline (1× PBS).
3. Liquid nitrogen.
4. 20-G needle.
5. 1 ml syringe.

2.2 RNase I Treatment, Sucrose Gradient and Isolation of Ribosome-Protected Fragments

1. RNase I (100 U/μl) (ThermoFisher Scientific).
2. RNase inhibitor, for example SUPERase-In RNase Inhibitor (ThermoFisher Scientific).
3. Sucrose.
4. Gradient buffer: 50 mM Tris–HCl, pH 7.2, 20 mM MgOAc, 80 mM NH_4Cl, 100 mM KCl.
5. TRIzol LS (ThermoFisher Scientific).
6. Polypropylene centrifuge tubes, 11 × 34 mm (Beckman Coulter).
7. TLS-55 swinging-bucket rotor (Beckman Coulter).
8. Gradient forming station (Biocomp).
9. Ultracentrifuge.
10. Nanodrop spectrophotometer.

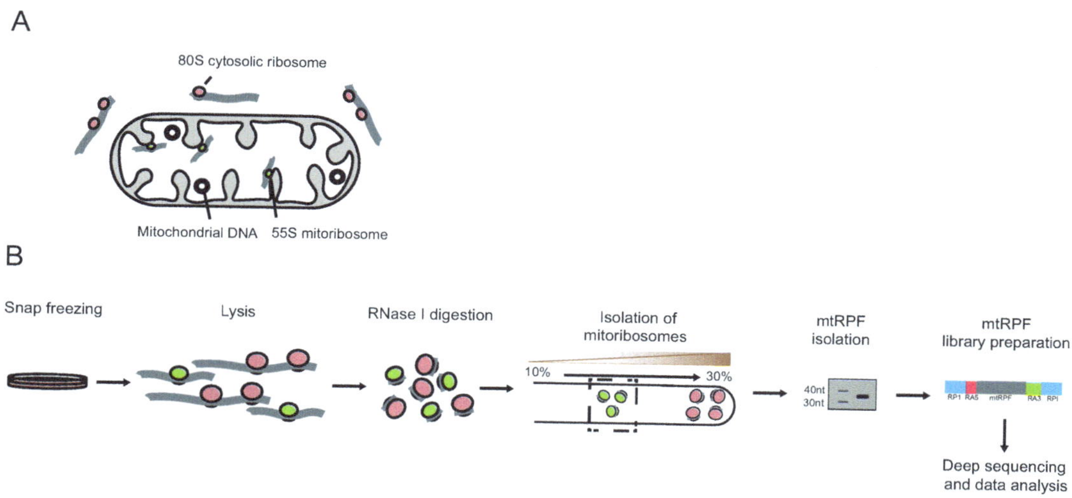

Fig. 1 Overview of mitoribosome profiling protocol. (**a**) Mammalian cells carry two distinct forms of ribosomes. 80S cytosolic ribosomes reside in the cytosol and translate mRNAs derived from nuclear gene expression, and 55S mitochondrial ribosomes (mitoribosomes), which are exclusively located in the mitochondrial matrix and translate the 11 mt-mRNAs derived from mtDNA. The distinct sedimentation coefficients of each ribosome species is utilized herein to enrich for mtRPFs of mt-mRNAs being translated. (**b**) Schematic representation of the MitoRibo-Seq pipeline. Cells are snap-frozen on liquid nitrogen before lysis, which releases mitochondrial and cytosolic ribosomes loaded with the mRNAs they are translating. Next, RNase I digestion of all ribosomes is performed, with RNase concentration optimized for degradation of exposed mRNA portions without damaging mitoribosome integrity. At this stage mitoribosomes are bound to mRNA fragments (footprints) representing the position and efficacy of translation. Lysates are fractionated across a 10–30% continuous sucrose gradient, and gradient fractions containing mitochondrial monosomes are collected for RNA isolation. Following extraction, RNA is resolved via polyacrylamide gel electrophoresis and RNA species between 30 and 40 nt in length are extracted, allowing for the protected mRNA footprints to be recovered. Following extraction, mtRPFs are treated with phosphatase to remove 3′ phosphate and a pre-adenylated 3′ DNA linker (RA3) is ligated, followed by 5′ kinase treatment of the mtRPF RNA and ligation of a 5′ RNA adaptor (RA5). Reverse transcription is performed, followed by PCR amplification using RP1 and RPI oligonucleotides to introduce sequences compatible with Illumina sequencing. Varying index sequences in the RPI oligonucleotides confer the ability of samples to be multiplexed during sequencing

2.3 Gel Purification of mtRPFs

1. Chloroform.
2. 3 M NaOAc, pH 5.5.
3. GlycoBlue coprecipitant, 15 mg/ml (Thermo Fisher Scientific).
4. 100% EtOH.
5. Gel Loading Buffer II (ThermoFisher Scientific).
6. 15% Novex TBE-Urea gel (ThermoFisher Scientific).
7. SYBR™ Gold Nucleic Acid Gel Stain, 10,000× Concentrate (ThermoFisher Scientific).
8. 1× TBE: 89 mM Tris base, 89 mM Boric acid, 2 mM EDTA.

9. 10 bp DNA ladder size markers (Invitrogen).
10. RNA gel extraction buffer: 300 mM NaOAc, pH 5.5, 1 mM EDTA, 0.25% SDS.

2.4 Adapter Ligation

1. T4 PNK (includes T4 PNK buffer) (NEB).
2. DNA gel extraction buffer: 300 mM NaCl, 10 mM Tris–HCl pH 8.0, 1 mM EDTA.
3. 5′ DNA adenylation kit (includes Mth RNA ligase) (NEB).
4. T4 RNA Ligase 2, truncated K227Q (includes T4 Rnl2 buffer and PEG 8000) (NEB).
5. 10 mM Tris–HCl, pH 7.5.
6. T4 RNA Ligase (includes 10× T4 RNA Ligase Reaction Buffer) (Promega).

2.5 Reverse Transcription and PCR Amplification

1. SuperScript III First-Strand Synthesis System for RT-PCR (ThermoFisher Scientific).
2. Phusion High-Fidelity PCR Master Mix with HF Buffer (NEB).
3. PCR purification kit.
4. 10% Novex TBE gel (ThermoFisher Scientific).
5. 1 kb DNA ladder size marker.
6. 10× DNA loading dye.
7. 10 mM Tris–HCl, pH 8.5.

3 Methods (*See* Note 3)

3.1 Cell Lysis

1. Culture cell line of choice to 80% confluency on 150 mm tissue culture plates. Typically, one 150 mm plate is required for the assay.
2. Aspirate media and wash cells with 5 ml of ice-cold PBS.
3. Aspirate all PBS to ensure minimal liquid carry over to the freezing process (*see* **Note 4**).
4. Submerge the closed dish in a reservoir of liquid nitrogen to a depth of 1 cm for 5 s.
5. Pour off any traces of liquid nitrogen from dish and transfer to dry-ice.
6. Dropwise, add 200 μl of lysis buffer evenly across the surface of the dish.
7. Transfer the dish to "wet ice" and use a cell scraper to collect the lysate and transfer to 1.5 ml microcentrifuge tube.

8. Using a 1 ml syringe coupled to a 20-G needle, triturate the sample ten times.
9. Centrifuge at 13,000 × *g* for 20 min at 4 °C and transfer supernatant to new 1.5 ml microcentrifuge tube (*see* **Note 5**).

3.2 RNase I Treatment, Sucrose Gradient Fractionation and Isolation of Ribosome-Protected Fragments

1. Prior to RNase treatment, set up linear 10–30% sucrose gradients for separation of monosomes containing mtRPFs using freshly prepared "gradient buffer."
2. Prepare 10% sucrose solution by dissolving 0.5 g of sucrose to a total volume of 5 ml "gradient buffer."
3. Prepare 30% sucrose solution by dissolving 1.5 g of sucrose to a total volume of 5 ml "gradient buffer."
4. To Beckman Coulter polypropylene centrifuge 11 × 34 mm tubes, add 1.1 ml of 10% sucrose solution.
5. Using a needle and 5 ml syringe, inject 1.1 ml of 30% sucrose solution below the 10% solution.
6. Use Gradient Station (settings: TLS-55—sucrose short—10–30%) to produce continuous 10–30% gradient (*see* **Note 6**).
7. To 200 μl of lysate, add 7 μl of 100 U/μl RNase I and incubate at room temperature (RT) for 30 min (*see* **Note 7**).
8. Add 5 μl of 20 U/μl RNase inhibitor to stop RNase I action.
9. Centrifuge RNase-treated lysate for 5 min at 5000 × *g* to remove any debris.
10. Overlay gradient with 200 μl of RNase I-treated lysate (*see* **Note 8**).
11. Centrifuge gradient at 39,000 rpm in a TLS-55 rotor for 2 h and 15 min at 4 °C.
12. Following centrifugation, take 100 μl fractions from top of gradient using micropipette and transfer each to individual microcentrifuge tubes (*see* **Note 9**).
13. Pool together the fractions that contain mitochondrial monosomes (typically, fractions 11–13, Fig. 2a) and add 900 μl TRIzol LS reagent. Split the collected gradient fractions into two tubes and perform extraction according to manufacturer's instruction, with the addition of 1 μl GlycoBlue during isopropanol precipitation. Resuspend the final RNA pellet in 20 μl 10 mM Tris–HCl, pH 7.5.
14. Measure RNA concentration using a Nanodrop spectrophotometer (*see* **Note 10**).

3.3 Gel Purification of mtRPFs

1. Take 1–2 μg of RNA obtained from ribosome purification, adjust volume with RNase-free water to 6 μl and add 6 μl of Gel Loading Buffer II.

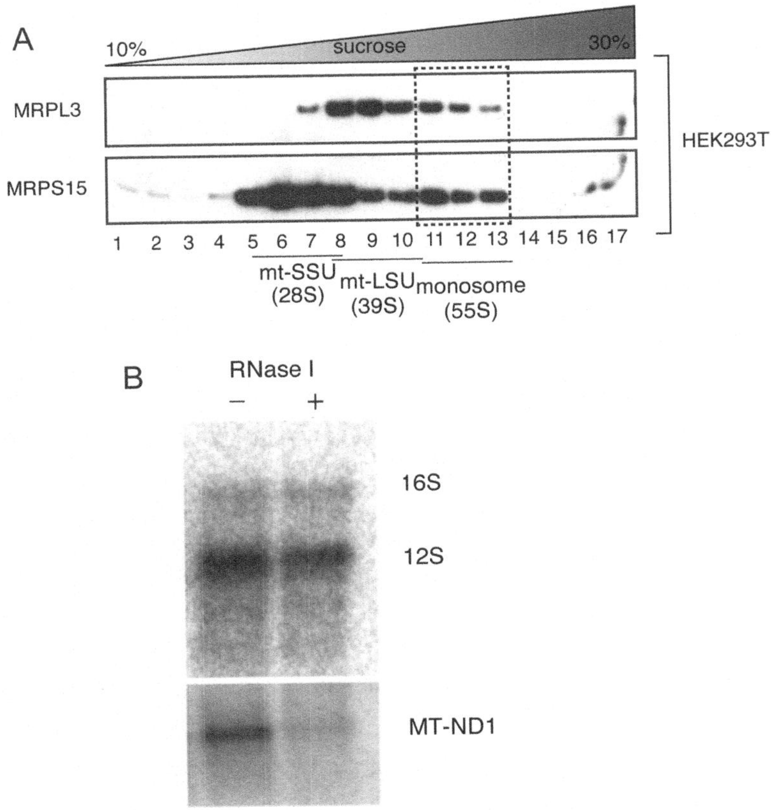

Fig. 2 Quality control analysis to assess integrity of mitoribosome and rRNA after RNAse treatment. (**a**) A sucrose gradient sedimentation analysis of mitoribosomes. Cell lysate was separated through a 10–30% sucrose gradient. Fractions were analyzed by western blot, using antibodies against mt-SSU (uS15m) and mt-LSU (uL3m). The positions of the mt-SSU (28S), mt-LSU (39S) and the monosome (55S) are indicated. (**b**) Northern blot analysis of mtRNA after RNase treatment. 3.5 U/μl RNase I treatment leads to digestion of the full length mitochondrial transcripts (MT-ND1), whereas mitochondrial rRNAs (16S and 12S) are protected under these conditions

2. Heat the samples at 80 °C for 3 min.
3. Place samples on ice for 1 min.
4. Set up 15% Novex TBE-Urea gel in suitable tank using 1× TBE as running buffer (*see* **Note 11**).
5. Load entire volume of each sample, separated by empty lanes, in addition to 10 bp DNA ladder (*see* **Note 12**).
6. Resolve samples until bromophenol blue dye front reaches the bottom of the gel.

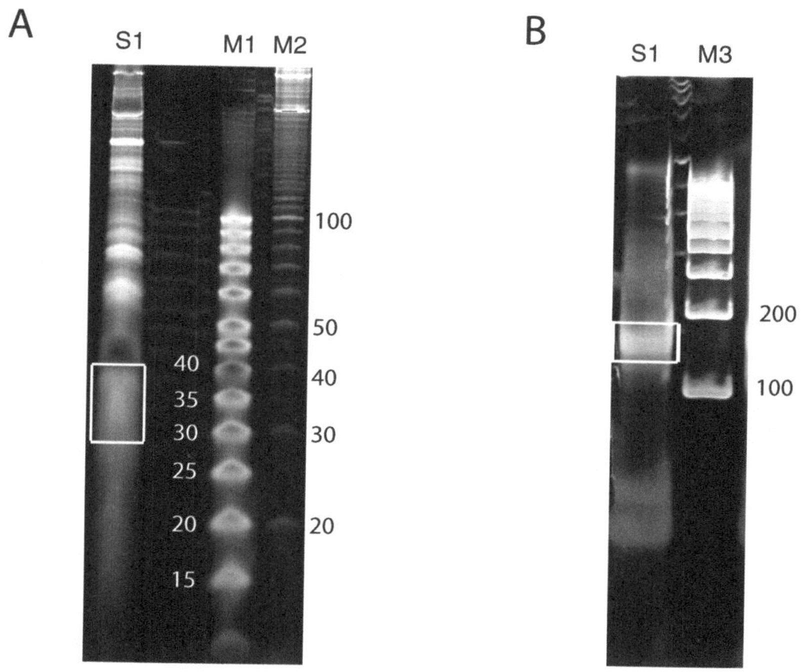

Fig. 3 Representative gels from purification steps. (**a**) Size selection of ribosome footprint fragments. Footprinting samples are derived from HeLa lysates with 1 μg input RNA. The white box indicates the gel region that should be excised. Lanes: S1—RNA sample; M1—5 bp ladder; M2—10 bp ladder. (**b**) Purification of PCR products. The white box indicates the ~155 nt product band to be purified. M3—100 bp ladder

7. Prepare 1× TBE:SYBR Gold by adding 10 μl SYBR Gold to 100 ml of 1× TBE buffer.
8. Following electrophoresis, stain the gel with 1× TBE:SYBR Gold solution for 5 min.
9. Visualize nucleic acids on a Blue light transilluminator and excise the required species using a scalpel blade, aligning to the outer edge of the 30 and 40 nt markers according to the 10 bp ladder and transfer to a 1.5 ml low-bind microcentrifuge tube (Fig. 3a) (*see* **Notes 13** and **14**).
10. To each gel slice, add 600 μl of RNA gel extraction buffer and incubate on a rotating wheel overnight at 4 °C.
11. Add 2 μl GlycoBlue reagent and 900 μl 100% ice-cold EtOH.
12. Place tube at −80 °C for 15 min to precipitate RNA (*see* **Note 15**).
13. Centrifuge at maximum speed for 20 min at 4 °C to pellet RNA.
14. Remove supernatant and wash pellet with 100% ethanol, followed by centrifugation again at maximum speed for 10 min at 4 °C to pellet RNA (*see* **Note 16**).
15. Resuspend the pellet in 10 μl 10 mM Tris–HCl, pH 7.5.

3.4 3′ Phosphatase Treatment of RNA

1. Take 5 μl of gel-purified RNA, add water to 15 μl and heat the sample at 80 °C for 2 min before placing on ice for 1 min (*see* **Note 17**).
2. Centrifuge tube to collect liquid at bottom.
3. To each tube, add 2 μl 10× T4 PNK buffer, 1 μl 20 U/μl RNase inhibitor and 1 μl T4 PNK (*see* **Note 18**).
4. Incubate samples at 37 °C for 2 h.
5. Heat-inactivate the reaction at 65 °C for 10 min.
6. To heat-inactivated sample, add 70 μl nuclease-free water, 2 μl GlycoBlue, 10 μl 3 M NaOAc and 300 μl ice-cold EtOH.
7. Place samples at −80 °C for 30 min to precipitate RNA (*see* **Note 19**).
8. Centrifuge at maximum speed for 20 min at 4 °C to pellet RNA.
9. Remove supernatant and wash pellet with 100% ethanol, followed by centrifugation again at maximum speed for 10 min at 4 °C to pellet RNA.
10. Resuspend the pellet in 7 μl 10 mM Tris–HCl, pH 7.5.

3.5 Preadenylation of 3′ Adaptor Primer RA3p′

1. To 6 μl of phosphorylated RA3 oligonucleotide (50 pmol/μl), add the following components from the NEB 5′ adenylation kit: 5 μl nuclease-free water, 2 μl of 10× 5′ DNA adenylation reaction buffer, 1 μl of 10 mM ATP, 6 μl Mth RNA Ligase.
2. Incubate samples at 65 °C for 1 h.
3. Heat inactivate at 85 °C for 5 min.
4. Add 180 μl of nuclease-free water.
5. Perform extraction of adenylated oligonucleotide by addition of 200 μl 1:1 phenol:chloroform.
6. Vortex samples for 1 min.
7. Centrifuge samples at maximum speed in a microcentrifuge at RT for 5 min.
8. Collect 100 μl upper aqueous phase and transfer to new Lo-Bind microcentrifuge tube.
9. Precipitate RNA by addition of 2 μl GlycoBlue, 20 μl 3 M NaOAc, pH 5.0 and 600 μl ice-cold 100% EtOH.
10. Precipitate at −80 °C for 30 min and centrifuge at maximum speed in 4 °C centrifuge for 10 min.
11. Discard supernatant and add 500 μl of 100% EtOH.
12. Centrifuge at maximum speed for 10 min.
13. Discard supernatant and resuspend final pellet in 13 μl 10 mM Tris–HCl, pH 7.5 (*see* **Note 20**).

3.6 Ligation of 3′ Adaptors to mtRPF Libraries

1. To 7 μl dephosphorylated RNA, add 2 μl adenylated RA3 primer from Subheading 3.5 above.
2. Heat mixture at 80 °C for 2 min and allow to cool to RT.
3. To total 9 μl volume of dephosphorylated RNA and RA3, add 2 μl 10× T4 RNA Ligase Reaction Buffer, 2 μl T4 Rnl2tr K227Q enzyme, 6 μl 50% PEG 8000, 1 μl SUPERase-In (*see* **Note 21**).
4. Incubate samples at 14 °C overnight.
5. To samples, add 160 μl nuclease-free H_2O, 2 μl GlycoBlue, 20 μl 3 M NaOAc, pH 5.5 and 600 μl ice-cold 100% EtOH.
6. Precipitate at −80 °C for 30 min and centrifuge at maximum speed in 4 °C centrifuge for 10 min.
7. Dissolve pellet in 5 μl 10 mM Tris–HCl, pH 7.5.
8. To samples, add 5 μl Gel Loading Buffer II.
9. Heat samples at 80 °C for 2 min and place directly on ice.
10. Set up 15% Novex TBE-Urea gel in the tank using 1× TBE as running buffer.
11. Load entire volume of each sample, separated by empty lanes, in addition to 10 bp DNA ladder.
12. Resolve samples until bromophenol blue dye front reaches the bottom of the gel.
13. Following resolution, stain the gel with 1× TBE:SybrGold solution for 5 min.
14. Visualize nucleic acids on a Blue light transilluminator and excise the required species using a scalpel blade (*see* **Note 22**).
15. To each gel slice, add 600 μl of RNA gel extraction buffer and incubate overnight at 4 °C.
16. To tube, add 2 μl GlycoBlue reagent and 900 μl 100% ice-cold EtOH.
17. Place tube at −80 °C for 15 min to precipitate RNA.
18. Centrifuge at maximum speed at 4 °C to pellet RNA.
19. Resuspend the pellet in 10 μl 10 mM Tris–HCl pH 7.5.

3.7 5′ Phosphorylation of Gel-Purified 3′ Adaptor Ligated Products

1. To the 5 μl of gel-purified RNA from Subheading 3.6, **step** 7, add 2 μl 10× T4 PNK buffer, 2 μl T4 PNK (10 U/μl), 2 μl 10 mM ATP, 1 μl 20 U/μl RNase inhibitor, 3 μl nuclease-free H_2O. Total volume should be 20 μl.
2. Incubate samples at 37 °C for 2 h.
3. To samples, add 2 μl GlycoBlue, 20 μl 3 M NaOAc, pH 5.0 and 600 μl ice-cold 100% EtOH, and precipitate at −80 °C for 30 min.
4. Centrifuge at maximum speed at 4 °C for 10 min.

5. Discard the supernatant and wash with 500 μl 100% EtOH by centrifugation at maximum speed at 4 °C for 10 min.
6. Discard supernatant and resuspend final pellet in 10 μl 10 mM Tris–HCl, pH 7.5.

3.8 Ligation of 5′ RNA Adaptor

1. To 10 μl of phosphorylated RNA from Subheading 3.7, **step 6**, add 2 μl 5′ Adaptor RA5 (50 pmol/μl) (*see* **Note 23**), 2 μl 10× T4 Rnl2 buffer, 2 μl T4 RNA Ligase, 1 μl 20 U/μl RNase inhibitor, 3 μl nuclease-free H_2O. Total volume should be 20 μl.
2. Incubate ligation at 25 °C for 6 h (*see* **Note 24**).
3. To each sample, add 160 μl nuclease-free water, 2 μl GlycoBlue, 20 μl 3 M NaOAc, pH 5.5 and 600 μl ice-cold EtOH and incubate at −80 °C for 30 min.
4. Centrifuge at maximum speed at 4 °C to pellet RNA.
5. Resuspend pelleted RNA in 3 μl 10 mM Tris–HCl pH 7.5.

3.9 Reverse Transcription

1. To 3 μl RNA from Subheading 3.8, **step 5**, add 1 μl RT primer (50 pmol/μl) and 0.5 μl 25 mM dNTPs.
2. Incubate at 65 °C for 5 min and transfer immediately to 55 °C.
3. Prepare the following mix for each sample: 2 μl 5× First-Strand buffer, 1 μl Superscript III, 2 μl 25 mM $MgCl_2$, 1 μl 100 mM DTT, 0.5 μl 20 U/μl RNase inhibitor.
4. Pre-warm cocktail to 55 °C and add 6.5 μl directly to RNA:RT primer mix. Total volume at this stage is 11 μl.
5. Incubate reaction at 55 °C for 50 min, followed by 85 °C for 5 min.

3.10 PCR Amplification of Library

1. To 2 μl of reverse transcription reaction, add 20 μl 2× Phusion High-Fidelity PCR Master Mix, 0.4 μl Primer RP1 (10 pmol/μl), 0.4 μl Primer RP2 (10 pmol/μl), 16.4 μl nuclease-free H_2O.
2. Conduct PCR using the following program: 98 °C—30 s, followed by 13 cycles of: 98 °C—10 s, 60 °C—30 s, 72 °C—15 s. Finally, 72 °C—10 min and hold at 10 °C.
3. Perform PCR clean-up using the QIAGEN PCR purification kit, eluting in 30 μl nuclease-free H_2O. Precipitate as usual and resuspend final pellet in 10 μl 10 mM Tris–HCl pH 7.5.
4. Resolve entire volume of sample on 10% Novex non-denaturing TBE gel (*see* **Note 25**) in a suitable tank using 1× TBE as running buffer. To prepare samples for loading, add 10 μl of water and 2 μl of 10× DNA loading dye and load samples across two lanes, loading 1 kb ladder as a size marker.

5. Following resolution, stain gel with SybrGold as described in Subheading 3.3, **step 8**. Excise the PCR product (Fig. 3b) (*see* **Note 26**).
6. Add 600 μl of DNA gel extraction buffer and incubate overnight at 4 °C with shaking in a thermomixer.
7. To tube, add 2 μl GlycoBlue reagent and 900 μl 100% ice-cold EtOH.
8. Place tube at −80 °C for 15 min to precipitate library, followed by centrifugation at maximum speed at 4 °C to pellet DNA.
9. Resuspend the PCR product in 10–15 μl 10 mM Tris–HCl pH 8.5 (*see* **Note 27**).
10. Concentration of libraries should be determined using a Qubit spectrophotometer or similar (*see* **Notes 28** and **29**).

4 Notes

1. All solutions should be prepared with nuclease-free water and molecular grade reagents. We recommend using low-bind 1.5 ml RNase-free microcentrifuge tubes during all stages of mtRPF purification and sequencing library generation. Note, however, that in such tubes, nucleic acid pellets can become loose and care must be taken when removing supernatants.
2. The oligonucleotide sequences are as for TruSeq Small RNA Illumina (Illumina). RA3 and RA5 should be ordered PAGE purified. Note, RA3 is 5′ phosphorylated. PCR primers 2 (RPI1–4) contain unique indexing sequences, so that samples can be pooled for sequencing. Adapters containing stretches of seven randomized bases can optionally be used. The inclusion of the randomized bases in amplicon libraries allows for computational removal of any PCR duplicates from the library therefore reducing artifacts arising from ligation biases. Note, however, that in our experience, the use of randomized primers can sometimes result in a small increase in adapter-only and too-short reads in the final library.
3. Unless otherwise stated, all steps should be performed on ice.
4. To capture a snapshot of ribosomes, it is essential to rapidly inhibit translation. If inhibition is slow, it may lead to the artificial pausing at specific positions [4]. Flash freezing is the most robust approach commonly used, however, the use of the translation inhibitors is also widely applied. Chloramphenicol can be used to inhibit mitochondrial translation at a final concentration of 100 μg/ml with incubation for 20 min prior to cell harvesting.

5. At this stage, samples can be flash-frozen and stored in liquid nitrogen.
6. Leave the gradient on ice during RNase I treatment. Handle gradient with care to avoid disturbing the content.
7. We advise optimization of the RNase I concentration prior to starting the experiments. The concentration used in this protocol has been optimized for HEK293 cells, however, we successfully used the same concentration in case of other cell lines (143B, HAP1, HeLa). It is important to use the highest concentration that does not disturb the integrity of the mitoribosome but efficiently degrades RNA that is not protected by the mitoribosome (Fig. 2b).
8. At this stage you should have approximately 250–300 μl of lysate. Use 200 μl for gradient centrifugation.
9. From these fractions, take 10 μl aliquots to perform western blotting using antibodies against mitochondrial ribosomal proteins to determine fractions where monosomes are present. We recommend to use anti-uL3m and anti-uS15m antibodies as reliable markers for the identification of fractions containing the mitochondrial monosome. The monosome can typically be found to fractionate in fractions 11–13.
10. The protocol typically yields 1–3 μg of RNA.
11. Clear urea from wells using syringe and needle. Fill all empty wells with Gel Loading Buffer.
12. Separate different samples from each other with one or more empty wells.
13. Use a fresh scalpel blade for each sample.
14. mtRPFs are longer than cytosolic ones. We have observed that excising fragments between 30 and 40 nt is sufficient, however we recommend the reader to determine empirically the desired size of the excised fragment that encompasses the mtRPFs.
15. At all further stages, you can stop the experiment at the RNA precipitation stage and store the samples at −80 °C.
16. The pellet can be loose, take extra care not to lose it during removal of the supernatant.
17. Store remaining 5 μl of gel-purified RNA at −80 °C, in case it is needed.
18. If using a PNK buffer other than that supplied by NEB, make sure the buffer is free of ATP to ensure phosphatase activity on RNA.
19. Set up preadenylation of the 3′ adaptor primer, described in Subheading 3.5, prior to final resuspension of precipitated RNA.

20. Adenylated RA3 can be stored at −20 °C for several months.
21. PEG 8000 is very viscous. Cut the end of a tip with a clean razor blade to pipette PEG 8000 to the reaction and mix thoroughly before overnight incubation.
22. If 30–40 nt fragments were excised in Subheading 3.3, **step 7**, the ligation product with RA3 should be of 51–61 nt.
23. A stock of 5′ Adaptor RA5 should be stored at −80 °C.
24. Alternatively, incubate ligation at 14 °C overnight.
25. Please note, it is non-denaturing TBE gel.
26. Expect the final product of ~155 bp in size. Avoid any lower product band resulting from unextended primer.
27. Double-stranded DNA may be stored at 4 °C or −20 °C.
28. We recommend using Qubit® dsDNA HS Assay Kit or Agilent BioAnalyzer, according to the manufacturer's protocol.
29. The resulting product is compatible for sequencing on Illumina platforms. PCR is performed with primers containing unique indexing sequences (RPI1–4 in Table 1). Therefore, samples can be pooled for sequencing. A single NextSeq 500/550 75SE high output run produces sufficient coverage across 4–5 indexed MitoRibo-Seq libraries.

Table 1
List of oligonucleotides (*see* Note 2)

Name	Sequence
3′ adapter (RA3)	5′ pTGGAATTCTCGGGTGCCAAGG 3′
3′ adapter (RA3r7)	5′ pNNNNNNNTGGAATTCTCGGGTGCCAAGG 3′
5′ adapter (RA5)	5′ GUUCAGAGUUCUACAGUCCGACGAUC 3′
5′ adapter (RA5r7)	5′ GUUCAGAGUUCUACAGUCCGACGAUCNNNNNNN 3′
RT primer	5′ GCCTTGGCACCCGAGAATTCCA 3′
PCR primer 1 (RP1)	5′ AATGATACGGCGACCACCGAGATCT ACACGTTCAGAGTTCTACAGTCCGA 3′
PCR primer 2 (RPI1) (index 1)	5′ CAAGCAGAAGACGGCATACGAGATCGTGAT GTGACTGGAGTTCCTTGGCACCCGAGAATTCCA 3′
PCR primer 2 (RPI2) (index 2)	5′ CAAGCAGAAGACGGCATACGAGATACATCG GTGACTGGAGTTCCTTGGCACCCGAGAATTCCA 3′
PCR primer 2 (RPI1) (index 3)	5′ CAAGCAGAAGACGGCATACGAGATGCCTAA GTGACTGGAGTTCCTTGGCACCCGAGAATTCCA
PCR primer 2 (RPI4) (index 4)	5′ CAAGCAGAAGACGGCATACGAGATTGGTCA GTGACTGGAGTTCCTTGGCACCCGAGAATTCCA

Index sequences are underlined

References

1. Ingolia NT, Ghaemmaghami S, Newman JR, Weissman JS (2009) Genome-wide analysis in vivo of translation with nucleotide resolution using ribosome profiling. Science 324 (5924):218–223. https://doi.org/10.1126/science.1168978
2. Wolin SL, Walter P (1988) Ribosome pausing and stacking during translation of a eukaryotic mRNA. EMBO J 7:3559–3569
3. Ingolia NT (2010) Genome-wide translational profiling by Ribosome footprinting. Methods Enzymol 470:119–142. https://doi.org/10.1016/S0076-6879(10)70006-9
4. Brar GA, Weissman JS (2015) Ribosome profiling reveals the what, when, where and how of protein synthesis. Nat Rev Mol Cell Biol 16:651–664. https://doi.org/10.1038/nrm4069
5. Rooijers K, Loayza-Puch F, Nijtmans LG, Agami R (2013) Ribosome profiling reveals features of normal and disease-associated mitochondrial translation. Nat Commun 4:1–8. https://doi.org/10.1038/ncomms3886
6. Pearce SF, Rorbach J, Van Haute L, D'Souza AR, Rebelo-Guiomar P, Powell CA, Brierley I, Firth AE, Minczuk M (2017) Maturation of selected human mitochondrial tRNAs requires deadenylation. eLife 6:1–22. https://doi.org/10.7554/eLife.27596
7. Morscher RJ, Ducker GS, Li SH-J, Mayer JA, Gitai Z, Sperl W, Rabinowitz JD (2018) Mitochondrial translation requires folate-dependent tRNA methylation. Nature 554:128–132. https://doi.org/10.1038/nature25460
8. Couvillion MT, Soto IC, Shipkovenska G, Churchman LS (2016) Synchronized mitochondrial and cytosolic translation programs. Nature 533:499–503. https://doi.org/10.1038/nature18015

Chapter 15

Application of Cryo-EM for Visualization of Mitoribosomes

Vivek Singh and Alexey Amunts

Abstract

Mitochondrial ribosomes (mitoribosomes) are specialized machineries that carry out the synthesis of a limited number of proteins encoded in the mitochondrial genome, including components of the oxidative phosphorylation pathway. They have incorporated several structural features distinguishing them from bacterial and eukaryotic cytosolic counterparts. Our current understanding of the assembly and functioning of mitoribosomes is limited, and recent developments in cryo-EM provide promising directions for detailed investigation. Here we describe methods to purify mitoribosomes from human embryonic kidney cells for cryo-EM studies.

Key words Mitochondria, Mitoribosome, Translation, Cryo-EM

1 Introduction

Mitoribosomes are compositionally distinct from bacterial and eukaryotic cytosolic ribosomes [1]. Mammalian mitoribosomes possess a twofold reduced mitochondrial ribosomal RNA (mt-rRNA) and at least 36 additional protein components [2–4]. Among the most pronounced features is the acquisition of a putative GTPase protein mS29 in the head region of the small mitoribosomal subunit (mt-SSU), while the large mitoribosomal subunit (mt-LSU) acquired mitochondrial transfer RNA (mt-tRNA) that serves as a replacement for the 5S rRNA. The incorporation of the mt-tRNA into the central protuberance is an example of structural "patching" that compensates instability by adopting pre-existing elements [5]. However, it is yet to be clarified how these unique elements contribute to the mitoribosomal function and how they are assembled into a single structural unit [6, 7]. The inter-subunit communication that drives the translation cycle has also been modified in mitoribosomes, and unusual degrees of conformational freedom of the mt-SSU have been reported [2, 3, 8]. Due to lack of functional information, the relevance of these features is not well understood.

Michal Minczuk and Joanna Rorbach (eds.), *Mitochondrial Gene Expression: Methods and Protocols*, Methods in Molecular Biology, vol. 2192, https://doi.org/10.1007/978-1-0716-0834-0_15,

A prerequisite for understanding how macromolecules function, is the knowledge of their atomic structures. Cryo-EM is now recognized as capable of providing direct crucial insights into the mechanism of action of biological processes. The main experimental advantage of the cryo-EM technique is that it requires very small amounts of material, up to four orders of magnitude less than for X-ray crystallography. In addition, a parallel computational progress allows to resolve protein complexes from a highly heterogeneous mixture, namely in silico purification based on coarse and fine angle alignment [9–12]. Therefore, it is possible to identify multiple protein conformations and functional states of biological molecules in solution through intense computational classification using masked 3D classification with signal subtraction of region of interest [12, 13]. This current methodology allows detailed analysis of subpopulations representing less than 1% of the total number of molecules, unraveling additional layers of complexity, degrees of freedom, and molecular dynamics.

The use of the cryo-EM in identifying different conformations of mitoribosomes is clearly exemplified in the structural studies of mammalian and yeast mitoribosomes [2, 3, 14]. 3D classification of human mitoribosome particles results in the sorting of particles into multiple classes that differ from each other in structural conformations [2, 3]. In addition, cryo-EM study of mitoribosomal assembly intermediates has been reported employing in silico sorting and focused classification of mt-LSU particles [15]. This allowed identification of the regulatory roles for the assembly factors MALSU1 (mitochondrial assembly of large subunit 1), mt-ACP (acyl carrier protein) and L0R8F8 (LYR-motif containing protein).

Here we present and discuss detailed protocols for carrying out cryo-EM studies of mitoribosomes from human embryonic kidney (HEK) cells in three steps: (1) Purification of human mitoribosomes; (2) Cryo-EM sample preparation and data collection; (3) Cryo-EM data processing.

2 Materials

2.1 Purification of Human Mitoribosomes

1. HEK293 501T cell line.
2. Supplemented Dulbecco's Modified Eagle Medium (DMEM) containing 10% tetracycline-free fetal bovine serum (FBS), 5 μg/mL blasticidin, and 200 μg/mL Azithromycin.
3. Freestyle 293 Expression Medium containing 5% tetracycline-free FBS.
4. T175, 1 L, 2 L, and 2.8 L vented flasks.
5. Mammalian cell culture incubator.

6. MIB buffer: 50 mM HEPES-KOH, pH 7.5, 10 mM KCl, 1.5 mM $MgCl_2$, 1 mM EDTA, 1 mM EGTA, 1 mM DTT, protease inhibitors.
7. SM4 buffer: 840 mM mannitol, 280 mM sucrose, 50 mM HEPES-KOH, pH 7.5, 10 mM KCl, 1.5 mM $MgCl_2$, 1 mM EDTA, 1 mM EGTA, 1 mM DTT, protease inhibitors.
8. MIBSM buffer: 3 volumes MIB buffer + 1 volume SM4 buffer.
9. Phosphate Buffered Saline.
10. SEM buffer: 250 mM sucrose, 20 mM HEPES-KOH, pH 7.5, 1 mM EDTA.
11. Stepwise sucrose density gradient stock solutions: 60%, 32%, 23%, and 15% sucrose in 20 mM HEPES-KOH, pH 7.5, 1 mM EDTA.
12. Lysis buffer: 25 mM HEPES-KOH, pH 7.5, 150 mM KCl, 50 mM MgOAc, 2% Polyethylene glycol octylphenyl ether, 2 mM DTT, protease inhibitors.
13. Sucrose cushion buffer: 1 M sucrose (34% w/v), 20 mM HEPES-KOH, pH 7.5, 100 mM KCl, 20 mM MgOAc, 1% Polyethylene glycol octylphenyl ether, 2 mM DTT.
14. Resuspension buffer: 20 mM HEPES-KOH, pH 7.5, 100 mM KCl, 20 mM MgOAc, 2 mM DTT.
15. Linear sucrose density gradient: 15–30% sucrose density gradient in resuspension buffer in TLS 55 polycarbonate tubes.
16. SW 40 tubes and rotor; TLA 120.2 tubes and rotor, TLS 55 (Ultra-clear) tubes and rotor (Beckman Instruments Inc.).
17. Gradient maker (Biocomp Instruments).
18. Precooled nitrogen cavitation chamber (Parr Instrument Company).
19. Cheesecloth.

2.2 Cryo-EM Sample Preparation and Data Collection

1. Cryo-EM grids, coated with 2–4 nm of carbon (Quantifoil Micro Tools); cryogenic grid boxes (Electron Microscopy Sciences).
2. Glow discharger (Ted Pella Inc.).
3. Plunge freezer (e.g., Vitrobot® from Thermo Fisher Scientific).
4. Clips and C-rings, grid clipping apparatus.
5. Liquid nitrogen and liquid ethane.

2.3 Cryo-EM Data Processing

1. RELION software package [9, 12, 13, 16, 17].
2. UCSF Chimera software [18].

3 Methods

3.1 Purification of Human Mitoribosomes

1. Culture HEK293 501T cells in Supplemented DMEM in a mammalian cell culture incubator, at 37 °C and 5% CO_2. Scale up to nine T175 flasks.
2. Upon achieving 90% confluency, harvest cells by centrifugation at 500 × *g* for 5 min and resuspend in Freestyle 293 Expression Medium containing 5% tetracycline-free FBS (about 300 mL) in a vented shaking flask to achieve a cell density of 1.5×10^6 cells/mL (*see* **Note 1**). Incubate cells at 37 °C and 5% CO_2 at 120 rpm.
3. Monitor the cell density and split the cells at a density of 3.0×10^6 cells/mL. This step should normally take 2 days. Pellet the cells as described above and resuspend in twice the volume used before to maintain an initial cell count of 1.5×10^6 cell/mL (two 300 mL cultures in 1 L vented flasks).
4. Scale up the culture following the same steps as above to reach a volume of 2 L split into two 2.8 L flasks.
5. Harvest the cells from 2 L culture when the cell count is between 3.0–4.0 × 10^6 cells/mL by centrifugation at 1000 × *g* for 7 min at 4 °C (*see* **Note 2**).
6. Resuspend and pool the pelleted cells in 200 mL PBS.
7. Spin down the cells at 1200 × *g* for 10 min at 4 °C and discard the supernatant.
8. Weigh the pellet and resuspend it in 120 mL of MIB buffer. Expected yield is ~20 g.
9. Leave the cells on ice for 10 min allowing them to swell in MIB buffer. Perform gentle stirring to keep the cells suspended.
10. Measure the volume of the resuspended swollen cells and pour them into a precooled nitrogen cavitation chamber kept on ice.
11. Add SM4 buffer (one-third of the resuspended cell volume) to give a final concentration of 70 mM sucrose and 210 mM mannitol.
12. Fill the sealed nitrogen cavitation chamber with nitrogen to reach a pressure of about 500 psi.
13. Leave the chamber on ice for 20 min, while, maintaining the pressure.
14. Release the nitrogen carefully from the chamber and recover the lysed material.
15. Clarify the lysate by centrifugation at 800 × *g* for 15 min at 4 °C, to separate the cell debris and nuclei.
16. While retaining the pellet, pass the supernatant through a cheesecloth into a beaker kept on ice.

17. Resuspend the pellet in half the previous volume (**step 11**) of MIBSM buffer. Use Teflon/glass Dounce homogenizer to homogenize the resuspended pellet. Pour the contents into the nitrogen cavitation chamber and repeat **steps 12–16**. Combine the supernatants thus collected.
18. Clarify the total supernatant by centrifugation at 1000 × *g* for 15 min 4 °C. Discard the pellet and filter the supernatant as in **step 16**.
19. To recover crude mitochondria from the supernatant, centrifuge at 10,000 × *g* for 15 min at 4 °C and resuspend the pellet in 10 mL MIBSM buffer (*see* **Note 3**).
20. Estimate protein concentration using a small volume of the sample. About 2 mg/mL of protein is typically obtained from a 2 L culture.
21. Add 200 U of RNase-free DNase and incubate on a roller in the cold room for 20 min to remove contaminating genomic DNA.
22. Recover mitochondria by centrifugation at 10,000 × *g* for 15 min at 4 °C and gently resuspend the pellet in 2 mL SEM buffer (*see* **Note 4**).
23. Prepare a stepwise sucrose density gradient, by pipetting 1.5 mL of 60% sucrose buffer into the bottom of an SW 40 (14 mL) tube, followed by gently adding 4.5 mL of 32% sucrose buffer, 1.5 mL of 23% sucrose buffer and 1.5 mL of 15% sucrose buffer, respectively. Make sure not to disturb the interface between the layers while preparing and handling the gradient.
24. Carefully, layer the mitochondrial suspension (approximately 3 mL) on top of the sucrose gradient.
25. Centrifuge in SW 40 rotor at 139,065 × *g* for 60 min at 4 °C.
26. Recover the brown band visible at the interface of 32% and 60% sucrose layers with a transfer pipette (Fig. 1).
27. For long-term storage, snap-freeze the isolated mitochondria using liquid nitrogen and transfer to −80 °C.
28. For purification of mitoribosome, thaw the frozen mitochondria in cold room or on ice.
29. Dilute the mitochondria by adding twice the volume of lysis buffer (mix 6 mL lysis buffer in 3 mL mitochondria). Invert the tube several times to mix.
30. Homogenize the solution using a small Teflon/glass Dounce homogenizer and incubate on ice for 5–10 min.
31. Clarify the lysate by centrifugation at 30,000 × *g* for 20 min at 4 °C. Collect the supernatant carefully and discard the pellet.

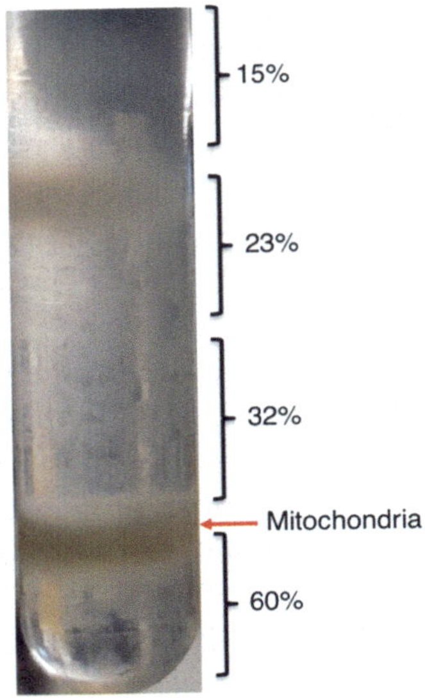

Fig. 1 Isolation of human mitochondria with sucrose density gradient centrifugation. Mitochondria accumulate at the 32–60% sucrose interface after density gradient centrifugation as a brown band indicted by the red arrow

32. Centrifuge the supernatant again at 30,000 × *g* for 20 min at 4 °C to ensure complete clarification. Pour the supernatant carefully into a fresh tube and discard the pellet.
33. To prepare a sucrose cushion, add 0.4 mL of sucrose cushion buffer per TLA 120.2 tube for 1 mL of the clarified lysate.
34. Load 1 mL of the mitochondrial lysate on top of the sucrose cushion in every TLA 120.2 tube to have a lysate:cushion ratio of 2.5:1.
35. Centrifuge at 231,550 × *g* for 45 min in a TLA 120.2 rotor at 4 °C.
36. Discard the sucrose cushion buffer and remove remaining sucrose and Polyethylene glycol octylphenyl ether by gentle washing with 100 μL resuspension buffer.
37. Resuspend the pellets sequentially, in a total volume of 100 μL resuspension buffer (*see* **Note 5**).
38. Dissolve the remaining aggregates by gentle, low speed vortexing for 30 s.
39. Clarify the sample by centrifugation at 18,000 × *g* for 10 min at 4 °C. Discard the pellet and clarify the supernatant once again.
40. Measure absorption of the supernatant at A_{260}. The yield from a 2 L prep is typically around 7 A_{260}, with A_{260}:A_{280} ratio of 1.3.

41. To prepare a linear 15–30% sucrose density gradient, first pipette 1.1 mL of 30% sucrose buffer into the bottom of a TLS 55 (Ultra-clear) tube, followed by carefully layering an equal volume of 15% sucrose buffer on top of it. From here on, a linear gradient can be easily produced using a gradient maker set to the appropriate program.
42. Apply the sample on top of a single linear 15–30% sucrose density gradient and centrifuge in a TLS 55 rotor at 213,626 × *g* for 120 min at 4 °C.
43. Fractionate the gradient into 50 μL volumes (Fig. 2). Measure the absorption at 260 nm and collect the fractions separately corresponding to mt-LSU peak and monosome peak. The typical A_{260}:A_{280} ratio of the peak fractions is ~1.6.
44. Perform buffer exchange, if needed. To calculate the final concentration, use the conversion, 1 A_{260} = 0.1 mg/mL.
45. For long-term storage, snap-freeze the purified mitoribosome in the resuspension buffer using liquid nitrogen and transfer to −80 °C.

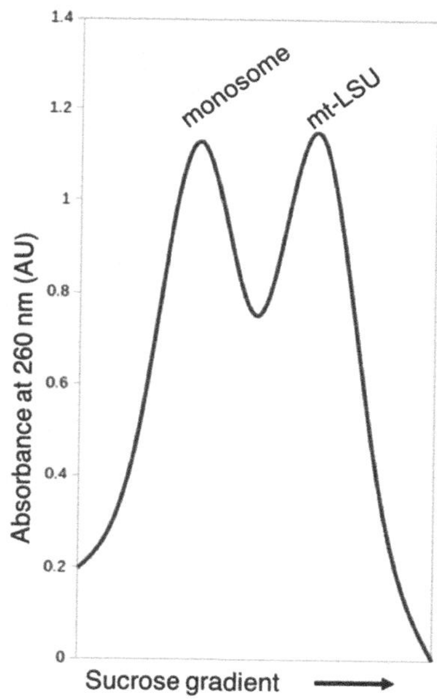

Fig. 2 Mitoribosome purification profile upon sucrose density gradient. A_{260} linear (15–30%) sucrose density gradient profile of mitoribosome (from bottom of the gradient to the top). The peaks corresponding to the 55S monosome (first peak) and the 39S mt-LSU (second peak) are indicated

3.2 Sample Preparation and Data Collection for Cryo-EM Studies

1. Dilute the sample to about OD 4 A_{260} in the resuspension buffer.
2. Prepare grids, freshly coated with 2–4 nm of carbon film and glow discharged at 20 mA for 30 s (*see* **Note 6**).
3. Load 3 μL of sample on the grid in an instrument like the Vitrobot® to maintain standard conditions of 4 °C temperature and 100% humidity.
4. Allow a waiting time of 30 s followed by 3 s blotting before vitrification in liquid ethane, for good results in terms of ice thickness and particle distribution.
5. Clip the grids and load them on the electron microscope. Perform an initial screening based on visual assessment of parameters such as, ice thickness, contaminations, particle distribution and density, to identify a good grid for further data collection (*see* **Note 7**).
6. Proceed to data collection using a satisfactory grid.
7. Collect 20–40 subframe movies with an exposure of about 30–40 electrons per micrograph (*see* **Note 8**), at a suitable magnification (*see* **Note 9**) and defocus range (e.g., −0.5 to −3.5 with step size of 0.5).
8. Collect the required number of movies (preferably more than 2000) depending on sample and grid quality and magnification (to have at least 100,000 monosome particles), for a reasonable 3D reconstruction.

3.3 Cryo-EM Data Processing

1. Perform motion correction of the movies and Contrast Transfer Function (CTF) estimation of motion corrected micrographs and discard all micrographs for which CTF could not be accurately determined by manual inspection of thon rings. Proceed with the remaining data for particle picking (*see* **Note 10**).
2. Reference-free autopicking can be used with a mask diameter of 320 Å for initial picking of particles (*see* **Note 11**) (Fig. 3).
3. Use the extracted particles for 2D classification (number of classes = 100, regularization parameter = 2, angular sampling = 6°, offset search range = 5 pixels, offset search step = 1 pixel, number of iterations = 30–40) and analyze the different orientations of the particles.
4. Select multiple classes, each one representing a distinct orientation of the mitoribosome and use the corresponding 2D class averages as reference to perform a reference-based particle picking (*see* **Note 12**).
5. Perform 2D classification using the extracted particles with the same parameters specified above (Fig. 4). Select only the mitoribosome classes and save the particles for further processing.

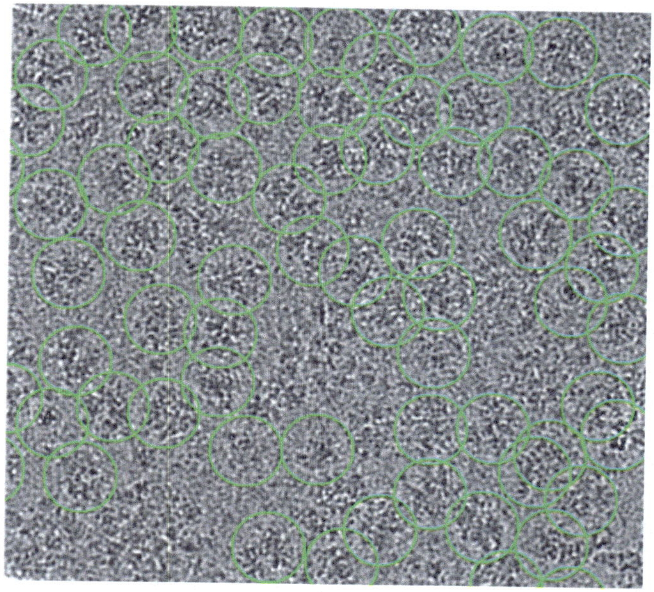

Fig. 3 Autopicking of mitoribosomal particles in a micrograph. The representative micrograph shows particles picked (in green circles) with reference-free Gaussian autopicking algorithm of Relion 2.1.0 with mask diameter = 360 Å

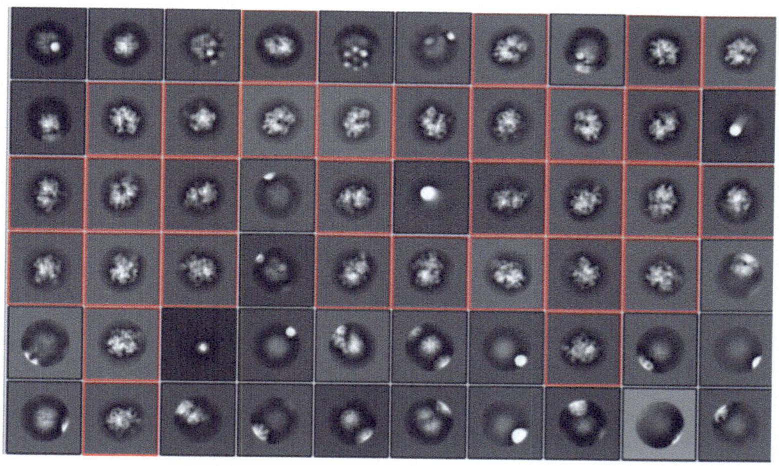

Fig. 4 2D classification of picked and extracted particles. 2D classification performed in Relion 2.1.0 aligns the particles and sorts them into distinct classes. Particles contributing to classes representing different orientations of the mitoribosome (marked by red squares) can be selected and saved for further processing, while other classes can be discarded

6. Create a reference map for 3D auto-refinement using the human mitoribosome map obtained from EMDB (EMD-2876) by rescaling it to the same pixel and box sizes as the extracted particle images.
7. Use this reference and the extracted particles for performing 3D auto-refinement (initial angular search step = 7.5°; initial offset range = 5 pixels and initial offset step = 1 pixel; local searches from 1.8°) to generate a 3D reconstruction of the mitoribosome (*see* **Note 13**).
8. Create a solvent mask around a low pass filtered monosome map generated in the previous step, providing a suitable extension (3–8 pixels), a soft edge of 3–10 pixels at a threshold which can be determined using UCSF chimera [18].
9. Perform 3D classification (number of classes = 6–8, regularization parameter = 4) using the map (low pass filtered to 10–20 Å) generated in **step 7** as reference and mask from **step 8** to identify heterogeneity in the data and sort out any unwanted particles such as the particles corresponding to mt-LSU, or poorly aligned classes, from complete monosomes (Fig. 5) (*see* **Note 14**).
10. Select only the high-resolution monosome enriched classes and proceed to further refinement.

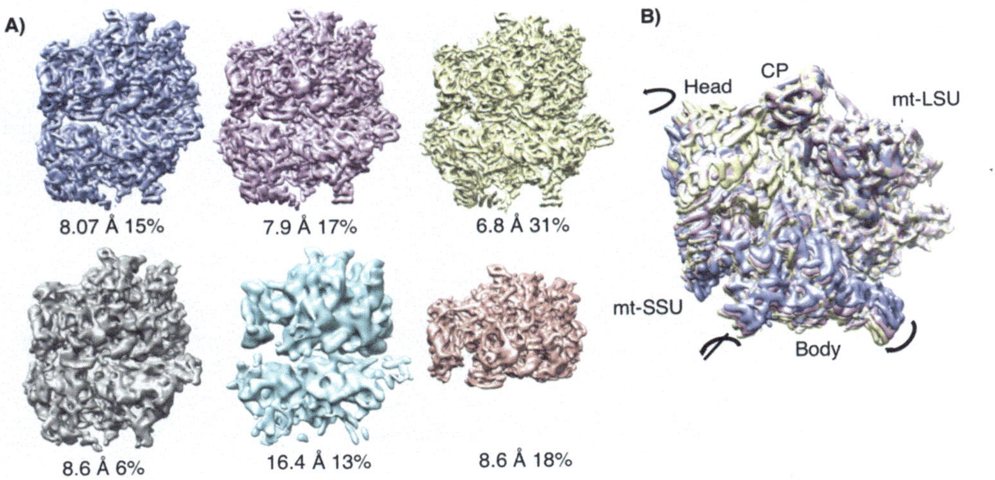

Fig. 5 3D classification of the mitoribosomal particles. (**a**) Mitoribosome particles sorted into six classes after 3D classification. Three classes colored in purple, magenta, and yellow containing 15%, 17%, and 31% particles, respectively, represent distinct conformational states of the mitoribosome. Classes shown in gray and cyan are comprised of poorly aligning bad particles (about 19%). The class colored in pink represents the mt-LSU particles (18%). (**b**) Superposition between the classes representing the complete monosome indicates the movement of the mt-SSU body and the head with respect to the mt-LSU

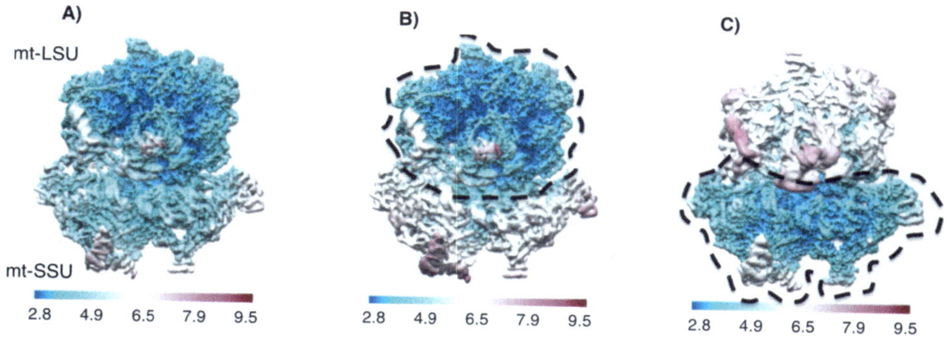

Fig. 6 Masked refinement of the map to improve local resolution. The unmasked cryo-EM map of the human mitoribosome (**a**). Focused refinement of the unmasked map using masks around mt-LSU (**b**) and mt-SSU (**c**) enhances the local resolution of the subunits. Map resolution from higher to lower values is colored in blue to red (2.8–9.5 Å) as indicated by the scale

11. Perform 3D auto-refinement on selected particles using a monosome solvent mask to produce a 3D reconstruction of the monosome (*see* **Note 15**).
12. Perform post-processing of the map thus obtained by applying the solvent mask and the MTF (∗.STAR) file of the cryo-EM direct electron detector used for data collection. A sharpening B-factor can be estimated automatically or manually assigned in this step to generate a sharpened map.
13. Create separate masks around the mt-LSU and mt-SSU in the same manner as explained in **step 8** and perform focused auto-refinement to produce maps of better local resolution (Fig. 6).

4 Notes

1. This will typically correspond to a starting volume of 300 mL in a 1 L vented flask.
2. The culture can be further scaled up, but 2 L is generally sufficient to provide a good yield of mitochondria for a mitoribosome preparation. It is recommended to perform the below steps quickly and on ice wherever possible.
3. The pellet will have a loose upper portion, which should be carefully washed away, and a tight lower portion which contains mitochondria and is to be resuspended in MIBSM buffer.
4. The pellet may form small aggregates. To resuspend the aggregates, homogenize gently using a small Teflon/glass Dounce homogenizer on ice. Do not perform more than five strokes to avoid damaging the mitochondria.

5. It is important to keep the tubes on ice while resuspending the pellet and ensure minimal frothing of the sample as it can denature mitoribosomes.
6. Copper or gold, 200–300 mesh grids, with holey carbon foil support, are regularly used in cryo-EM experiments and are suitable for mitoribosome structural studies. For achieving high resolution, it is recommended to use a finer mesh as they provide greater support to the carbon film. It is advised to use a thin continuous carbon film on the grids. Even though, carbon can reduce the contrast of the micrographs, it typically results in better particle orientation and distribution compared to ice alone. Another problem associated with carbon coating is cryo-crinkling of carbon upon cooling. A gold foil support on gold mesh has been found to reduce cryo-crinkling and beam-induced disturbances associated with carbon-coated grids [19, 20]. For the purpose of this experiment, 300 mesh copper or gold grids coated with ~3 nm of continuous carbon, give good results.
7. A small data set can be collected to monitor parameters such as degree of homogeneity, number of particles of interest, and their distribution. This can be achieved by carrying out a 2D classification of the particle images as explained in the Methods (Subheading 3.3).
8. Collecting movies with multiple subframes is useful in correcting beam-induced motion and accounting for radiation damage. The amount of electron exposure used for data collection is decided as a trade-off between contrast and radiation damage. 30–40 electrons per movie and 1.5–1.6 electrons per movie frame for mitoribosomes produces good contrast images.
9. A higher magnification on one hand allows access to higher frequency information, on the other hand it limits the exposure area and therefore, more time (and also more hard drive space) is needed to collect the same amount of data in terms of number of particles.
10. Initial steps of data processing can be performed on-the-fly as the movies are being collected. This is useful for assessing the quality of data. Bad micrographs such as those with ice contaminations, broken carbon, anisotropic thon rings should be manually checked and removed.
11. Mask diameter for picking and extraction should be higher than the longest mitoribosome diameter and the box size should be reasonably bigger than the longest particle diameter (1.5–2 times). It is a good idea to rescale the particles during extraction by a factor of up to 6, to reduce computational usage and time. The particles will need to be re-extracted without downscaling later, after removal of unwanted particles for generation of map.

12. Particle picking must be performed rigorously so that a maximum number of particles and orientations can be identified.
13. The reference map used for refinement must be low pass filtered to around 40 Å as inclusion of high-resolution information could lead to biasing. Perform local angular searches starting from 1.8° (within ±6 times the sampling rate) to make the angular searching less computationally intensive.
14. If a reasonably high angular accuracy could be achieved in the previous 3D auto-refinement step, a fine angular sampling rate (typically 1.8° or less) may be used for 3D classification within a local angle search range ±3–4 times the sampling rate. Typically, up to 40 iterations are enough to achieve stable classification. 3D classification may have to be repeated a few times, using particles from the best classes identified from the previous run as input, to end up with good quality data.
15. If the particles had been rescaled during extraction, the particles need to be re-extracted without rescaling (or with the final desired scaling factor) before this step and auto-refined with the correctly scaled reference.

Acknowledgements

We thank Juni Andréll and Shintaro Aibara for contributing to Figs. 2 and 6, respectively. This work was supported by the Swedish Foundation for Strategic Research (FFL15:0325), Ragnar Söderberg Foundation (M44/16), Swedish Research Council (NT_2015-04107), Cancerfonden (CAN 2017/1041), H2020-MSCA-ITN-2016 (REMIX). The cryo-EM data was collected at the Swedish national cryo-EM facility funded by the Knut and Alice Wallenberg, Family Erling Persson, and Kempe Foundations. We thank M. Carroni, J-M de la Rosa Trevin and S. Fleischmann for the smooth running of the data collection and processing.

References

1. Ott M, Amunts A, Brown A (2016) Organization and regulation of mitochondrial protein synthesis. Annu Rev Biochem 85:77–101
2. Amunts A, Brown A, Toots J, Scheres SH, Ramakrishnan V (2015) The structure of the human mitochondrial ribosome. Science 348 (6230):95–98
3. Greber BJ, Bieri P, Leibundgut M, Leitner A, Aebersold R, Boehringer D, Ban N (2015) The complete structure of the 55S mammalian mitochondrial ribosome. Science 348 (6232):303–308
4. Greber BJ, Ban N (2016) Structure and function of the mitochondrial ribosome. Annu Rev Biochem 85:103–132
5. Petrov A, Wood E, Bernier C, Norris A, Brown A, Amunts A (2019) Structural patching fosters divergence of mitoribosomes. Mol Biol Evol 36(2):207–219
6. Rorbach J, Gao F, Powell CA, D'Souza A, Lightowlers RN, Minczuk M, Chrzanowska-Lightowlers ZM (2016) Human mitochondrial ribosomes can switch their structural RNA composition. Proc Natl Acad Sci U S A 13(43):12198–12201

7. Chrzanowska-Lightowlers Z, Rorbach J, Minczuk M (2017) Human mitochondrial ribosomes can switch structural tRNAs–but when and why? RNA Biol 14(12):1668–1671
8. Englmeier R, Pfeffer S, Förster F (2017) Structure of the human mitochondrial ribosome studied in situ by cryoelectron tomography. Structure 25(10):1574–1581
9. Scheres SH (2012) RELION: implementation of a Bayesian approach to cryo-EM structure determination. J Struct Biol 180:519–530
10. Bai XC, Fernandez IS, McMullan G, Scheres SH (2013) Ribosome structures to near-atomic resolution from thirty thousand cryo-EM particles. Elife 2:e00461
11. Jonić S (2016) Cryo-electron microscopy analysis of structurally heterogeneous macromolecular complexes. Comput Struct Biotechnol J 14:385–390
12. Scheres SH (2016) Processing of structurally heterogeneous cryo-EM data in RELION, Methods in enzymology, vol 579. Academic, San Diego, pp 125–157
13. Bai X-C, Rajendra E, Yang G, Shi Y, Scheres SHW (2015) Sampling the conformational space of the catalytic subunit of human γ-secretase. Elife 4:e11182
14. Desai N, Brown A, Amunts A, Ramakrishnan V (2017) The structure of the yeast mitochondrial ribosome. Science 355(6324):528–531
15. Brown A, Rathore S, Kimanius D, Aibara S, Bai XC, Rorbach J et al (2017) Structures of the human mitochondrial ribosome in native states of assembly. Nat Struct Mol Biol 24(10):866
16. Fernandez-Leiro R, Scheres SHW (2017) A pipeline approach to single-particle processing in RELION. Acta Crystall D Struct Biol 73 (6):496–502
17. Zivanov J, Nakane T, Forsberg B, Kimanius D, Hagen WJ, Lindahl E, Scheres SH (2018) RELION-3: new tools for automated high-resolution cryo-EM structure determination. bioRxiv 421123
18. Pettersen EF, Goddard TD, Huang CC, Couch GS, Greenblatt DM, Meng EC, Ferrin TE (2004) UCSF Chimera—a visualization system for exploratory research and analysis. J Comput Chem 25(13):1605–1612
19. Russo CJ, Passmore LA (2016) Progress towards an optimal specimen support for electron cryomicroscopy. Curr Opin Struct Biol 37:81–89
20. Russo CJ, Passmore LA (2014) Ultrastable gold substrates for electron cryomicroscopy. Science 346(6215):1377–1380

Chapter 16

Sucrose Gradient Sedimentation Analysis of Mitochondrial Ribosomes

Austin Choi and Antoni Barrientos

Abstract

Mitochondria contain ribosomes (mitoribosomes) specialized in the synthesis of a handful of proteins essential for oxidative phosphorylation. Therefore, mitoribosome integrity and function are essential for the life of eukaryotic cells and lesions that affect them result in devastating human disorders. To broadly analyze the integrity and assembly state of mitoribosomes it is useful to start by determining the sedimentation profile of these structures by sucrose gradient centrifugation of mitochondrial extracts. During centrifugation, mitoribosome subunits, monosomes and polysomes, and potentially accumulated assembly intermediates will sediment through the gradient at different rates. Sedimentation will depend on the centrifugal force applied and the density and viscosity of the gradient. Importantly, it will also depend on the size, shape, and density of the mitoribosome particles present in the samples under study. Variations of this technique, often coupled with additional downstream approaches, have been used to analyze the process of mitoribosome biogenesis, the composition of assembly intermediates, or to monitor the interaction of extraribosomal proteins with individual mitoribosome subunits or monosomes.

Key words Sucrose gradient, Mitochondrial ribosome, Mitoribosome profile, Gradient maker, Gradient master, Gradient fractionation, Immunoblotting

1 Introduction

1.1 Mitochondrial Ribosomes

Mitochondria are vital eukaryotic organelles thought to be derived from a prokaryotic ancestor based on the presence of numerous remnants of their once independent life [1]. These vestiges include a compacted mitochondrial genome (mtDNA) maintained in the mitochondrial matrix and a mitochondrial ribosome (mitoribosome), which is more closely related to the bacterial ribosome than to its cytosolic counterpart [2, 3]. The mitoribosome is solely dedicated to the translation of a handful of mtDNA-encoded genes; 8 in yeast *Saccharomyces cerevisiae* and 13 in mammals. With the exception of a single yeast mtDNA product that is a ribosomal protein, all other mtDNA-encoded proteins in yeast and mammalian cells are subunits of the enzymes that form the

Michal Minczuk and Joanna Rorbach (eds.), *Mitochondrial Gene Expression: Methods and Protocols*,
Methods in Molecular Biology, vol. 2192, https://doi.org/10.1007/978-1-0716-0834-0_16,

oxidative phosphorylation (OXPHOS) system. These proteins are co-translationally inserted into the membrane where they assemble with nuclear DNA-encoded proteins to form four of the OXPHOS enzymes.

Though involved in numerous critical cellular functions, mitochondria are best known for their role in the production of ATP through OXPHOS. This pathway is the primary source of cellular ATP, and it is therefore not surprising that OXPHOS dysfunction is causative or strongly associated with a plethora of human diseases. Mutations in either the nuclear or mitochondrial genome that produce primary defects in OXPHOS are responsible for the relatively rare, highly heterogeneous, and often devastating collection of syndromes known as mitochondrial diseases [4]. Further, mitochondrial dysfunction and the accompanying decline in OXPHOS efficiency is implicated in the progression and phenotype of aging-related diseases including societally costly and increasingly prevalent neurodegenerative diseases like Alzheimer's and Parkinson's [5]. Relevant to the topic of this chapter, mutations in mitochondrial translation factors and ribosome components have also been revealed to be causal of mitochondrial disorders, mainly producing cardio- and encephalomyopathies [6]. Furthermore, mitoribosomes and mitochondrial translation have emerged as a target for therapeutic interventions to combat several types of cancer [7].

The interest in mitochondria and their role in disease have grown steadily in recent decades. However, much remains to be discovered about the underlying processes that directly influence productive assembly and regulation of the OXPHOS complexes, such as the assembly and structure–function relationship of the mitoribosome and its protein components. The complete mitoribosome is a massive complex of two distinct large (LSU) and small (SSU) subunits composed of a total of 80 (mammals) proteins and 3 rRNAs, which have been resolved to a high resolution by cryo-EM [2, 3]. These structures provide a trove of invaluable information about the fully assembled mitoribosome but reveal little about how it progresses from individual proteins to a structured multimeric complex. Recently, studies tracking the effects on assembly of systematic deletion of each LSU protein in yeast [8] and incorporation kinetics of labeled mammalian mitoribosomal proteins (MRPs) into the mitoribosome [9] have revealed that mitoribosome assembly initiates near the inner mitochondrial membrane [8, 10] and proceeds by incorporation of preassembled modules with groups of proteins preferentially incorporating at early, middle, or late stages of the overall assembly process [8, 9]. These studies provide a broad foundation from which a more specific understanding of how mitoribosome assembly occurs can be built.

1.2 Density Gradient Centrifugation: General Concepts and Applications to the Study of Mitoribosomes

The biological and biomedical arguments provided in the previous paragraphs highlight the importance of establishing standardized methods to analyze mitoribosome profiles and assess their assembly status. For this chapter, we focus on a classical approach to the study of mitoribosome assembly: density gradient sedimentation analysis.

Density gradient ultracentrifugation is a powerful technique for the fractionation of particle mixtures, purification of subcellular organelles, or isolation of macromolecules. The method involves the layering of a sample containing a mixture of macromolecules of different size and mass on the surface of a vertical column of liquid (e.g., an ultracentrifuge tube containing a solution of sucrose, glycerol, or the chemical of choice) whose density increases from top to bottom forming a gradient. The two main types of density gradient centrifugation are rate-zonal separation and isopycnic separation. In rate-zonal separation, particles are separated based on their size and mass, such as in most sucrose gradient sedimentation analyses. The density of the particles is greater than the density of the gradient, and if centrifugation is continued long enough, all particles will end up as one pellet at the bottom of the tube. In isopycnic separation, the particles migrate through the solvent gradient until they reach the point where their buoyant density is equal to that of the gradient, such as in the separation of nucleic acids in cesium chloride gradients, or of complex macromolecular protein mixtures using gradients of iodixanol, a nonionic polymer. In this case, the density of the gradient medium must be higher than the density of the particles to be separated. According to the means of preparation, density gradients may be either step gradients or continuous gradients. Step gradients are prepared by successively layering solutions of different density in the centrifuge tube and then layering the sample to be fractionated on top of the last "step." Sucrose or Nicodenz step gradients are useful for example to purify organelles of similar density. In continuous density gradients, the density changes smoothly and continuously, either linearly or exponentially, from one extreme to another. Continuous gradients can be produced from step gradients by allowing sufficient time for diffusion to smooth out the steps, but they are usually prepared directly by using dedicated gradient makers.

Rate-zonal separation in linear sucrose gradients [11–13] and isopycnic separation in iodixanol gradients [9] are both commonly used for the study of mitoribosome assembly profile. Here, we will focus exclusively on explaining the experimental details of sucrose density gradient sedimentation analysis. This method is prevalent in current literature, and we have used it extensively to analyze mammalian [11, 13, 14] and, with some modifications, *S. cerevisiae* mitoribosomes [8, 15, 16]. It is useful in identifying factors associating with the mitoribosome in wild-type cells and to determine the consequences on mitoribosome assembly of gene ablation and/or complementation of cells depleted of individual MRPs or mitoribosome assembly factors with modified versions. The body of the method is written for use with mammalian cell lines and is based in large part on previously published methods [17, 18] with minor modifications. Here, we have combined those methods to a single protocol, which covers mitochondrial isolation, sucrose gradient formation, sedimentation, and subsequent analysis by immunoblotting to determine mitoribosome composition through immunoblot of candidate proteins. Though not covered in this method, the total composition of co-sedimenting mitoribosomal proteins and/or associated factors can then be identified in an unbiased manner by mass spectrometry analysis. Due to the availability of a large number of approaches and commercial options for gene editing in mammalian cell lines that frequently require extensive optimization, the generation of gene-edited cell lines is beyond the scope of this method, and it assumes the user has already procured cell lines with genetic modifications of interest. *S. cerevisiae* yeast cells are far more amenable to genetic modification for which we suggest the approaches described in a recent publication by our group [8]. Overall, the method yields consistent results and is simple and manageable with numerous potential pause points. In addition to the elaboration of individual steps, Subheading 4 details alternative approaches useful in fitting the protocol to the question, timing, and economic constraints of the user.

The usefulness of the methodology is exemplified with the recent observation by our group that the mitochondrial DEAD-box helicase DDX28 co-sediments with the mitoribosome large subunit and the monosome in a salt-dependent manner (Fig. 1). This information was an essential step in guiding subsequent experiments that led us to conclude that DDX28 resides in mitochondrial RNA granules and functions in mitoribosome large subunit biogenesis [11].

2 Materials

All solutions are prepared in double distilled water (ddH_2O) and should be made fresh unless otherwise noted. Chill solutions to 4 °C before use to minimize potential protein degradation. $MgCl_2$ or EDTA, as well as KCl or other salts, are used at different concentrations in extraction buffers and sucrose solutions depending on the purpose of the experiment (*see* **Notes 1** and **2**).

2.1 Isolation of Mitochondria

1. T-K-Mg Buffer: 10 mM Tris–HCl pH 7.4, 10 mM KCl, 0.5 mM $MgCl_2$ (Stock solution can be filtered and stored at room temperature (RT)).

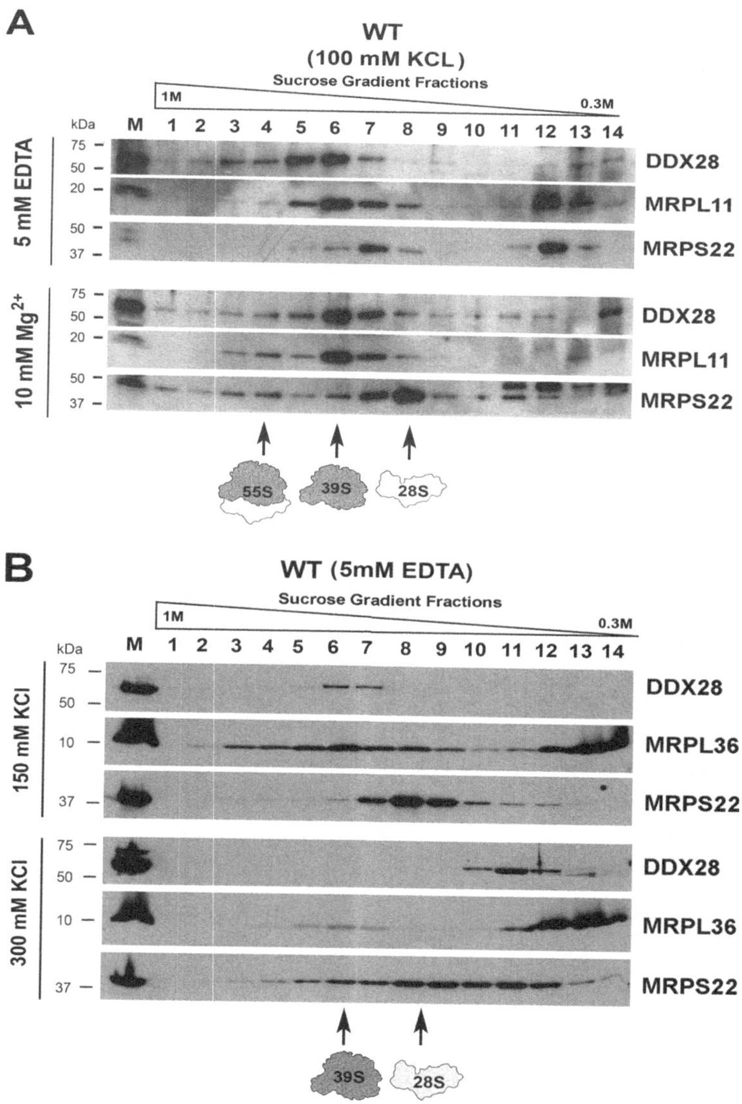

Fig. 1 Sucrose gradient sedimentation analyses of the mtLSU assembly factor DDX28 and mitoribosomal proteins from wild-type (WT) HEK293T mitochondrial extracts. (**a**) Sedimentation profile of mitoribosomes extracted in 5 mM EDTA or 10 mM $MgCl_2$. (**b**) Sedimentation profile of mitoribosomes extracted in 5 mM EDTA and 150 or 300 mM KCl. (Reproduced and modified from Tu and Barrientos, 2015 [11] with permission from Elsevier (license # 4470451296140))

2. Trypsin-EDTA solution: 0.5 g/l porcine trypsin and 0.2 g/l EDTA·4Na in Hank's Balanced Salt Solution with phenol red (commercially available and can be stored long-term at −20 °C or a few weeks at 4 °C).
3. 1 M Sucrose Stock solution: 1 M sucrose, 10 mM Tris–HCl pH 7.4.

2.2 Preparation of a 10–30% Linear Sucrose Gradient with Biocomp Gradient Master

1. 10% sucrose solution: (10 mM $MgCl_2$ *or* 5 mM EDTA), 20 mM HEPES pH 7.4, 100 mM KCl, 0.1 M PMSF, 0.1% Digitonin, 1× EDTA-free protease inhibitor, 10% w/v sucrose.
2. 30% sucrose solution: (10 mM $MgCl_2$ *or* 5 mM EDTA), 20 mM HEPES pH 7.4, 100 mM KCl, 0.1 M PMSF, 0.1% Digitonin, 1× EDTA-free protease inhibitor, 30% w/v sucrose.
3. Polypropylene ultracentrifuge tube (13 × 51 mm).
4. Marker block (Provided with Gradient Master).
5. 4 mm tube caps (Provided with Gradient Master).
6. Sucrose layering cannula—syringe attachment (Provided with Gradient Master).
7. Tube holder (Provided with Gradient Master).
8. Air bubble leveling tool.

2.3 Mitoribosome Extraction and Sedimentation Analysis

1. Extraction Buffer: 20 mM HEPES pH 7.4, 100 mM KCl, (10–20 mM $MgCl_2$ *or* 5 mM EDTA), 0.5 mM PMSF, 0.8% (w/v) high purity Digitonin, 1× EDTA-free protease inhibitor (*see* **Notes 1–3**).

2.4 Sodium Dodecyl Sulfate-Polyacrylamide Gel Electrophoresis (SDS-PAGE) and Immunoblotting

1. 12% SDS-PAGE polyacrylamide gel (homemade gels or gels commercially available from multiple sources—e.g., Biorad, GeneScript—can be used).
2. Wash Buffer: 10 mM Tris pH 8, 1 mM EDTA, 150 mM NaCl, 0.1% (v/v) Triton X-100.
3. Blocking Buffer: 5% (w/v) nonfat dry milk in Wash Buffer.
4. Ponceau protein staining solution: 0.2 g Ponceau in 3% (w/v) TCA (Trichloroacetic acid).
5. Laemmli sample buffer 4× (LB 4×): 200 mM Tris–HCl pH 6.8, 4% SDS, 40% glycerol, 4% β-mercaptoethanol, 0.05% (w/v) bromophenol blue.
6. Antibodies against mitoribosome large and small subunit proteins: A large number of antibodies raised against each mitoribosomal protein are commercially available, for example anti-mL45 (Abcam-ab113786), anti-uL16m (Sigma-HPA054133), anti-mS27 (Proteintech-17280-1-AP), anti-mS29 (ab155499).

3 Methods

3.1 Isolation of Mitochondria

1. Minimum starting material ranges between 2 and 4 × 10^8 adherent mammalian cells grown on 15 × 150 mm cell culture plates (*see* **Note 4**).

2. Aspirate culture media from plates, wash with 10 ml PBS and add 1.5 ml trypsin to each plate. Tilt plates back and forth to ensure trypsin has passed over entire plate surface area. Incubate for 2 min (*see* **Note 5**).
3. Completely dislodge adherent cells from plate surface by firmly tapping each plate against the hand.
4. Inactivate trypsin by resuspending cells in 5 ml complete DMEM and combine cell suspension in 50 ml conical tubes.
5. Pellet cells by centrifugation at 600 × *g* for 3 min and aspirate media. All subsequent steps are performed on ice, at 4 °C, and in prechilled buffers.
6. Resuspend cell pellet in 10 ml PBS (if cell suspension is spread across multiple tubes, combine to a single 50 ml conical tube).
7. Pellet cells by centrifugation at 600 × *g* for 3 min and aspirate PBS.
8. Repeat **steps 6** and 7.
9. Determine the weight of cell pellet and gently resuspend cells in 1 ml of the hypotonic T-K-Mg buffer per 0.15 g cells.
10. Incubate cells for 5 min to allow swelling of the cells. Avoid incubation over 10 min (*see* **Note 6**).
11. Homogenize cells with a glass/Teflon tissue grinder Dounce homogenizer equipped with a serrated PTFE (polytetrafluoroethylene, a.k.a. Teflon) pestle (10 ml capacity). Homogenize the cells using 10–25 strokes of the pestle of a tight-fitting Dounce (*see* **Note 7**).
12. Immediately bring cell homogenate to 0.25 M sucrose with 1 M Sucrose Stock (1:3 homogenate: 1 M Sucrose Stock) to make it isotonic.
13. Return homogenate to 50 ml conical tube and centrifuge for 3 min at 1200 × *g* to pellet unbroken cells, nuclei, and other cellular debris.
14. Collect supernatant in a new 50 ml conical tube and centrifuge again for 3 min at 1200 × *g*. If any pellet is observed, repeat this step (*see* **Notes 8** and **9**).
15. Collect supernatant (containing mitochondria) and aliquot into 1.5 ml microcentrifuge tubes with 1 ml per tube (*see* **Note 10**).
16. Centrifuge tubes at 15,000 × *g* for 5 min.
17. Wash pellets by resuspending in STE buffer and combine suspension into a single tube.
18. Pellet suspension at 15,000 × *g* for 5 min.
19. Optional: Repeat **steps 17** and **18** for increased mitochondrial purity.

20. Resuspend pellet in minimal STE buffer (use a volume of STE buffer roughly equivalent to the volume of the mitochondrial pellet). This sample contains isolated mitochondria.
21. Determine mitochondrial protein concentration by Lowry, Bradford, or preferred method (*see* **Note 11**).
22. Keep mitochondria on ice until used or immediately flash-freeze aliquots by submerging in liquid N_2 and storing at −80 °C for long-term storage (*see* **Note 12**).

3.2 Preparation of a 10–30% Linear Sucrose Gradient with Biocomp Gradient Master

1. Prepare the master sucrose solutions in the same buffer as the mitochondrial extraction is performed, although devoid of detergent. The two sucrose solutions must be of the maximum and minimum concentrations wanted (e.g., 10–30% is useful to fractionate the mitoribosome components and the monosome) (*see* **Note 13**).
2. To prepare the gradient using the Gradient Master from Biocomp Instruments, start by reading the Operator's Manual at http://www.biocompinstruments.com.
3. Place the ultracentrifuge tube inside the marker block and use a fine tip marker to mark at the upper, 4 mm cap level, which will indicate the "stop point" when filling the tube with sucrose solution (Fig. 2a). *See* **Notes 14** and **15** for alternative methods to gradient formation requiring little to no equipment.
4. Using the cannula attached to a syringe or simply by pipetting, fill the ultracentrifuge tube with 0.3 M sucrose solution until the volume of solution in the tube is just past the stop point.
5. Using a cannula-attached syringe filled with 1 M sucrose solution, insert the cannula tip to the bottom of the tube and slowly inject the 1 M sucrose solution. An interface between the 0.3 and 1 M sucrose solutions should be visible. Continue adding 1 M sucrose solution until the interface is just past the stop point.
6. Remove the cannula quickly but smoothly.
7. Cap the ultracentrifuge tube with the 4 mm tube cap. Use a pipette to remove any excess sucrose from the top of the cap. Ensure no bubble is present between the sucrose solution and the cap. If a bubble is present, remove the cap, add sufficient 0.3 M sucrose solution on top of the gradient and recap the tube.
8. Insert the tube into the gradient holder.
9. Ensure the Gradient Master base plate is level using the digital leveling controls and an air bubble level.

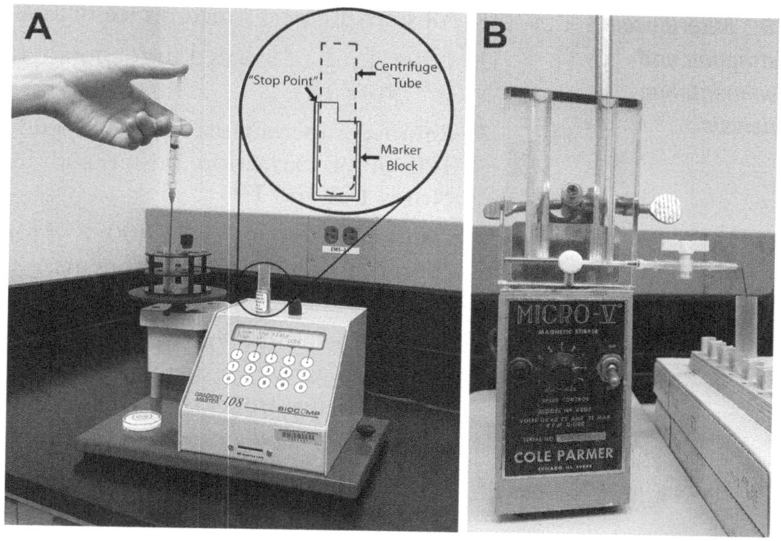

Fig. 2 Preparation of a continuous sucrose gradient using gradient makers. (**a**) The automatized BioComp Instruments Gradient Master. This instrument is programmable, capable of producing six identical, linear gradients in less than 1 min by utilizing tilted tube rotation technology. Inset depicts marker block described in Subheading 3.2, **step 3**. (**b**) A classical manual gradient maker (C.B.S. Scientific). The device is linear with side outlets and has two chambers where the two sucrose solutions (of maximum and minimum concentrations) are placed. Gradient flow is controlled by a valve centered between the two chambers. The outflow channel is fitted with a male luer adapter, which can be used with any needle or luer valve to facilitate continuous and smooth flow into the ultracentrifugation tube. Only one gradient can be prepared at a time in some 10 min. The system includes a tubing adapter kit with a valve, tubing adapters, butterfly set, and silicone tubing. This kit can be used to adapt your gradient maker for either a gravity gradient or a pumping gradient

10. Gently place the gradient tube holder containing the sucrose gradient directly onto the center of the Gradient Master base plate.
11. "Balance" the tube holder as you would a centrifuge, such that each tube is placed directly across from a tube filled with similar density material.
12. Select on digital gradient master controls: "Grad" → "List" → "SW50", scroll down until "10–30%" is displayed then select "Use" → "Run".
13. The Gradient Master will now mix the sucrose solutions to produce the 0.3–1 M linear sucrose gradient in approximately 1 min (*see* **Note 16**).
14. Remove the cap. The gradient is now ready and should be kept on ice until used (*see* **Note 17**).

3.3 Mitoribosome Extraction and Sedimentation Analysis

1. All steps are performed on ice or at 4 °C in prechilled buffers.
2. Pellet 4 mg of isolated mitochondria at 10,000 × *g* for 5 min (*see* **Note 18**).
3. Remove supernatant and resuspend mitochondrial pellet in 400 μl of extraction buffer and incubate for 10 min (*see* **Notes 1–3** and **19**).
4. Centrifuge extract at 24,000 × *g* for 15 min to pellet mitochondrial membrane components.
5. Collect the supernatant containing the mitoribosome and soluble mitochondrial proteins and aliquot 40 μl (10%) for later use in Western blot analysis as "total extract". The pellet can either be discarded or resuspended in sample buffer as an alternative "total extract".
6. Gently add the supernatant onto the top of the 10–30% sucrose gradient. If the volume of sample is large, 100–200 μl of sucrose solutions can be removed from the top of the sucrose gradient to make space (*see* **Note 20**).
7. Place the sucrose gradient tubes into an SW55Ti swinging rotor bucket and cap the bucket tightly.
8. Hook the bucket into the SW55Ti rotor.
9. Ensure the rotor is balanced by ultracentrifuge tubes filled with sucrose stock solution loaded into rotor buckets.
10. Centrifuge at 40,000 rpm (Average RCF = 151,693) for 3 h and 10 min (*see* **Note 21**).
11. Cut the tip of a standard 1000 μl micropipette tip so that the tip mouth is approximately 0.3–0.4 cm wide.
12. Using the modified tip and a 1000 μl pipette, place the top just under the gradient surface at the middle of the tube and collect 260 μl into a microcentrifuge tube.
13. Repeat **step 11** until the entire gradient has been collected for a total of ~14 fractions.
14. Consecutively label the collected fractions.
15. The fraction samples can then be immediately used for western blot, protein precipitation, or stored at −80 °C for later use (*see* **Note 22**).

3.4 Sodium Dodecyl Sulfate-Polyacrylamide Gel Electrophoresis (SDS-PAGE) and Immunoblotting

1. Prepare samples for western blot analysis by adding 13 μl of 4× LB to 40 μl "Total extract" and 37.5 μl 4× LB to 112.5 μl from each fraction #1–14 in microcentrifuge tubes and mix thoroughly.
2. Load a 12% SDS-PAGE gel starting with a pre-stained protein ladder, total extract, and then 100 μl of each of the 14 fractions in sequential order.

3. Separate sample proteins by electrophoresis at 80 V for 30 min to allow samples to enter the resolving portion of the gel, and then increase the voltage to 150 V until Laemmli sample buffer dye front reaches the bottom of the gel.
4. Transfer proteins from gel to nitrocellulose membrane using, for example, an Owl™ HEP Series Semidry Electroblotting System (ThermoFisher Scientific). Any alternative semidry or wet transfer systems can be used.
5. To assess a normal distribution of proteins throughout the gradient and the absence of protein degradation, incubate membrane in Ponceau protein staining solution for 15 min or until protein bands are visible.
6. Using the protein ladder and protein staining as a guide, cut out horizontal strips of membrane corresponding to the molecular weight of proteins to be blotted against.
7. Wash membrane strips by incubation in washing buffer for 5 min with agitation on a rocker to remove the Ponceau protein stain.
8. Incubate membrane strips in blocking buffer for 30 min at room temperature with agitation.
9. Incubate membranes with antibodies against mtLSU or mtSSU markers, or mitoribosome interacting factors of interest at a dilution of 1:250–1000 (depending on manufacturer recommendations or optimization) for 3 h at RT or 4 °C overnight with agitation (*see* **Note 23**).
10. Wash membrane for 5 min with agitation in washing buffer three times.
11. Incubate membrane with horseradish peroxidase (HRP)-conjugated secondary antibodies with agitation for 1–3 h at RT or overnight at 4 °C.
12. Wash membrane for 15 min in washing buffer three times.
13. Develop membrane by enhanced chemiluminescence (ECL) reagents followed by exposition X-ray films or luminescence detection of choice. *See* Fig. 1 for representative mitoribosome sedimentation profiles.

4 Notes

1. $MgCl_2$ (usually 10–20 mM) maintains mitoribosome LSU and SSU interactions to preserve the fully formed monosome while EDTA chelates Mg^{2+} causing disassociation of the monosome into separated LSU and SSU. In some mutant cell lines, EDTA could disrupt unstable intermediates and labile interactions; therefore, simply 0–1 mM should be used instead. Salt

concentration in extraction buffer and sucrose gradient solutions can be varied between 10–300 mM KCl to preserve or interrupt a substantial number of mitoribosome–protein interactions. Integral mitoribosome components are not disrupted even at 300 mM KCl [19]. Figure 1 portrays an example of how the associations of mitoribosome subunits and interacting proteins are affected by inclusion of EDTA, Mg^{2+}, or increasing salt concentrations in the extraction buffer and sucrose solutions.

2. Efficient purification of intact mitoribosomes requires optimized conditions in which the ratio of monovalent to divalent cations is crucial [20, 21]. For that purpose, the ideal buffer would contain 50 mM NH_4Cl and 10 mM $MgCl_2$.
3. The choice of detergent in the mitochondrial extraction buffer is essential. Avoid strong detergents that can disrupt mitoribosome integrity. Nonionic detergents such as n-Dodecyl-β-D-Maltoside (lauryl maltoside) or digitonin are especially useful for solubilizing membrane proteins or large complexes such as mitoribosomes to preserve their integrity and activity. It is strongly advised to perform preliminary mitoribosome extraction tests in-house by titrating the detergent of choice to the optimal concentration. 0.5–0.8% (w/v) digitonin or 0.5% (w/v) lauryl maltoside are useful reference concentrations. Further, some optimization is necessary for every detergent batch, as purity can vary between lots.
4. For larger scale preparations of isolated mitochondria, cells capable of non-adherent growth (like 293T) can be grown in suspension by liquid culture methods, which can be less laborious and make more efficient use of culture media. Our usual yield is 4 g of cells per liter. If using liquid cultures, start at **step 5** of Subheading 3.1.
5. Trypsinization efficiency can be increased by placing cells in 37 °C incubator or rinsing cells with PBS an extra time before adding trypsin. As an alternative to trypsinization, after washing adherent cells in PBS, they can also be collected by adding 5 ml PBS, scraping cells from culture plate surface with a cell scraper, collecting PBS with the scraped cell suspension, and continuing at **step 5** of Subheading 3.1.
6. Do not allow excessive incubation of cells in the T-K-Mg buffer to avoid rupture of the outer mitochondrial membrane.
7. Appropriate homogenization technique involves full insertion of a pestle to bottom of a homogenizer vessel and slow withdrawal of pestle such that a vacuum is generated just below the pestle which forces the sample volume past pestle. Do not overload the homogenizer, as the entire sample will not be exposed to vacuum homogenization with each stroke. Sample volume should not exceed 75% nominal capacity of the

homogenizer. If the sample volume is large, sample aliquots can be homogenized in multiple rounds or in a larger volume homogenizer.

8. To increase the total mitochondrial yield, the pellet from **step 13** can be resuspended, re-homogenized, cleared according to **steps 13** and **14**, Subheading 3.1, and the supernatant combined with the original low-speed supernatant.
9. If working with large volumes of homogenate (>10 ml) the given spin times are insufficient. It is advised to increase spin time to 10–15 min or aliquot 10 ml homogenate per 50 ml conical tube before spinning.
10. Larger 50 ml tubes can be used (for substantial reduction of labor) if your lab possesses centrifuges/rotors capable of loading large tubes, refrigeration, and speeds of 15,000 × *g*.
11. Isolated mitochondria can be further purified using Sucrose [22] or Nicodenz [23] step gradients. For example, use the following steps based on the protocol described by Meisinger et al. [22]. Prepare a 60%/32%/23%/15% sucrose step gradient in TE buffer (10 mM Tris–HCl, 1 mM EDTA pH 7.4) by gently layering 1 ml 60% sucrose, 2 ml 32% sucrose, 1 ml 23% sucrose, and 1 ml 15% sucrose on top of one another (densest to lightest: bottom to top) in a 13 × 51 mm ultracentrifuge tube. Load the isolated mitochondria onto the top of the gradient and centrifuge for 1 h at 4 °C at 134,000 × *g*. Collect mitochondria from a minimal volume at the 60%/32% sucrose interface which should contain 70–80% of the starting material (at least 2 mg starting material is recommended). Dilute sample with 2–3 volumes of STE buffer. Pellet mitochondria at 10,000 × *g* for 10 min, discard sup, and resuspend pellet in a minimal volume of STE buffer (~2–3 packed pellet volume). Measure protein concentration of the sample and use it immediately or flash-freeze in liquid nitrogen for long-term storage.
12. Mitochondria prepared and stored in this way have intact outer and inner membranes, are electrochemically competent, and capable of transmembrane protein transport. They can be used for measurements of oxygen consumption and oxidative phosphorylation, *in organello* DNA synthesis, *in organello* transcription, *in organello* tRNA aminoacylation, *in organello* protein synthesis, *in organello* protein import, and *in organello* mtDNA footprinting as described by Fernandez-Vizarra et al. [17]. If you intend to perform any of these assays use of freshly isolated mitochondria is highly recommended as mitochondrial competence can decrease dramatically with freezing. Further, 0.1% fatty acid-free BSA should be added to homogenization media to prevent fatty acid-induced mitochondrial membrane uncoupling as electrochemically competent mitochondria are required for normal mitochondrial function.

13. After preparing the sucrose solutions, allow to sit for 5–10 min to allow any air bubbles to dissipate from the sucrose solution. Air bubbles are disruptive to the gradient making process. The solutions could also be degassed by vacuum. For that purpose, place the solution in a side-arm flask and use a rubber stopper to seal off the top. Place the flask on a stir plate and turn the plate on so the stir bar is spinning at a medium speed. Apply vacuum until all the gas is released.
14. A gradient maker (like Thomas-Scientific CAT# 1186V98; Fig. 2b) can also be used to generate a 10–30% gradient. In this case, the addition of 0.1% Digitonin to both 10% and 30% sucrose solutions is recommended to lubricate the passage of solutions through this apparatus and into the ultracentrifuge tube with a constant and smooth flow.
15. Gradients can also be formed by simple diffusion with no additional equipment [24, 25]. In detail: 2.5 ml 30% sucrose solution is added to the 13 × 51 mm ultracentrifuge tube. 2.5 ml of 10% solution is then layered on top. An interface between the two sucrose solutions should be visible. The tube is then sealed with a cap or parafilm and *slowly and gently* inverted horizontally. The solutions then mix by diffusion and the gradient forms throughout 1 h at room temperature or 3 h at 4 °C. The tube is then *slowly and gently* returned to a vertical position, the seal removed, and stored at 4 °C until used, preferably on the same day. Gradients formed in this way are not perfectly linear but are consistent between batches as well as cost and time efficient.
16. If an air bubble is present and moves through the gradient during the mixing process, the gradient should be discarded, as moving bubbles will disrupt the gradient.
17. Handle gradients with care to prevent disturbing the contents.
18. Significantly less isolated mitochondria (1–2 mg) can be used if a protein precipitation step is added after gradient fraction collection. For a preliminary and cost-effective alternative to using isolated mitochondria, whole cells collected from a single 80–90% confluent 150 mm culture plate can be extracted and used for sedimentation analysis exactly as described for isolated mitochondria. A minimum of 1 mg whole cell extract should be loaded onto the sucrose gradient for sedimentation. Following gradient fractionation, fraction proteins should be precipitated before immunoblot analysis. Proteins loosely associated with the mitoribosome or with low stoichiometry may not be detectable with this approach. Further, large protein complexes from other cellular compartments will be present in extract and may confound results.

19. RNase inhibitors can be added to the extraction buffer if excessive mitoribosome degradation is observed. A cost-effective option is to use ribonucleoside vanadyl complexes at 10 mM.

20. The sample volume to be loaded onto the gradient is approximately 10% of the total gradient volume, since deviations of this proportion can compromise the fractionation resolution.

21. Slow acceleration and deceleration centrifuge settings are recommended to avoid disturbing gradient.

22. Protein precipitation can be performed on each fraction for greater resolution in immunoblotting or subsequent analysis by mass spectrometry. For immunoblotting, immunoprecipitation can be performed with final 25% trichloroacetic acid (TCA) followed by washes of the precipitate first with 0.5 M Tris-Base and subsequently with water, before solubilization of the protein pellet in 25 μl of loading Laemmli buffer for loading onto an SDS-polyacrylamide gel. For mass spectrometry analysis of fraction protein composition, the samples are best precipitated by a method based on a defined methanol-chloroform-water mixture for the quantitative precipitation of soluble as well as hydrophobic proteins from dilute solutions [26]. Practically, 4 volumes (V) methanol and 1 V chloroform are added to 1 V of the sample. A phase separation is achieved by the addition of 3 V water whereby the protein is precipitated at the chloroform-methanol-water interphase. The addition of an excess (4 V) of methanol and subsequent centrifugation results in a protein pellet which is free of interfering substances [26].

23. Primary antibodies can be kept in the immunoblotting blocking solution at −20 °C and reused extensively until no longer effective, or solution spoils.

Acknowledgements

We thank Dr. Priyanka Maiti for critical reading of the manuscript. This research was supported by NIH R35 Grant GM118141 (to A. B.) and MDA Grant MDA-381828 (to A.B.).

References

1. Margulis L (1975) Symbiotic theory of the origin of eukaryotic organelles; criteria for proof. Symp Soc Exp Biol 29:21–38
2. Amunts A, Brown A, Toots J, Scheres SHW, Ramakrishnan V (2015) The structure of the human mitochondrial ribosome. Science 348:95–98
3. Greber BJ, Bieri P, Leibundgut M, Leitner A, Aebersold R, Boehringer D, Ban N (2015) Ribosome. The complete structure of the 55S mammalian mitochondrial ribosome. Science 348:303–308
4. Lightowlers RN, Taylor RW, Turnbull DM (2015) Mutations causing mitochondrial

disease: what is new and what challenges remain? Science 349:1494–1499
5. Murphy MP, Hartley RC (2018) Mitochondria as a therapeutic target for common pathologies. Nat Rev Drug Discov 5:174
6. De Silva D, Tu YT, Amunts A, Fontanesi F, Barrientos A (2015) Mitochondrial ribosome assembly in health and disease. Cell Cycle 14:2226–2250
7. Kim HJ, Maiti P, Barrientos A (2017) Mitochondrial ribosomes in cancer. Semin Cancer Biol. https://doi.org/10.1016/j.semcancer.2017.1004.1004
8. Zeng R, Smith E, Barrientos A (2018) Yeast mitoribosome large subunit assembly proceeds by hierarchical incorporation of protein clusters and modules on the inner membrane. Cell Metab 27:645–656
9. Bogenhagen DF, Ostermeyer-Fay AG, Haley JD, Garcia-Diaz M (2018) Kinetics and mechanism of mammalian mitochondrial ribosome assembly. Cell Rep 22:1935–1944
10. Bogenhagen DF, Martin DW, Koller A (2014) Initial steps in RNA processing and ribosome assembly occur at mitochondrial DNA nucleoids. Cell Metab 19:618–629. https://doi.org/10.1016/j.cmet.2014.1003.1013
11. Tu YT, Barrientos A (2015) The human mitochondrial DEAD-box protein DDX28 resides in RNA granules and functions in mitoribosome assembly. Cell Rep 10:854–864
12. Lavdovskaia E, Kolander E, Steube E, Mai MM, Urlaub H, Richter-Dennerlein R (2018) The human Obg protein GTPBP10 is involved in mitoribosomal biogenesis. Nucleic Acids Res 46:8471–8482
13. Maiti P, Kim HJ, Tu YT, Barrientos A (2018) Human GTPBP10 is required for mitoribosome maturation. Nucleic Acids Res 46:11423–11437
14. Kim H-J, Barrientos A (2018) MTG1 couples mitoribosome large subunit assembly and intersubunit bridge formation. Nucleic Acids Res 46(16):8435–8453
15. De Silva D, Fontanesi F, Barrientos A (2013) The DEAD-Box protein Mrh4 functions in the assembly of the mitochondrial large ribosomal subunit. Cell Metab 18:712–725
16. De Silva D, Poliquin S, Zeng R, Zamudio-Ochoa A, Marrero N, Perez-Martinez X, Fontanesi F, Barrientos A (2017) The DEAD-box helicase Mss116 plays distinct roles in mitochondrial ribogenesis and mRNA-specific translation. Nucleic Acids Res 45:6628–6643
17. Fernandez-Vizarra E, Ferrin G, Perez-Martos-A, Fernandez-Silva P, Zeviani M, Enriquez JA (2010) Isolation of mitochondria for biogenetical studies: an update. Mitochondrion 10:253–262
18. Horn D, Fontanesi F, Barrientos A (2008) Exploring protein-protein interactions involving newly synthesized mitochondrial DNA-encoded proteins. Methods Mol Biol 457:125–139
19. Kehrein K, Schilling R, Moller-Hergt BV, Wurm CA, Jakobs S, Lamkemeyer T, Langer T, Ott M (2015) Organization of mitochondrial gene expression in two distinct ribosome-containing assemblies. Cell Rep 12: S2211–S1247
20. Couvillion MT, Soto IC, Shipkovenska G, Churchman LS (2016) Synchronized mitochondrial and cytosolic translation programs. Nature 533:499–503
21. Vignais PV, Stevens BJ, Huet J, Andre J (1972) Mitoribosomes from *Candida utilis*. Morphological, physical, and chemical characterization of the monomer form and of its subunits. J Cell Biol 54:468–492
22. Meisinger C, Pfanner N, Truscott KN (2006) Isolation of yeast mitochondria. Methods Mol Biol 313:33–39
23. Glick BS, Pon LA (1995) Isolation of highly purified mitochondria from *Saccharomyces cerevisiae*. Methods Enzymol 260:213–223
24. Davies E, Abe S (1995) Methods for isolation and analysis of polyribosomes. Methods Cell Biol 50:209–222
25. Stone AB (1974) A simplified method for preparing sucrose gradients. Biochem J 137:117–118
26. Wessel D, Flugge UI (1984) A method for the quantitative recovery of protein in dilute solution in the presence of detergents and lipids. Anal Biochem 138:141–143

Chapter 17

The Analysis of Yeast Mitochondrial Translation

Andreas Carlström, Magdalena Rzepka, and Martin Ott

Abstract

The mitochondrial genome encodes only a handful of proteins, but methods to track their synthesis are highly limited. *Saccharomyces cerevisiae* is a model organism that offers possibilities to expand the classical systems to analyze mitochondrial translation. In this chapter, we present two approaches of monitoring mitochondrial protein synthesis. Labeling of mitochondrially translated products with radioactive amino acids can be performed either in intact cells or in isolated mitochondria. However, these classical methods have disadvantages that can affect cell physiology and hence are not suitable for all types of research questions. Some of these limitations can be overcome by the use of reporter genes that are inserted into yeast genetic screens mitochondrial DNA via biolistic transformation. These reporter genes can be used for yeast genetic screen and to monitor regulation and efficiency of mitochondrial translation with a variety of methods.

Key words Translation, Mitochondria, Yeast, Reporter genes, Protein synthesis

1 Introduction

The mitochondrial proteome consists of proteins synthesized in both the cytoplasm and the mitochondrial matrix. In contrast to the 13 protein coding genes found in the human mitochondrial genome, the mtDNA of the baker's yeast *Saccharomyces cerevisiae* (*S. cerevisiae)* encodes only eight proteins [1]. This can be explained by the fact that *S. cerevisiae* lack complex I of the respiratory chain. Hence, the membrane-anchored mitochondrial ribosome (mitoribosome) in yeast is responsible for synthesizing seven hydrophobic core subunits of the respiratory chain, namely Cyt*b* of complex III, Cox1, Cox2 and Cox3 of complex IV, Atp6, Atp8 and Atp9 of the ATP synthase as well as Var1, a protein of the small mitoribosomal subunit [1].

Andreas Carlström and Magdalena Rzepka contributed equally to this work.

Michal Minczuk and Joanna Rorbach (eds.), *Mitochondrial Gene Expression: Methods and Protocols*, Methods in Molecular Biology, vol. 2192, https://doi.org/10.1007/978-1-0716-0834-0_17,

Even though there are only a few proteins expressed from the mtDNA, the approaches enabling to study their synthesis are limited. The high hydrophobicity of the translated membrane proteins together with the difficulty to purify translationally active mitoribosomes has prevented the design of functional in vitro assays [2]. Radioactive labeling of mitochondrial translation products has been the classical approach to study mitochondrial translation [3, 4]. Depending on the research question asked, either whole cells (in vivo) or isolated mitochondria (*in-organello*) are incubated with radioactive [^{35}S]-methionine which is then incorporated into newly synthesized polypeptide chains. Labeled polypeptides are separated through SDS-PAGE and visualized through autoradiography. This enables to study the synthesis of mitochondrially encoded proteins and possible differences in their expression, membrane insertion, assembly and degradation. However, to distinguish the signal from mitochondrially and nuclear encoded proteins in in vivo experiments, it is a prerequisite to inhibit cytosolic translation. This interference in cell physiology can potentially affect mitochondrial translation [5–8]. On the contrary, radiolabeling of mitochondrial translation products in isolated mitochondria does not necessitate inhibition of cytosolic translation, but there are other factors to consider regarding *in-organello* experiments, such as that proteins synthesized in the cytoplasm cannot be transported into the organelle, which could disturb protein insertion, assembly and potential feedback loops [6]. Therefore, labeling performed either in vivo or *in-organello* can be affected by impaired cytosolic protein synthesis, import to mitochondria or changes in cell metabolism that might affect results.

Due to these potential drawbacks of the radiolabeling methods on cell physiology, other types of methods to monitor mitochondrial translation have been developed in yeast. One such method is to use mitochondrially encoded reporter genes, like green fluorescent protein [9, 10] or proteins acting as auxotrophic markers [11–13]. Unlike radioactive labeling, the use of reporter proteins provides the possibility to monitor mitochondrial protein synthesis in unperturbed cells. Construction of mtDNA containing reporter genes is achieved through biolistic transformation. DNA-coated macro-carrier particles are used to deliver DNA into mitochondria, where it will be inserted into mtDNA through homologous recombination [11]. Substituting authentic mitochondrial genes with a reporter construct makes the cell respiratory deficient. As an alternative, these reporter constructs can be inserted in silent regions of the yeast mtDNA as an additional ninth protein expressed in yeast mitochondria under control of a native *COX2* promoter [9, 13]. This approach allows to monitor mitochondrial translation in various applications without affecting or disturbing the overall physiology of the cell.

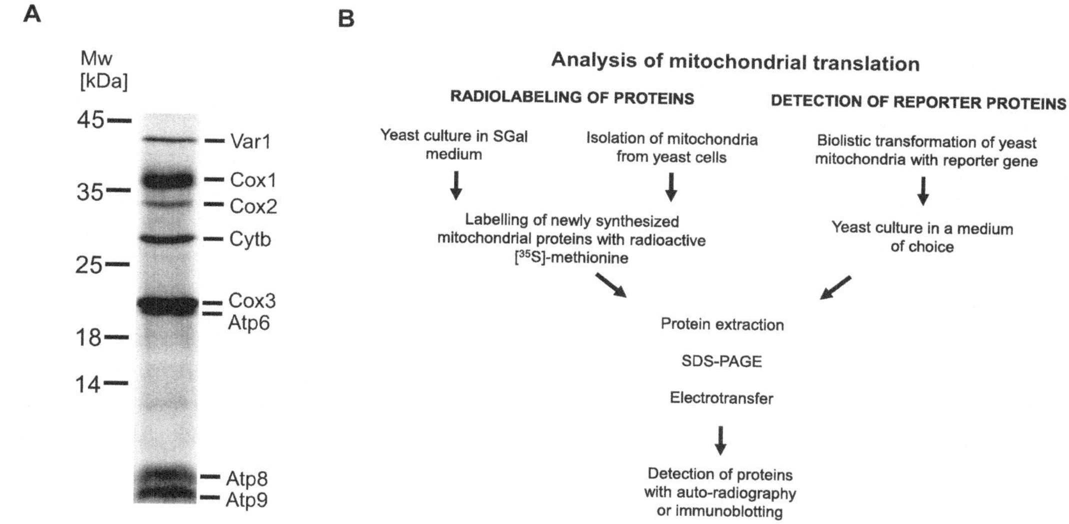

Fig. 1 Analysis of mitochondrially encoded translation products. (**a**) The mitochondrial genome of the yeast *Saccharomyces cerevisiae* encodes eight proteins; the mitoribosomal protein Var1 and the seven core subunits of the respiratory chain Cox1, Cox2, Cytb, Cox3, Atp6, Atp8 and Atp9. Here bands corresponding to the molecular weight of these proteins are shown after *in-organello* radiolabeling followed by separation through SDS-PAGE, transfer to a nitrocellulose membrane and detection by autoradiography. (**b**) Schematic description of the overall procedure of the two main methods to analyze mitochondrial translation presented in this chapter

In the following chapter, we present protocols for performing in vivo and *in-organello* pulse-chase labeling of mitochondrially encoded translation products as well as a method to monitor mitochondrial translation with the mitochondrially encoded reporters *sf*GFP and Arg8 (Fig. 1).

2 Materials

All solutions are dissolved in sterile and deionized H_2O unless stated otherwise.

2.1 In Vivo Labeling of Mitochondrial Translation

1. SGal with amino acids: 1.7 g/l yeast nitrogen base, 5 g/l $(NH_4)_2SO_4$, 2% galactose, 20 mg/l adenine, 20 mg/l uracil, 30 mg/l leucine, 30 mg/l lysine, 15 mg/l tryptophan, 15 mg/l histidine, 20 mg/l arginine (*see* **Note 1**). Pre-mix 8.5 g of yeast nitrogen base and 25 g of $(NH_4)_2SO_4$ in 1 l H_2O and autoclave to make a 5× S-medium stock. For 500 ml SGal with amino acids, mix 100 ml 5× S-medium, 33.3 ml galactose (30% stock) 5 ml adenine (stock 2 mg/ml), 5 ml uracil (2 mg/ml), 1.5 ml leucine (10 mg/ml), 1.5 ml lysine (10 mg/ml), 5 ml arginine (2 mg/ml), 750 μl tryptophan (10 mg/ml), 750 μl histidine (10 mg/ml) and 347 ml of H_2O.

2. SGal without amino acids: 1.7 g/l yeast nitrogen base and 5 g/l $(NH_4)_2SO_4$ dissolved in 250 ml H_2O.
3. [^{35}S]-Methionine, 10 mCi/ml.
4. 200 mM cold methionine solution: dissolve 0.3 g of methionine in 10 ml H_2O. Divide in aliquots and store at −20 °C.
5. SH-buffer: 0.6 M sorbitol and 20 mM HEPES-KOH, pH 7.4 dissolved in H_2O. Mix 12 ml of autoclaved 2.4 M sorbitol with 1 ml of 1 M HEPES-KOH, pH 7.4, and 37 ml of H_2O to make a 50 ml solution.
6. Amino acid mix: 2 mg/ml alanine, arginine, aspartic acid, asparagine, glutamic acid, glutamine, glycine, histidine, isoleucine, leucine, lysine, phenylalanine, proline, serine, threonine, tryptophan, and valine dissolved in 10 ml H_2O. Aliquot and store at −20 °C.
7. 1 mg/ml tyrosine dissolved in H_2O.
8. 10 mM cysteine solution dissolved in H_2O.
9. 7.5 mg/ml cycloheximide dissolved in H_2O. Preferably prepare fresh before use.
10. Stop mix: For 1 ml, mix 185 μl of 10 M NaOH, 74 μl of 14.3 M β-mercaptoethanol and 100 μl of 200 mM PMSF in 641 μl of H_2O.

2.2 In Organello Labeling of Mitochondrial Translation

1. Snap-frozen or freshly prepared isolated yeast mitochondria according to standard procedures (e.g., [13]).
2. 1.5× translation buffer: 0.6 M sorbitol, 150 mM KCl, 15 mM phosphate buffer pH 7.4, 20 mM HEPES-KOH pH 7.4, 12.7 mM $MgSO_4$, 4 mM ATP, 0.5 mM GTP, 5 mM α-ketoglutarate, 25 μM creatine phosphate, 0.6 U/ml creatine kinase, 66.7 μM cysteine, and 12.13 μg/ml of all other proteogenic amino acids except methionine.

   For 1.5 ml 1× translation buffer, mix 375 μl of 2.4 M sorbitol, 225 μl of 1 M KCl, 22.5 μl of 1 M phosphate buffer pH 7.4, 30 μl of 1 M HEPES-KOH pH 7.4, 19 μl of 1 M $MgSO_4$, 9.1 μl of proteogenic amino acid mix (2 mg/ml alanine, arginine, aspartic acid, asparagine, glutamic acid, glutamine, glycine, histidine, isoleucine, leucine, lysine, phenylalanine, proline, serine, threonine, tryptophan and valine dissolved in 10 ml H_2O, as also described in Subheading 2.1 above), 18.2 μl of 1 mg/ml tyrosine, 10 μl of 10 mM cysteine, 30 μl of 200 mM ATP, 15 μl of 50 mM GTP, 15 μl of 500 mM α-ketoglutarate, 30 μl of 1.25 mM creatine phosphate, 1.5 μl of 600 U/ml creatine kinase and 700 μl of H_2O.
3. [^{35}S]-methionine, 10 mCi/ml.
4. 200 mM methionine dissolved in H_2O.

5. SH-buffer: 0.6 M sorbitol and 20 mM HEPES-KOH, pH 7.4 dissolved in H_2O.
6. Reducing sample buffer: 50 mM Tris pH 6.8, 2% SDS, 10% glycerol, 0.1% bromophenol blue, 50 mM DTT.

2.3 Analysis of Mitochondrial Translation using Mitochondrially Encoded Reporter Genes

1. Yeast strains with mitochondrially encoded reporter genes for superfolder GFP (sfGFP) or acetylornithine aminotransferase (Arg8) (*see* **Note 2**).
2. YP medium: 1% yeast extract, 2% peptone. Mix 10 g of yeast extract and 20 g of bactopeptone in 1 l of water. Adjust pH to 5.5 with HCl and autoclave.
3. 40% glucose: fill about 600 ml of H_2O into a beaker and stir with a magnetic stirrer. Slowly add 400 g glucose until it is dissolved and fill up to 1 l with H_2O. Autoclave.
4. 30% glycerol: mix 700 ml of H_2O with 300 ml of 100% glycerol and stir with magnetic stirrer. Autoclave.
5. YPD medium: mix under sterile conditions 950 ml of autoclaved YP medium with 50 ml of 40% glucose to a final concentration of 2%.
6. YPG medium: mix under sterile conditions 943 ml of autoclaved YP medium with 67 ml of 30% glycerol to a final concentration of 2%.
7. Protein extraction buffer: mix 741 μl of H_2O, 185 μl of 10 M NaOH and 74 μl of β-mercaptoethanol.
8. Tris-buffered saline (TBS): 50 mM Tris–HCl and 0.15 M NaCl. For 1 l mix 6.05 g of Tris base and 8.76 g of NaCl and add 600 ml of H_2O. Adjust pH to 7.4 with HCl and bring up to 1 l with H_2O.
9. 5% Milk in TBS: mix 5 g of skimmed milk powder in 100 ml of TBS.
10. Sodium azide 20%, 2 g in 10 ml H_2O.
11. Primary antibodies (*see* **Note 3**).
    (a) α-GFP (Roche) diluted 1:1000 in 5% milk in TBS. For 10 ml mix 10 μl of the α-GFP antibody.
    (b) α-Arg8 diluted 1:500 in 5% milk in TBS. For 10 ml mix 20 μl of the α-Arg8 antibody.
12. Horse radish peroxidase (HRP)-conjugated secondary antibodies (*see* **Note 4**).
    (a) α-mouse (Sigma) diluted 1:3000 in 5% milk in TBS. For 10 ml use 3.3 μl of α-mouse antibody.
    (b) α-rabbit (BioRad) diluted 1:3000 in 5% milk in TBS. For 10 ml use 3.3 μl of α-rabbit antibody.
13. Western Bright Quantum HRP substrate solutions (Advansta).

2.4 Protein Extraction, SDS-PAGE and Electrotransfer

1. 72% Trichloroacetic acid (TCA) solution: Dissolve 72 g of TCA in 100 ml of H_2O.
2. Isopropanol.
3. 1 M Tris–HCl pH 6.8: Dissolve 12.1 g of Tris in 100 ml of H_2O. Adjust pH to 6.8 with HCl.
4. Reducing sample buffer: 100 mM Tris–HCl pH 6.8, 4% SDS, 20% glycerol, 100 mM DTT, 0.2% bromophenol blue. For 50 ml, mix 5 ml of 1 M Tris–HCl pH 6.8 stock, 2 g of SDS, 20 ml of 100% glycerol and 10 mg of bromophenol blue. Fill up to 50 ml with H_2O.
5. 30%/0.2% acrylamide/bis-acrylamide solution: dissolve 1 kg of acrylamide powder in 2 l of H_2O, add 6.7 g of bis-acrylamide and fill up to 3.3 l with H_2O. Filtrate solution through a folded filter paper (*see* **Note 5**).
6. 0.6 M Tris–HCl pH 8.8: Dissolve 227 g of Tris base in 800 ml of H_2O. Adjust pH to 8.8 with HCl. Bring up to 1 l.

   0.6 M Tris–HCl pH 6.8: Dissolve 227 g of Tris base in 800 ml of H_2O. Adjust pH to 6.8 with HCl. Bring up to 1 l.
7. 10% SDS: Resuspend 1 g of sodium dodecyl sulfate (SDS) in 10 ml of H_2O.
8. Running gel solution: 16% acrylamide, 400 mM Tris–HCl pH 8.8, 0.1% SDS. For 500 ml mix 276 ml of 30%/0.2% acrylamide/bis-acrylamide solution, 107 ml of 0.6 M Tris–HCl pH 8.8, 5 ml of 10% SDS and 121 ml of H_2O.
9. Stacking gel solution: 5% acrylamide, 60 mM Tris–HCl pH 6.8, 0.1% SDS. For 500 ml mix 84 ml of 30%/0.2% acrylamide/bis-acrylamide solution, 50 ml of 0.6 M Tris–HCl pH 6.8, 5 ml of 10% SDS and 361 ml of H_2O.
10. 10% Ammonium persulfate (APS) solution: Resuspend 1 g of APS in 10 ml of H_2O.
11. *N*,*N*,*N'*,*N'*-Tetramethylethylenediamine (TEMED).
12. SDS-PAGE running buffer: 25 mM Tris, 0.192 M glycine, 0.1% SDS. For 1 l mix 3 g of Tris base, 14.4 g of glycine and 1 g of SDS in 1 l of H_2O. pH will be 8.3 and do not adjust.
13. 10× blotting buffer: 250 mM Tris base, 1.92 M glycine. For 1 l mix 30.3 g of Tris and 144 g of glycine and dissolve in 1 l of H_2O. pH will be 8.3, do not adjust.
14. Transfer buffer: 1× blotting buffer, 20% methanol. For 1 l mix 200 ml of methanol and 100 ml of 10× blotting buffer. Add 700 ml of H_2O.
15. Ponceau staining solution: for 200 ml, mix 200 mg of Ponceau S, 10 ml of acetic acid and 190 ml of H_2O.

3 Methods

All steps should be performed at room temperature unless stated otherwise.

3.1 In Vivo Labeling of Mitochondrial Translation

Radiolabeling of mitochondrially encoded translation products in vivo requires addition of a cytoplasmic translation inhibitor, such as cycloheximide. In this section, a protocol for performing in vivo pulse-chase radiolabeling is described, where the synthesis and stability of mitochondrial translation products are followed over time.

3.1.1 Yeast Culturing

1. Start an overnight culture of chosen yeast strain from a single colony in 5 ml of SGal medium with amino acids.
2. Let the culture grow until an optical density (OD_{600}) of 1.5–2 (*see* **Note 6**).
3. Dilute the cultures to an OD_{600} of 0.4 in 20 ml media and grow them further for 1–2 h to reach an OD_{600} of 0.5–1 (*see* **Note 7**).
4. Harvest the cells by centrifugation at 3000 × *g* for 3 min (*see* **Note 8**).
5. Remove the supernatant and wash the cells in 5 ml deionized H_2O.
6. Pellet the cells by centrifugation at 3000 × *g* for 3 min and wash them once with 5 ml SGal without amino acids.
7. Pellet the cells again and resuspend them in 1 ml SGal without amino acids. Measure the OD_{600} and transfer the volume equivalent to an OD of 4 to a 1.5–2 ml tube.

3.1.2 Radiolabeling

1. Pellet the cells, remove the supernatant and resuspend in 1.5 ml SGal without amino acids (*see* **Note 9**).
2. Add 9 μl of amino acid mix (2 mg/ml of each amino acid in the solution), 18 μl of 1 mg/ml tyrosine and 9.6 μl of 10 mM cysteine and incubate the cell suspension at 30 °C for 10 min in a benchtop heat block, shaking at 700–800 rpm.
3. Add 30 μl of 7.5 mg/ml cycloheximide to a final concentration of 150 μg/ml to inhibit cytosolic translation. This prevents incorporation of radiolabeled methionine into cytosolic translation products which otherwise will overshadow the mitochondrial proteins.
4. Incubate the cells at 30 °C for 2.5 min and add 3 μl of [^{35}S]-methionine.

5. Take 200 μl aliquots from each cell suspension after 5, 10 and 15 min (*see* **Note 10**) to follow the mitochondrial translation over time (called pulse). Immediately add 50 μl of the Stop mix and 10 μl of 200 mM cold methionine to each sample (*see* **Note 11**). Vortex shortly and put samples on ice.
6. To follow stability of the newly synthesized mitochondrial translation products over time (called chase), add 40 μl of 200 mM cold methionine and incubate the cells at 37 °C (*see* **Note 12**).
7. Immediately take out 200 μl as the starting sample for the chase at 0 min and mix with 50 μl of the Stop mix and 10 μl of 200 mM cold methionine (again *see* **Notes 10** and **11**).
8. Take out 200 μl aliquots after 30, 60 and 90 min and immediately mix with 50 μl of the Stop mix and 10 μl of 200 mM cold methionine.
9. After aliquoting, leave samples on ice for 10 min.

3.1.3 Protein Extraction and Analysis

1. Add 72 μl of 72% TCA to the samples for a final concentration of 12% and mix by vortexing (*see* **Note 13**).
2. Leave the samples on ice for 20 min or store the samples at −20 °C overnight (*see* **Note 14**).
3. Pellet proteins by centrifugation at 25,000 × *g* for 30 min at 4 °C.
4. Carefully remove the supernatant without disrupting the pellet.
5. Add 1 ml of cold acetone to the pellet and mix by vortexing.
6. Centrifuge samples at 25,000 × *g* for 15 min at 4 °C.
7. Remove the supernatant and dry the pellet by leaving the lid open to let the residual acetone evaporate.
8. Resuspend the protein pellet in 70 μl of reducing sample buffer.
9. Incubate for 15 min at 70 °C at 1400 rpm in a benchtop shaker. If the pellet has not dissolved, prolong incubation for another 30 min at 45 °C (*see* **Note 15**).
10. Load 30 μl of each sample on a 16%/0.2% SDS polyacrylamide/bis-acrylamide gel and run the gel until completion (*see* Subheading 3.4 of this chapter).
11. Transfer the separated proteins to a nitrocellulose membrane by electrotransfer before analysis and visualization through autoradiography (*see* Subheading 3.4 of this chapter) (Fig. 2). Alternatively, the gel can be dried and directly used for autoradiography.

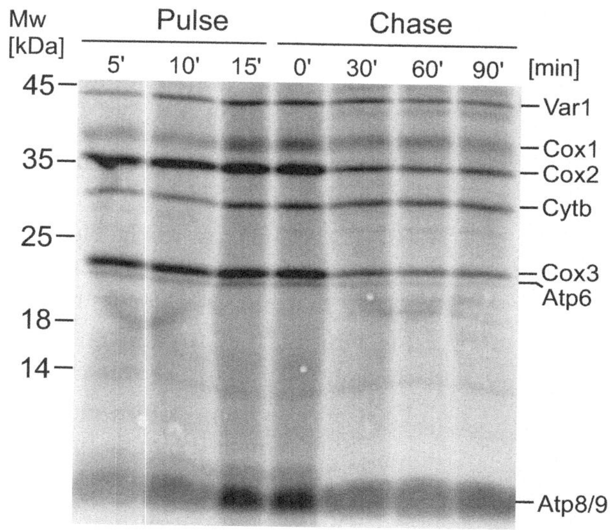

Fig. 2 Example of an in vivo pulse-chase labeling experiment. The synthesis of mitochondrial translation products (pulse) is followed by incubating yeast cells at 30 °C with radioactive [^{35}S]-methionine and taking samples at 5 min intervals. After 15 min, the stability of the newly synthesized mitochondrial translation products (chase) is monitored by adding an excess of non-radioactive methionine while increasing the temperature to 37 °C and taking samples with 30 min intervals. Samples are then TCA-precipitated, separated on a 16%/0.2% SDS polyacrylamide/bis-acrylamide gel, transferred to a nitrocellulose membrane through electrotransfer and visualized by autoradiography. *Mw [kDa]* molecular weight in kilodalton

3.2 In-Organello *Labeling of Mitochondrial Translation*

The following section describes a protocol for performing an *in-organello* pulse-chase radiolabeling to follow the synthesis and stability of mitochondrial translation products in isolated mitochondria.

1. Before the start of this experiment, mitochondria need to be isolated from yeast cells according to a standard protocol for mitochondrial preparation (e.g., [13]) (*see* **Note 16**). The organelles can be used freshly after isolation or after snap-freezing in liquid N_2 and storage at −80 °C.
2. Freshly prepare 1.5× Translation buffer (*see* **Note 17**).
3. Thaw isolated and intact mitochondria (450 μg per strain) in a 1.5 ml tube on ice.
4. Pellet the mitochondria through centrifugation at 10,000 × *g* for 10 min at 4 °C.
5. Carefully remove the supernatant and resuspend the mitochondrial pellet in 450 μl 1.5× Translation buffer.
6. Incubate the mitochondrial suspension in a heat block shaker for 5 min at 30 °C, shaking at 700 rpm.

7. Start the labeling of mitochondrial translation products (pulse) by adding 2 μl of [^{35}S] methionine (*see* **Note 18**) and incubate the samples for an additional 15 min (*see* **Note 19**).
8. Stop the labeling by adding 10 μl of 200 mM cold methionine.
9. Take out 200 μl pulse samples and immediately dilute them 1:1 with 200 μl SH-buffer.
10. The stability of the labeled mitochondrial translation products is then monitored (chase) by incubating the mitochondrial suspension for 30 min at 30 or 37 °C (*see* **Note 20**).
11. During the 30 min chase, centrifuge the pulse samples at 10,000 × *g* for 10 min at 4 °C to pellet the mitochondria.
12. Carefully remove the supernatant and resuspend the pellet in 70 μl reducing sample buffer.
13. Take out 200 μl chase samples and immediately dilute them 1:1 with 200 μl SH-buffer.
14. Pellet the mitochondria through centrifugation at 10,000 × *g* for 10 min at 4 °C.
15. Resuspend the resulting mitochondrial pellet in 70 μl sample buffer.
16. Incubate the pulse and chase samples resuspended in sample buffer for 15 min at 30 °C (*see* **Note 21**).
17. Load 30 μl of each sample on a 16%/0.2% SDS polyacrylamide/bis-acrylamide gel and run the gel until completion before analysis with electrotransfer and visualization through autoradiography (*see* Subheading 3.4 of this chapter).

3.3 Analysis of Mitochondrial Translation Through Mitochondrially Encoded Reporter Genes

3.3.1 Yeast Culturing

1. Start an overnight 5 ml culture of a yeast strain with mitochondrially encoded reporter genes like *sfGFP* or *ARG8* in YPD at 30 °C with shaking 220 rpm.
2. In the morning, check the OD of the yeast culture after thoroughly mixing the cells in the culture tube or flask. Blank with YPD medium and measure the OD_{600}.
3. Dilute the cells to OD_{600} of 0.2 in 5 ml YPG.
4. Incubate the cells for 3–4 h until they reach the exponential growth phase (OD_{600} of 0.6–0.8) at 30 °C, shaking at 220 rpm.
5. Measure the OD_{600} of the cell culture as before.
6. Harvest a cell amount equivalent of $OD_{600} = 2$ by centrifugation 1 min, 5000 × *g* in a microcentrifuge tube and carefully remove supernatant without disrupting the pellet.
7. Resuspend the cell pellet in 200 μl of H_2O.
8. Add 50 μl of protein extraction buffer.
9. Mix by inverting the tube ten times and incubate 10 min on ice.

3.3.2 Protein Extraction and Separation

1. Add 60 μl of 72% TCA to the samples for a final concentration of 12% and mix by vortexing.
2. Leave the samples on ice for 20 min or store the samples at −20 °C overnight (*see* **Note 14**).
3. Pellet proteins by centrifugation at 25,000 × *g* for 30 min at 4 °C.
4. Carefully remove the supernatant without disrupting the pellet.
5. Add 1 ml of cold acetone to the pellet and mix by vortexing.
6. Centrifuge samples at 25,000 × *g* for 15 min at 4 °C.
7. Remove the supernatant and dry the pellet by leaving the lid open to let the residual acetone evaporate.
8. Resuspend the protein pellet in 50 μl of reducing sample buffer.
9. Incubate for 15 min at 70 °C shaking at 1400 rpm in a benchtop shaker. If the pellet has not dissolved, prolong incubation for another 30 min at 45 °C (*see* **Note 15**).
10. Load 25 μl of the samples on a 16%/0.2% SDS polyacrylamide/bis-acrylamide gel and run the gel until completion. Transfer the separated proteins to a nitrocellulose membrane (*see* Subheading 3.4 of this chapter).

3.3.3 Immunoblotting

1. Block the nitrocellulose membrane for 60 min in 5% milk diluted with TBS in room temperature while shaking.
2. Incubate the membrane overnight at 4 °C in 10 ml of primary antibody α-GFP or α-Arg8 while shaking.
3. Wash the membrane three times for 10 min in 10 ml of TBS.
4. Incubate the membrane for 1 h in 10 ml of secondary antibody. Use α-mouse for the membrane incubated with the α-GFP antibody and α-rabbit for the one with the α-Arg8 antibody.
5. Wash the membrane three times for 10 min in 10 ml of TBS.
6. Develop the signal on the membrane with Western Bright Quantum HRP substrates (or equivalent ECL solution) according to the manufacturer manual.
7. Record the chemiluminescence with ChemiDoc or a similar imaging system and analyze the results (Fig. 3).

3.4 SDS-PAGE, Electrotransfer and Autoradiography

3.4.1 Sodium Dodecyl Sulfate-Polyacrylamide Gel Electrophoresis (SDS-PAGE)

1. Assemble the gel cast system by placing plastic spacers between two clean glass plates and fixing them tightly in a designated gel cast holder or chamber (*see* **Note 22**).
2. Prepare the running gel by mixing 8 ml of running gel solution, 43 μl of 10% APS and 6.5 μl of TEMED in a 15 ml falcon tube and pour the solution between the glasses in the caster. Cover

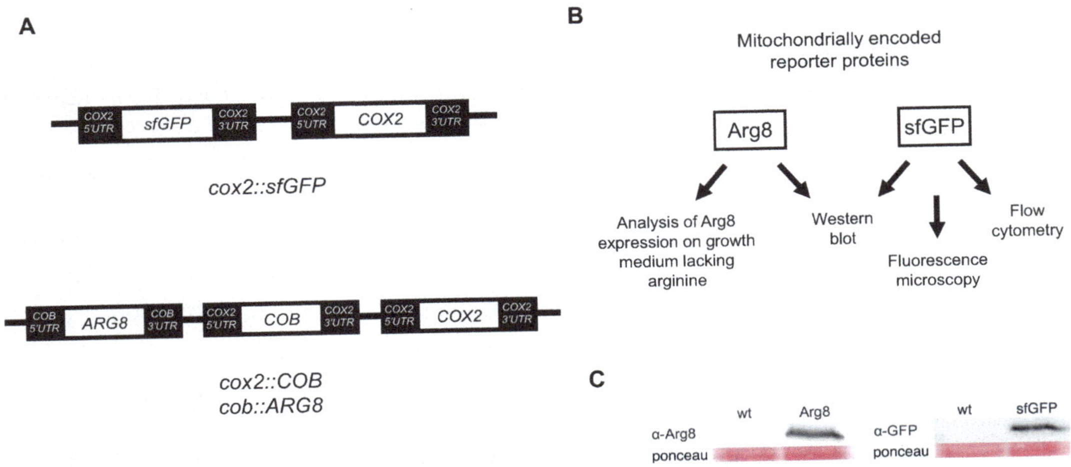

Fig. 3 Analysis of mitochondrial translation through the mitochondrially encoded reporter proteins *sf*GFP [9] and Arg8 [13]. (**a**) Schematics of the manipulated mitochondrial genomes of the yeast strains with mitochondrially encoded reporter proteins. The coding sequences of the reporter proteins were integrated by biolistic transformation and homologous recombination into the mtDNA. *sfGFP* is expressed as an additional gene via the UTRs of cytochrome c oxidase 2 (*COX2*). *ARG8* is expressed through the UTRs of cytochrome b (*COB*) while *COB* itself is cloned and expressed through the UTRs of *COX2*. (**b**) Possible ways of analyzing expression of mitochondrially encoded reporter proteins in yeast cells include plating on selective media plates, immunoblotting, fluorescence microscopy and flow cytometry measurements. (**c**) Immunoblots obtained following SDS-PAGE and electrotransfer of proteins extracted from yeast strains, either wild type (wt) or mutants with mitochondrially encoded Arg8 or *sf*GFP. Ponceau staining of the nitrocellulose membranes served as a loading control

the top of the running gel with isopropanol. Let polymerize for 45 min.

3. Pour out the isopropanol from the gel caster.
4. Prepare the stacking gel by mixing 3 ml of stacking gel solution, 11 μl of 10% APS and 2.2 μl of TEMED in a 15 ml falcon tube and pour in the solution into the caster on top of the running gel. Immediately insert the comb. Let polymerize for 45 min.
5. When the gel has polymerized, remove the comb and put the gel cassette into the gel running chamber.
6. Pour the SDS-PAGE running buffer to cover the gel and wash wells with running buffer to remove the residual polymerized acrylamide with a pipette tip.
7. Centrifuge the samples for 10 s in 10,000 × *g*.
8. Load 30 μl of samples and 10 μl of unstained protein marker into the wells.
9. Run the electrophoresis until the dye front reaches the bottom of the gel.

3.4.2 Electrotransfer

1. Disassemble the gel cassette using a spatula. The gel should stay on one of the glass plates. Cut out and discard the stacking gel and put the running gel into a box with transfer buffer.
2. Assemble the wet transfer sandwich submerged in a box filled with Transfer buffer. In the following order, place two sponges on the bottom followed by one Whatman filter paper, the acrylamide gel, a nitrocellulose membrane, another Whatman filter paper and finally two sponges on the top.
3. Put the sandwich into the blotting chamber with the nitrocellulose membrane closer to the anode and the gel closer to the cathode.
4. Run the transfer for 1.5 h according to the instrument at hand.
5. Disassemble the sandwich and put the nitrocellulose membrane into a small container.
6. Rinse the nitrocellulose membrane with ddH_2O.
7. Cover the membrane with 10 ml of Ponceau staining solution and incubate shaking for 5 min to stain the membrane.
8. Remove the Ponceau solution and rinse away the excess of stain from the membrane with ddH_2O to visualize bands for the extracted proteins (*see* **Note 23**). Take a picture.

3.4.3 Autoradiography

1. For detection of the marker bands during autoradiography, mark the marker bands with diluted [^{35}S]-methionine with the help of a pipette tip (*see* **Note 24**).
2. Dry the now radioactive nitrocellulose membrane at room temperature or with the help of a blow-dryer.
3. Place an autoradiography/phosporimager screen in a cassette holder and put the membrane face down on to the screen with a Whatman filter paper on top to cover it. Close the cassette holder.
4. Expose the membrane to the autoradiography screen for a couple of days before developing the screen in a phosphorimager machine (*see* **Note 25**).

4 Notes

1. Prepare and autoclave all the stock solutions of yeast nitrogen base with $(NH_4)SO_4$ (5× S-medium), amino acids, nucleotides and sugars separately before mixing them together into the SGal medium.
2. The yeast strains with mitochondrially encoded reporter genes were prepared using biolistic transformation [11]. The method to insert *GFP* into mtDNA was first established by Cohen and Fox [10]. The original strain with the *COB* gene replaced by an

ARG8 reporter [12] was a gift from Tom Fox (Cornell University). In the protocol described in this chapter, we use strains constructed within our group according to Suhm et al. [9] and Gruschke et al. [13], with help regarding both discussion and materials from Tom Fox (Cornell University) and Alexander Tzagoloff (Columbia University).

3. To prevent microbial contamination, 0.02% sodium azide can be added to the primary antibody dilutions. The antibody solutions can then be stored in −20 °C and re-used.
4. Do not add sodium azide to secondary antibody solutions since it will inhibit the HRP enzymatic reaction. Prepare the secondary antibody solution fresh every time.
5. Acrylamide is poisonous. Work under the fume hood and use a mask to avoid inhalation of the powder during preparation of acrylamide stocks.
6. OD_{600} is measured in a spectrophotometer set at the wavelength $\lambda = 600$ nm. It may take 2–3 days to grow the yeast culture to a sufficiently high OD_{600} when it is possible to dilute the culture to $OD_{600} = 0.4$ in 20 ml media.
7. Yeast cells should be in logarithmic growth phase (OD_{600} of 0.5–1) when harvested.
8. For harvesting and subsequent washing steps, we transfer the 20 ml cell culture to a 50 ml Falcon tube. The cells are pelleted through centrifugation and the supernatant is poured out carefully from the tube.
9. Caution should be used during the last step of washing, since it is easy to disrupt the pellet and lose cells when removing the supernatant from the microcentrifuge tube. It is important that 4 OD_{600} units of cells are taken out for each strain, otherwise comparisons of mitochondrial translation levels between strains will not be possible.
10. Alternatively, take out a 400 μl sample at the 15 min time point where 200 μl can serve as the starting sample at 0 min for the chase. This can facilitate the experiment.
11. You can prepare and label all the sample tubes with the Stop mix and cold methionine before starting the experiment.
12. Addition of 40 μl of 200 mM cold methionine will effectively stop incorporation of radiolabeled [^{35}S]-methionine into new translation products since we are adding a large excess of non-labeled methionine.
13. Final percentage of TCA in the sample should not exceed 14% due to the high amount of NaOH used. Remember to add twice the amount of 72% TCA (144 μl) to the 15 min sample if you earlier decided to take out double the amount (400 μl) to use it for both the 15 min pulse and 0 min chase time points.

14. After addition of TCA the sample can be stored at −20 °C in the freezer overnight or longer.
15. It is important to not boil the samples at too high temperature (≥75 °C) as this can lead to aggregation of the highly hydrophobic translation products. When the protein pellet has been properly dissolved the samples can be separated through SDS-PAGE or be stored at −20 °C for later analysis.
16. Each mitochondrial preparation is different. Therefore, it is good to perform the *in-organello* experiments on mitochondria from at least three different mitochondrial preparations to confirm and validate results.
17. Prepare the 1.5× translation buffer fresh. Stocks used for the translation buffer should be stored in −20 °C, except for 2.4 M Sorbitol (stored at 4 °C) and salts (can be kept at room temperature).
18. The amount of [^{35}S]-methionine added depends on how old the stock is. If the signal after exposure and developing of the membrane is weak and it is not possible to use more radioactivity, try exposing the membrane for a few more days.
19. Time for incubation during the labeling phase can vary between 5 and 30 min depending on the conditions that are being investigated. For example, when adding certain translational inhibitors, it can be good to incubate for a longer time. However, isolated mitochondria usually only translate efficiently for 30–60 min.
20. Time for incubation during the chase of the experiment can also vary and should be adjusted to the protein degradation rate in the used strain.
21. Do not boil the samples in 95 °C as this could affect the labeling intensity, but instead incubate them in lower temperatures such as 30 or 42 °C for a longer time.
22. Different sizes of polyacrylamide gels and different types of gel systems can be used. However, it is important to remember that the separation and running behavior of the mitochondrial translation products varies greatly between gel sizes and systems. In our hands, a 16%/0.2% acrylamide/bis-acrylamide gel works well to separate the translation products in a reproducible fashion.
23. Document the Ponceau-stained membrane to use it as a loading control.
24. The unstained protein marker bands are not visible on the membrane. Mark the bands corresponding to the differently sized protein marker standards with a pen when they are stained with Ponceau S. This way it is possible to estimate the size of the proteins visualized through autoradiography or immunoblotting.

25. Depending on the radioactivity of the samples, expose the membrane for 3–7 days for in vivo labeling and 1–3 days for *in-organello* labeling before developing.

References

1. Ott M, Amunts A, Brown A (2016) Organization and regulation of mitochondrial protein synthesis. Annu Rev Biochem 85:77–101
2. Lightowlers RN, Rozanka A, Chrzanowska-Lightowlers ZN (2014) Mitochondrial protein synthesis: figuring the fundamentals, complexities and complications, of mammalian mitochondrial translation. FEBS Lett 588 (15):2496–2503
3. Douglas MG, Butow RA (1976) Variant forms of mitochondrial translation products in yeast: evidence for location of determinants on mitochondrial DNA. Proc Natl Acad Sci U S A 73:1083–1086
4. McKee EE, Poyton RO (1984) Mitochondrial gene expression in Saccharomyces cerevisiae. I. Optimal conditions for protein synthesis in isolated mitochondria. J Biol Chem 259:9320–9331
5. Dai CL, Shi J, Chen Y, Iqbal K, Liu F, Gong CX (2013) Inhibition of protein synthesis alters protein degradation through activation of protein kinase B (AKT). J Biol Chem 288 (33):23875–23883
6. Couvillion MT, Soto IC, Shipkovenska G, Churchman LS (2016) Synchronized mitochondrial and cytosolic translation programs. Nature 533(7604):499–503
7. Suhm T, Ott M (2017) Mitochondrial translation and cellular stress response. Cell Tissue Res 367(1):21–31
8. Loewith R, Hall MN (2011) Target of rapamycin (TOR) in nutrient signalling and growth control. Genetics 189(4):1177–1201
9. Suhm T, Habernig L, Rzepka M, Kaimal JM, Andreasson C, Buttner S, Ott M (2018) A novel system to monitor mitochondrial translation in yeast. Microbial Cell 5:158–164
10. Cohen JS, Fox TD (2001) Expression of green fluorescent protein from a recoded gene inserted into Saccharomyces cerevisiae mitochondrial DNA. Mitochondrion 1(2):181–189
11. Bonnefoy N, Fox TD (2007) Directed alteration of Saccharomyces cerevisiae mitochondrial DNA by biolistic transformation and homologous recombination. Methods Mol Biol 372:153–166
12. Ding MG, Butler CA, Saracco SA, Fox TD, Godard F, di Rago JP, Trumpower BL (2008) Introduction of cytochrome b mutations in Saccharomyces cerevisiae by a method that allows selection for both functional and non-functional cytochrome b proteins. Biochim Biophys Acta 1777:1147–1156
13. Gruschke S, Römpler K, Hildenbeutel M, Kehrein K, Kühl I, Bonnefoy N, Ott M (2012) The Cbp3–Cbp6 complex coordinates cytochrome b synthesis with bc1 complex assembly in yeast mitochondria. J Cell Biol 199(1):137–150

Chapter 18

In Situ Studies of Mitochondrial Translation by Cryo-Electron Tomography

Robert Englmeier and Friedrich Förster

Abstract

Cryo-electron tomography (cryo-ET) enables the three-dimensional (3D) visualization of macromolecular complexes in their native environment (in situ). The ability to visualize macromolecules in situ is in particular advantageous for complex, membrane-associated processes, such as mitochondrial translation. Mitochondrial translation occurs almost exclusively associated with the inner mitochondrial membrane, giving rise to the mitochondrial DNA-encoded subunits of oxidative phosphorylation machinery. In cryo-ET, the 3D volume is reconstructed from a set of 2D projections of a frozen-hydrated specimen, which is sequentially tilted and imaged at different angles in a transmission electron microscope. In combination with subtomogram analysis, cryo-ET enables the structure determination of macromolecular complexes and their 3D organization. In this chapter, we summarize all steps required for structural characterization of mitochondrial ribosomes in situ, ranging from data acquisition to tomogram reconstruction and subtomogram analysis.

Key words Cryo-electron tomography, Mitochondria, Mitochondrial ribosomes, Translation

1 Introduction

Cryo-electron tomography (cryo-ET) enables the three-dimensional (3D) visualization of frozen-hydrated biological specimens in a close-to-native state at molecular resolution [1]. In order to obtain a 3D image, the sample is sequentially tilted in the transmission electron microscope (TEM) and projection images are acquired, resulting in a tilt series. In contrast to classical electron microscopy (EM) of dehydrated, heavy metal stained and plastic-embedded specimens, vitrification by rapid cooling (cryo-preparation) preserves the molecular structure of the specimen and enables the detailed analysis of macromolecular complexes [2].

While cryo-EM single particle analysis (SPA) allows for the structure determination of macromolecular complexes at atomic resolution, this method requires purification of the respective molecules, thus isolating them from their native context. In contrast,

Michal Minczuk and Joanna Rorbach (eds.), *Mitochondrial Gene Expression: Methods and Protocols*, Methods in Molecular Biology, vol. 2192, https://doi.org/10.1007/978-1-0716-0834-0_18,

cryo-ET can be applied to isolated organelles or even whole cells, enabling the visualization of macromolecules in situ. Therefore, this imaging modality is suitable for the structural analysis of membrane-associated processes. Mitochondrial translation belongs to this category: mitochondrial mRNA is translated by the membrane-bound mitochondrial ribosome (mitoribosome), and the product is typically co-translationally inserted into the inner mitochondrial membrane (IMM) [3].

Application of cryo-ET to isolated mitochondria can visualize mitoribosomes *in organello*. Due to the beam sensitivity of vitrified biological samples tomograms are acquired with low doses (typically $<100\ e^-/\text{Å}^2$). The resulting low signal-to-noise ratio (SNR) limits the resolution of the tomograms to approximately 5 nm [4]. Key to quantitative analysis of mitoribosomes in noisy tomograms is a process called template matching, which can localize and identify copies of the target macromolecule based on its known structural signature. By aligning and averaging multiple copies of the macromolecule, i.e., subtomogram averaging, the SNR improves, allowing subnanometer and even atomic resolution in selected cases [5, 6]. Classification allows for disentangling different conformational or compositional states, e.g., separating fully-assembled mitoribosomes from smaller species.

In this method chapter we cover cryo-ET sample preparation, data acquisition, and processing in the context of mitochondrial translation. For data processing we also describe the software packages TOM [7] and PyTom [8].

2 Materials

2.1 Isolation of Mitochondrial Vesicles

The precise purification protocol will ultimately depend on the biological question, which may require different levels of enrichment or ultrastructural preservation. We achieved a fairly pure sample of yeast mitochondria with a previously described protocol [9]. For human mitochondria, we previously used a protocol [10] adapted from Frezza et al. [11]. Both protocols employ differential centrifugation, and show sufficient enrichment for cryo-ET analysis despite notable contamination by multivesicular vesicles and ER. Here, the protocol that we employed for the purification of mitochondria from Freestyle™ 293-F cells grown in suspension is described [10].

1. Freestyle™ 293-F cells grown in Freestyle medium.
2. PBS buffer: Dissolve 8 g of NaCl, 0.2 g of KCl, 1.44 g of Na_2HPO_4 and 0.2 g of KH_2PO_4 in 800 ml of H_2O. Adjust pH to 7.4 with HCl and fill up to 1 l with H_2O.

3. Isolation buffer: 10 mM Tris, 150 mM sucrose, 1 mM EGTA, pH 7.4. Prepare 200 mM Tris stock solution by resolving 2.64 g of Trizma HCl and 0.38 g of Trizma Base in 100 ml. Prepare 0.5 mM EGTA stock solution by resolving 1.9 g EGTA in 8 ml. Adjust pH to 8.0 with KOH and fill up to 10 ml. Prepare 2 M Sucrose stock solution by resolving 18 g in 35 ml H_2O. Fill up to 50 ml with H_2O. Pipette 5 ml of the 200 mM Tris stock solution with 100 μl of 0.5 M EGTA solution, 3.85 ml of the 2 M sucrose solution and 41.15 ml of H_2O.
4. Glass-Teflon homogenizer.

2.2 Preparation of Cryo-EM Grids

1. Mechanical or automated grid-plunger (Vitrobot™, Thermo-Fisher Scientific) including all the required accessories, i.e., container with separate cup for liquid nitrogen and cryogen and a tweezer-mount with appropriate tweezer.
2. Ethane or Ethane-Propane mixture as a cryogen.
3. Ice-free liquid nitrogen.
4. Holey or lacey carbon coated grids (Quantifoil).
5. Glow discharger (e.g., Pelco Easiglow).
6. Filter paper (Whatman, Grade 595).
7. 10 nm BSA-coated gold beads (e.g., UMC Utrecht). Dilute them at the half of the recommended value (usually 1:40 to 1:50) in 20 mM Hepes pH 7.4 buffer to achieve a 2× gold buffer for on-grid dilution.
8. EM grid storage boxes (e.g., Ted Pella).

2.3 Electron Microscopy

The crowded environment of the mitochondrial matrix as well as the thickness of mitochondria both result in low contrast in tomograms and make the identification of mitoribosomes difficult. The minimum requirement to obtain interpretable data of the interior of isolated mitochondria is a 200 kV cryo-TEM, equipped with a field-emission gun, energy filter, and direct electron detector. With this equipment, the vitrified mitochondria should not exceed 200 nm thickness along the normal of the EM grid. A 300 kV TEM in combination with a phase plate maximizes penetration depth of electrons and hence the resulting contrast.

2.4 Software

The following software is required to perform the protocols described in this method chapter:

- Current version of SerialEM [12] for tilt series acquisition (here we use version 3.6) (http://bio3d.colorado.edu/SerialEM/).
- motioncor2 [13], for alignment of dose-fractionated movies.

- TOM and AV3 toolbox [5, 7]; for localization of gold markers required for tilt series alignment (https://bitbucket.org/FridoF/av3).
- Matlab R2014a or earlier; to run the TOM/AV3 toolbox. Add TOM and av3 directories to the Matlab search path, i.e., by the "`Set path`" button or the "`addpath`" command.
- PyTOM v0.971 [8]; for tomogram reconstruction, template matching, subtomogram alignment, and classification (http://pytom.org).
- UCSF Chimera 1.10 or higher [14]; for data visualization.
- "Chooser" plugin for Chimera; available on the PyTom website [15].

Regarding the processing of tomographic data, the TOM/AV3 toolbox is only required for the gold marker clicking. It includes all required functions for the processing of 2D and 3D images (e.g., filtering, downscaling, cropping, reconstruction of tomograms, and averaging of subtomograms) and enables the integration of standard Matlab functions and external Matlab packages for data analysis. Template matching, subtomogram alignment, and classification are implemented in PyTOM, which provides more functionalities for subtomogram processing, higher interpolation accuracy, and higher computational speed. We will therefore focus on the application of PyTom and mention the usage of TOM/AV3 functions where required.

3 Methods

3.1 Purification of Crude Mitochondrial Vesicle from Human Suspension Cells

1. Grow the cells to a cell density of approximately 1×10^6 cells/ml.
2. Collect the cells by centrifugation for 5 min at $360 \times g$ and 4 °C. All subsequent steps should be carried out at 4 °C.
3. Wash the cells twice by resuspending the cell pellet in 1× PBS buffer and repeating the centrifugation from **step 2**.
4. Resuspend the cell pellet in homogenization buffer (5 ml/g cell pellet).
5. Transfer the cell suspension to a Glass-Teflon Potter and homogenize it by 120 up- and downstrokes (*see* **Note 1**).
6. Clear the lysate for 10 min at $800 \times g$.
7. Transfer the supernatant to a new tube and centrifuge for 10 min at $9000 \times g$.
8. Resuspend the mitochondrial pellet in 1 ml/g homogenization buffer and centrifuge it again at $9000 \times g$ for 10 min.

9. Resuspend the mitochondrial pellet to a concentration of 10 mg/ml in homogenization buffer. Store it at −80 °C upon flash-freezing in liquid nitrogen or use it directly for grid preparation by diluting it to 1.5 mg/ml (*see* **Note 2**).

3.2 Cryo-EM Grid Preparation of Mitochondrial Vesicles

To analyze purified biological sample in the cryo-TEM, the sample needs to be applied to a specimen carrier, the EM grid, and vitrified by plunge-freezing into a cryogen (ethane or ethane-propane). The EM grid is a thin, circular (Ø 3 mm) specimen container with a regular grid-mesh (e.g., copper or molybdenum), and a support film (usually carbon) to accommodate the sample. Due to the hydrophobicity of carbon, EM grids are generally made hydrophilic by a plasma treatment in a glow discharger just prior to grid preparation. Due to the relatively short inelastic mean free path of electrons in vitreous ice (~400 nm at 300 kV [16], ~250 nm at 120 kV [17]), the EM grid is blotted after applying the sample and just prior to plunge-freezing resulting in a thin the water-film containing the sample (~200 nm).

1. Glow discharge an adequate amount of Quantifoil holey or lacey carbon-coated grids.
2. Cool the container down with liquid nitrogen.
3. Make sure that the container is dry and condense the cryogen in the cooled container (*see* **Note 3**).
4. Pick up the glow discharged grid with the tweezers and mount it on the manual or automated grid-plunger.
5. Pipette 3 μl of your mitochondrial sample (1.5 mg/ml) on to the EM grid, followed by 3 μl of the 2× gold buffer (*see* **Note 4**).
6. Blot the EM grid, either one-sided with a manual plunger or from both sides with an automated plunger.
7. Plunge the grid into the cryogen.
8. Transfer the grid into a grid storage box, repeat for the desired number of grids and store them in liquid nitrogen.

3.3 Data Acquisition with SerialEM

SerialEM is an open-source, academic software, which includes all functionalities required for cryo-ET data acquisition [12]. In addition to a low-dose mode that allows the setup of five different imaging modes and the exposure of separate areas to minimize radiation damage during acquisition, it has an implemented mapping functionality ("Navigator"), supports the execution of scripts, and provides control over all the necessary detector and energy filter parameters. We will briefly cover the data acquisition with SerialEM, but the considerations of imaging parameters apply to any cryo-ET data acquisition irrespective of the software. Before starting, make sure to optically align the TEM and perform all essential calibrations in SerialEM (e.g., pixel size on specimen level, image-, beam-, stage-shift, beam-tilt, etc.; see Serial EM home page [18] for detailed instructions on installation and calibration). Here we will focus on using the Navigator to acquire grid montages and multiple tilt series. For additional details concerning the operation of SerialEM, the reader is referred to the SerialEM documentation.

3.3.1 Fast and Systematic: Using the Navigator and Montage-Maps in SerialEM

The initial parameters that need to be defined are the magnifications at which the sample will be screened (View and Search modes), as well as the magnification at which tilt series will be recorded (Record, Focus, and Trial modes). The lateral size of mitochondrial vesicles ranges from 300 to 800 nm (depending on the isolation conditions). The field of view (FOV) in Record mode should cover that area. Once the settings are defined, it is useful to map the entire EM grid to obtain a low magnification overview that will aid targeting regions of appropriate ice thickness. SerialEM provides the option to acquire montage-maps (i.e., stitched images), at an intermediate magnification that minimizes the electron dose applied to the sample and can be used to interactively select features and move to them from the Navigator window. This function expedites the screening process and also helps to document samples, facilitating the identification of mitochondria within heterogenous samples.

1. Set up the magnification of the five modes (View, Search, Focus, Trial, Record) to cover the useful ranges (the values in the brackets correspond to the approximate pixel sizes of the K2 Summit Direct Electron Detector): View: ~5 μm FOV (~1.5 nm/pixel), Search: ~500 μm FOV (~120 nm/pixel), Record/Focus/Trial: ~700 nm FOV (~0.22 nm/pixel) (*see* **Note 5**).
2. Adjust the exposure time and acquisition mode of the detector (Super-resolution mode, Dose fractionation and frame rate) for your five acquisition modes, and the file options for your record parameter ("`Setup`" in the Camera control panel) so that they match your requirements (*see* **Note 6**).
3. For a full grid montage, open the navigator and go to "`Navigator/Montage/Full Grid montage`." Make sure to have the desired low magnification settings (~500 μm FOV) saved to the View parameters. If calibrated correctly, SerialEM will automatically choose the correct number of patches to acquire a full grid montage and the covered area will be displayed below (~2.5 × 2.5 mm^2).
4. To map the area around the current location (adjust to above magnification for the View mode if you have changed it for a full grid montage), select "`File/New Montage`." The number of tiles which also defines the covered area can be specified.

5. Start the acquisition of the map from the "`Montage`" floating window by clicking "`Start.`"
6. After the acquisition, load the map into the Navigator window by clicking "`New map.`"
7. To add points of interest to the navigator, click on "`Add points`" in the navigator floating window and then click on the area of interest on the map. You can add comments to the points in the Navigator and assign them different colors for easy identification on the map.

3.3.2 Tilt Series Acquisition

During the tilt series acquisition, the specimen is sequentially tilted, and projection movies are acquired. Despite high mechanic accuracy of the stage, the sample is never completely eucentric during the tilt. To compensate for the residual lateral and horizontal motion, tracking and focusing are usually performed after each tilt. In order to prevent the sample from unnecessary exposure both are performed on user-defined areas that are translated with away from the exposure area along the tiltaxis ("low dose").

1. Once you have found and centered a suitable region at intermediate magnification (View mode), move the sample to eucentric height by running the routine "`Tasks/Eucentric rough.`" For high magnification also run "`Tasks/Eucentric fine.`"
2. Define the position of the Focus and Trial area in the "Low Dose" control panel (*see* **Note 7**).
3. Open the Tilt series dialog box.
4. Check and define all the parameters of the tilt series. The major parameters are the tilt scheme (uni-, bidirectional, or dose-symmetric), tilt range, tilt increment, starting angle, settling time, and criteria for tracking and focusing (*see* **Note 8**).
5. Press "`GO`" to start the acquisition of the tilt series.

3.3.3 Setting Up a Batch Acquisition

The option to set up a batch acquisition is implemented via the Navigator window. SerialEM requires two maps per position, one at low (View mode) and one at high magnification (Record mode). The reference maps are stored in two different files, and the function "Realign to Item" is used by SerialEM to find back areas of interest based on the stored stage coordinates and by cross-correlation of the images.

1. Open two new files for the high and low magnification maps (e.g., "`maps.mrc`" and "`anchors.mrc`") by clicking "`File/Open New.`"
2. Navigate to the area of interest. If you have stored them in the navigator, locate them using the "`Go To XYZ`" button.

3. Acquire a preview picture of the feature of interest. If necessary, center it and acquire another preview picture. Make sure that the image shift is low (<0.5 FOV).
4. Toggle to the "`maps.mrc`" file from the "`Buffer Control`" panel and click "`New Map`."
5. Acquire a View image.
6. Toggle to the "`maps.mrc`" file from the "`Buffer Control`" panel and click "`New Map`."
7. Check the boxes "`Acquire at position`" and "`New file at item`" for the high magnification? item in the navigator window.
8. Repeat this procedure for all your points/areas of interest.
9. After having created high and low magnification maps at all points, open the batch acquisition window by "`Navigator/ Acquire at points...`."
10. Select the desired operations to execute at each point. If the eucentricity has not been refined at all points, this option should be checked.
11. Start the batch acquisition by pressing "`GO`."

3.4 Reconstructing a 3D Tomogram from 2D Micrographs

In order to reconstruct a 3D tomogram from the 2D projections of a tilt series, several mechanical and optical distortions that arise during the acquisition of a projection at near-atomic resolution have to be corrected for. The first major step is the alignment of the subframes, to account for mechanical and beam-induced motion of the sample during the exposure. For this task we recommend motioncor2 [13]. The second major step is the alignment of the tilted images to a common 3D coordinate system. If the images contain gold beads (following Subheading 3.1), the following steps will cover the tilt series alignment with TOM/PyTOM. If this is not the case, we recommend IMOD for alignment by patch tracking (not covered here, see IMOD web site for more information [19]).

1. Run motioncor2 by executing the following command in the terminal (*see* **Note 9**):

```
motioncor2 -InTif 'path to your frames' -OutMrc 'targetpath'
-Patch 5 5
```

2. PyTOM and TOM read projections in the *.em format based on a basename followed by an index ascending according to the tilt angle (i.e., projection1.em corresponds to −60°, the maximum negative tilt). To sort the motion-corrected frames according to the tilt series and the tilt angle in ascending order (e.g., "tomogram1/sorted/sorted[1- 61].em," run av3_sortTSbymdoc) (*see* **Note 10**):

```
av3_sortTSbymdoc(numtomo, mdocdir, mdocprefix, rawframesuf-
fix, framedir, projdir, dim, scale)
```

The information of the corresponding angles is derived from the SerialEM *.mdoc file. Here, numtomo is the index of the tomogram (in the above example 1), mdocdir and mdocprefix specify the mdoc logfile, rawframesuffix and framedir the raw frames, projdir the location of the sorted and aligned projections and dim the lateral size of the generated images (in pixels). Define a downscaling factor (e.g., 4: scale = 4) to generate downscaled projections, which will accelerate and facilitate the tilt series alignment.

3. Start the GUI for gold marker by typing "tom_setmark" in the Matlab shell.
4. Load the tilt series by clicking "New" and selecting the last projection in the directory of the scaled projections (Fig. 1, label 1). Four new windows will open.
5. Choose the first gold marker by clicking "ADD" in the main panel (Fig. 1, label 2), and then clicking on your desired gold marker in the working images (Fig. 1, label 3) and the magnified image (Fig. 1, label 4).
6. Check the "Turbo" box (Fig. 1, label 5) to automatically load the next projection, and click the marker for all projections of the tilt series.
7. After clicking one marker for the whole tilt series, add new markers by clicking "NEW" and adding them as before. Click at least three gold markers in all projections and compute the alignment. The residual error should ideally be below 1.5 pixels.
8. Write a markerfile corresponding to the full-sized images by multiplying the values in the created markerfile with the previously applied downscaling factor from **step 4** of this section (e.g., factor 2).
9. Refine the marker positions using av3_finelocate (matlab) using the full-sized projections and write out the corresponding markerfile.

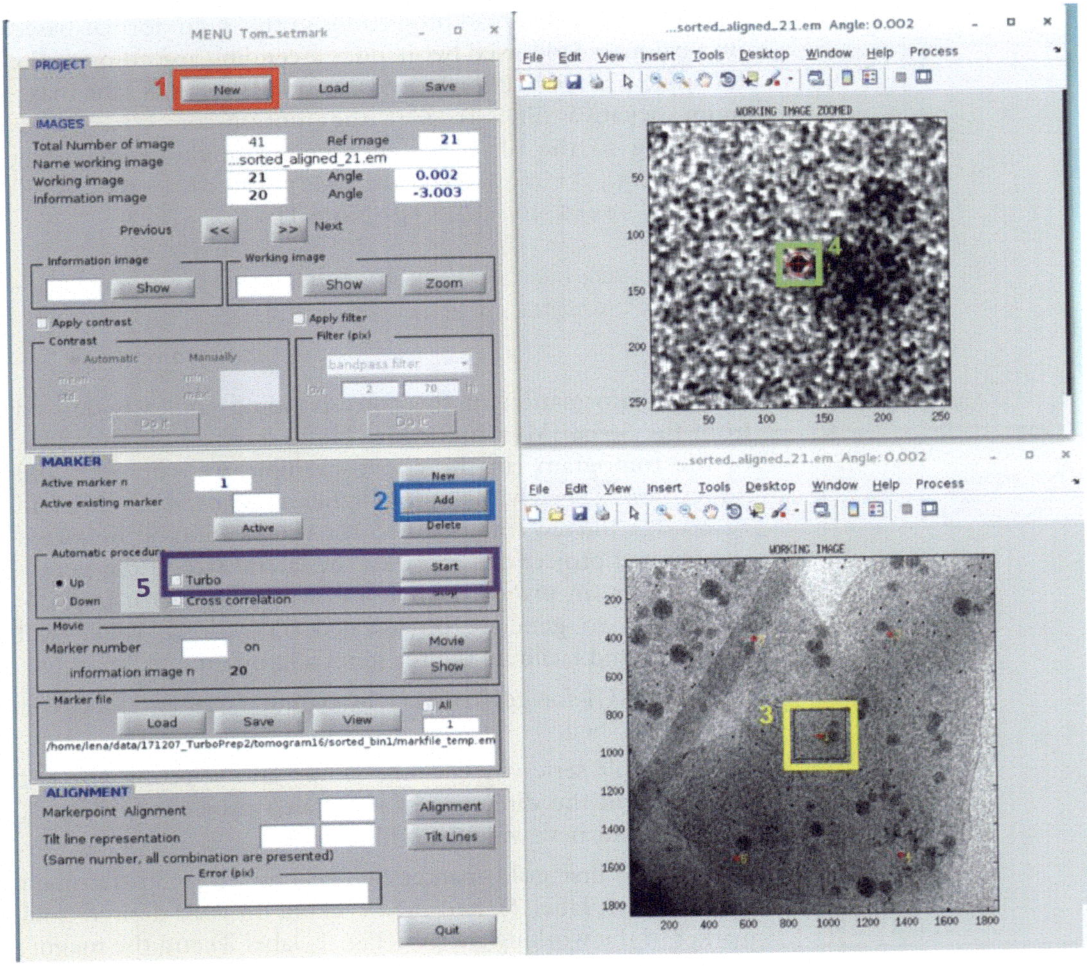

Fig. 1 Interface of the `tom_setmark` GUI. Load a new tilt series from the Project tab (1). Add the first marker by clicking "`ADD`" (2), and then selecting the area containing your first marker in the working image (bottom right, 3). Then click on the gold marker in the zoomed image (top right, 4). Check the box "`Turbo`" (5) and click "`Start`"

10. Run the function "`reconstructTomogram.py`" with the desired parameters to align the projections and reconstruct the tomogram by weighted backprojection. Type "`reconstructTomogram.py --help`" to display all parameters. Choose the 0° projection as the reference index, the refined markerfile as markerfile ("`markerfile_refined.em`") and the most central marker as reference marker (*see* **Note 11**).

3.5 Subtomogram Averaging

The resolution of a tomogram is typically not limited by the sampling (=voxel size on specimen level), but rather by the SNR. Similar to SPA, subtomogram averaging (STA) enables the reconstruction of a high-resolution density by aligning and averaging

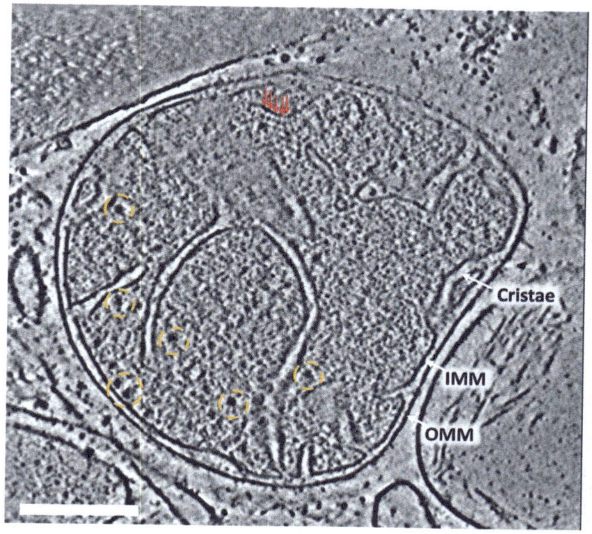

Fig. 2 Slice from a reconstructed tomogram of a human mitochondrion (data acquired with the Volta Phase Plate at 300 kV). In the resulting tomogram of the mitochondrion, the outer and inner mitochondrial membranes (OMM and IMM), as well as cristae, membrane-associated mitoribosomes and ATP synthases can be identified

multiple subtomograms each depicting copies of the macromolecule. A common approach to STA is to (1) interactively localize copies of the macromolecule of interest in a few tomograms, (2) to align and average the corresponding subvolumes by fast rotational matching allowing exhaustive orientation sampling [20], (3) to localize more copies in the remaining datasets by template matching, and (4) to determine a higher resolution average of different classes of the molecule using real space methods. In order to select initial candidates, exclude template bias and select for true positives, the complex of interest should be visible in the tomogram. For mitochondria, the ATP synthases and mitoribosomes can be identified in a high-quality tomogram (Fig. 2).

3.5.1 Creating an Initial, Reference-Free Average from Manually Picked Particles by FRM Alignment

1. Open chimera and load the reconstructed tomogram (*see* **Note 12**).
2. Open the Volume tracer in the Volume Viewer Panel ("Tools/ Volume Tracer," Fig. 3).
3. Choose how to place a marker (e.g., using middle + control button).
4. Set the color of the marker by clicking on it and choose an opacity of 0.1–0.2 to facilitate particle selection. Make sure that within the Viewing panel (Favorites/Side View/Effects), the box "`single layer`" (under transparency) is unchecked.

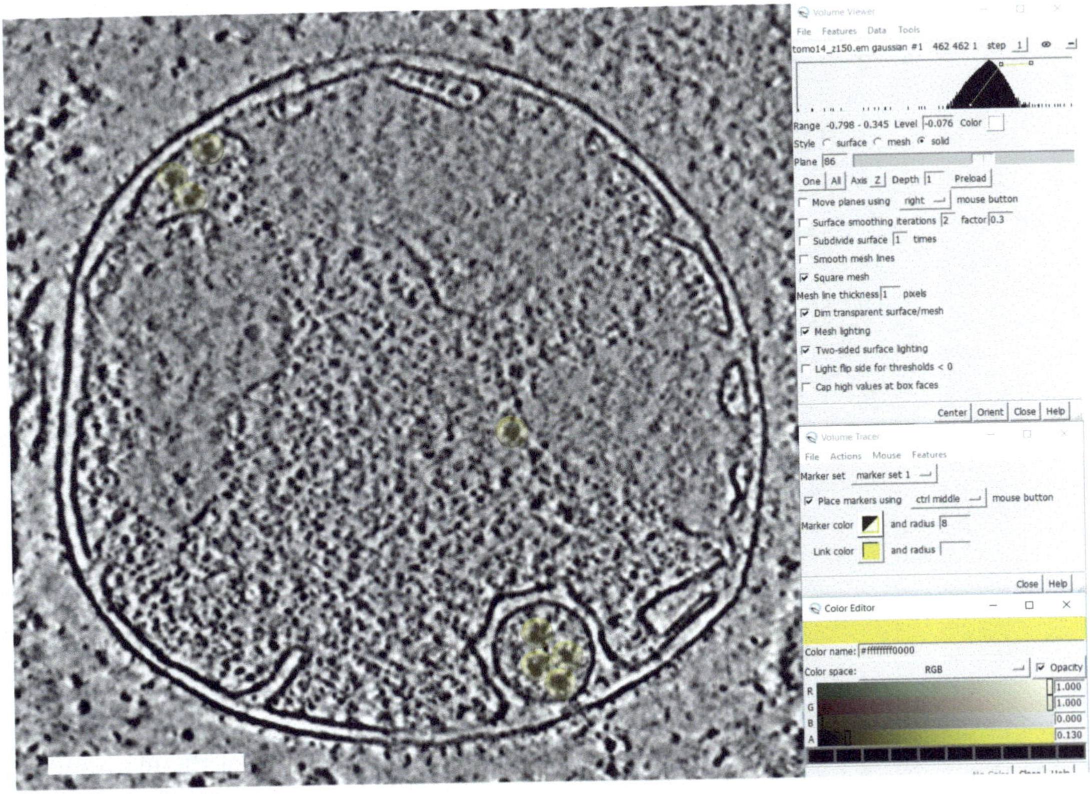

Fig. 3 Manual particle picking in Chimera. Use the Volume filter and/or adjust the histogram to get sufficient contrast. Open the Volume Tracer dialog box (bottom right) and choose the color and radius of your marker. Place markers by clicking on the data planes

5. Use the slider to go through your z-slices to locate your particles. For each particle you wish to pick, place a marker on top of it to record its location. When you are done, save the marker file ("File/Save current marker set as," e.g., `tomogram1/reconstruction/man_picked.cmm`).
6. Use the matlab script av3_cmm2particlelist to read the *xyz* coordinates from the "`.cmm`" marker file (textfile) and write a Pytom compatible particle list in `.xml` format (*see* **Note 13**).
7. Run the `reconstruct_subtomos_INFR.py` function to reconstruct subvolumes with the INFR method (*see* **Note 14**). In this example full-magnification subvolumes of 256 × 256 × 256 voxels are reconstructed:

```
pytom PathToPytom/reconstruction/reconstruct_subvolume-
s_INFR.py -d [Path_to_unweighted_projections/] -s 256 -b 1 -o
0,0,0 -p path_to_particleList.xml
```

8. Check that your subtomograms indeed depict particles using with tom_dspcub (matlab) or Chimera. In case of a mitoribosome, you should clearly see a central density in the lowpass-filtered subtomogram.
9. Make a directory for your FRM alignment.
10. For an initial alignment, it is advisable to scale down the subvolumes to 5–10 Å voxel size. Use either `tom_rescale` (matlab) or `resize` (pytom) to write downscaled versions of the reconstructed full-size subtomograms (*see* **step 7**).
11. Generate a particleList for your resized particles (*see* **step 6**).
12. Create an average from your particles created with `tom_average` (matlab) or `average.py` (pytom). Display the average with `tom_dspcub` (matlab) or in Chimera and check that there is a clear density in the center.
13. Generate a mask with `tom_spheremask` (matlab) or `initSphere.py` (pytom). Check that the mask encompasses the structure of interest (Fig. 3).
14. The FRM alignment requires a jobfile (e.g., "`job.xml`") format specifying the parameters (**bold** parameters need to be adjusted to your environment and data) (*see* **Note 15**). To this end, execute "av3_createFRMjobfile" in the matlab shell to create the jobfile with the respective parameters. These are the lower (here: 8) and upper (64) limits of spherical harmonics, lowpass for initial iteration (6), number of iterations (30), maximum offset of peaks (30), name of resulting average ("`average.em`"), mask ("`maskfile.em`"), pixelsize (5.24 Å), particle diameter (250 Å) and particlelist ("`particleList.xml`"):

```
av3_createFRMjobfile('job.xml', 8, 64, 6, 30, 30, 'average.
em', 'maskfile.em', 5.24, 250.0, 'particleList.xml')
```

15. Run the FRM alignment:

```
pytom PathToPytom/frm/FRMAlignment.py -j job.xml -v
```

After each iteration, an unfiltered average, as well as an average filtered to the determined resolution and an updated particleList will be written out (*see* **Note 16**) (Fig. 4).

3.5.2 Template Matching

During the template matching, the cross-correlation of a masked template structure is computed at different orientations and at each voxel coordinate. Therefore, the tomographic volume, a template, a mask, and a list of rotations are required. Due to the noise within the tomogram and to speed up the computation, template matching is usually performed on downscaled tomograms. Depending on the macromolecule of interest, we recommend an effective voxel

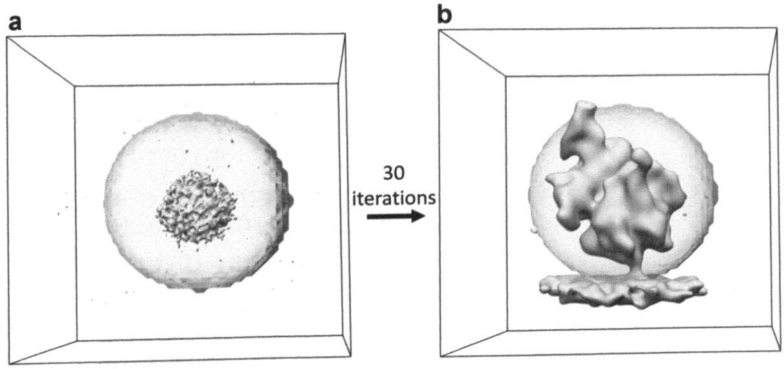

Fig. 4 FRM alignment of manually picked particles. (**a**) The average of the subtomograms (gray) with randomly assigned angles should have a spherical shape, and the mask transparent should encircle it. (**b**) After 30 rounds of alignment, the spherical shape should ideally converge to a structure resembling your molecule of interest, a human mitoribosome computed from 231 subtomograms in this case

size of 1–2 nm (the example of the human Mitoribosome was performed at 2 nm).

1. Generate a template by applying the appropriate scaling factor to either your reference-free average or external structure (*see* **step 10**, Subheading 3.4) (*see* **Note 17**).
2. Generate a mask with same dimensions as the template (*see* **step 12**, Subheading 3.5.1).
3. If computational time is scarce, crop the tomogram in *z* to only capture the sample (note down the *z* offset!). Use either `read` (pytom) or `tom_emread` (matlab) to read and write a subvolume of the tomogram.
4. Execute `av3_createTMjobfile` in the matlab shell to create the jobfile with the respective parameters (tomogram "`tomogram.em`," template "`template.em`," mask "`mask.em`," missing wedge of 30°, 7112 angles specified in "`angles_12.85_7112.em`") (*see* **Note 18**):

```
av3_createTMjobfile('JobInfo.xml', 'tomogram.em', 'template.em', 'mask.em', 30, 'angles_12.85_7112.em')
```

5. Start the Job with the following function that supports message passing interface (MPI). The precise MPI syntax might vary depending on your system (*see* **Note 19**):

```
mpiexec --tag-output -n 16 pytom/path_to_pytom/bin/localization.py JobInfo.xml 4 4 1
```

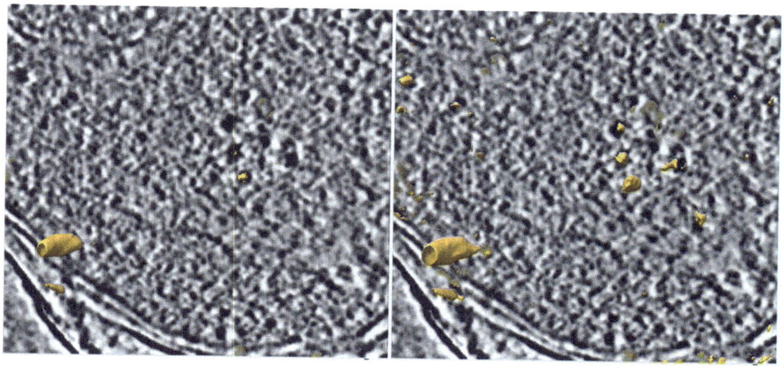

Fig. 5 Tomogram with superimposed cross-correlation peaks from template matching. The volume file containing the scores ("`scores.em`," orange density) obtained by template matching was superimposed with the tomogram (shown as slice). At a high threshold (left), the most significant correlation peaks superimpose with mitoribosomes (center) as well ice contamination (left). Reducing the threshold reveals less significant correlation peaks that superimpose with mitoribosomal densities (right image; center and top left part), as well as false-positive matches with the membrane (edges)

6. Inspect the resulting correlation function by opening the "`scores.em`" file and superimposing it with your tomogram. Adjust the histogram to show the highest scores (Fig. 5) (*see* **Note 20**).

3.5.3 Particle Extraction and Subtomogram Reconstruction

Prior to subtomogram reconstruction, the resulting correlation ("`scores.em`") and angle ("`angles.em`") volumes obtained by template matching need to be converted into a list (paricleList in PyTom, motiflist in TOM) containing the particle coordinates, orientation, and correlation values. During the particle extraction step, the voxels around the high correlation peaks are zeroed within a defined radius to exclude multiple entries of the same particle. To separate false positives from true-positive particles in your template matching results, it is usually necessary to manually filter the identified correlation peaks. This can be done with "Chooser," a Chimera plugin available on the PyTom website.

1. Extract the particle coordinates into an .xml file and a motiflist with the following function (*see* **Note 21**):

```
pytom PathToPyTom/bin/extractCandidates.py -j job.xml -n
700 -s 8 -r scores.em -o angles.em -p pl.xml -m targetpath.em
-t pathToNewParticles
```

2. Open Chimera and load the tomogram that was used for template matching. Load the corresponding particlelist with the Chooser.

3. The Chooser will display all the entries from the particlelist, starting from the highest correlation values. Inspect all the correlation peaks and assign class indices (e.g., 1 for correct and 0 false-positive matches; more than two class labels can be assigned if desired) (*see* **Note 22**).
4. Save the class labels by clicking "Save" and close the Chooser. Each line in the resulting text file corresponds to the respective entry in the particle-/motifList.
5. Filter the particle-/motifList by excluding the entries according to the assigned classLabels by executing `av3_filterClassLabels` (*see* **Note 23**):

```
av3_filterClassLabels(motlin, labelfile, class, motlout,
zheight, scaling, rawsize)
```

6. Run the INFR subtomogram reconstruction (*see* **step 7**, Subheading 3.4), or use the weighted back projection algorithm with the filtered particleList as input (*see* **Note 24**):

```
reconstructWB.py -p particleList.xml --projectionDirectory
../reconstructTomo/alignedProjections/ -s 128 -b 1 -o 0,0,192
```

7. Check the correct reconstruction by looking at the subtomograms. Depending on the downscaling factor and pixel size, it might be necessary to apply a strong filter to see features (*see* **Note 25**).
8. Average the particles with the following function (*see* **Note 26**):

```
pytom PathToPyTom/bin/average.py -p particleList.xml -a Aver-
age.em
```

3.5.4 Gold Standard Subtomogram Alignment in Real Space

In addition to the FRM alignment (*see* Subheading 3.4), PyTom also provides the option to perform the subtomogram alignment in real space. The real space alignment tends to be more accurate because it simultaneously samples rotational and translational degrees of freedom, but due to the higher computational requirements the rotational search is restricted. Thus, the method requires initial starting angles, which were at this point either determined from the template matching or by a previous round of FRM alignment. The following steps will cover the gold standard real space alignment, which splits the dataset into two independent halves used for the alignment against independent references to reduce over-fitting.

1. Create a directory for the real space alignment.

2. For an initial alignment, it is advisable to downscale the particles to 5–10 Å voxel size. Use either `tom_rescale` (matlab) or `resize` (pytom) to write downscaled particles (*see* Subheading 3.3.1, **step 4**), or use a downscaling parameter ("`-b`") for reducing volumes on the fly during the alignment (*see* **step 6**).
3. Generate a particleList for your resized particles (*see* Subheading 3.4, **step 6**).
4. Create an average from your particles with `tom_average` (matlab) or `average.py`. Open the average and check that there is a clear density in the center (*see* Subheading 3.4, **step 12**).
5. Generate a spherical mask (*see* **step 13**, Subheading 3.4). Check that the mask encompasses the structure of interest (Fig. 3).
6. Run the "gold standard" Real Space local alignment. In this example, ten iterations of alignment are performed with the data downscaled on the fly by a factor of 2 using an initial rotational sampling of 3° increment (subsequently adjusted according to resolution) in three shells:

```
mpirun -n numberOfCPUs pytom PathToPytom/bin/GLocalJob.py -p
particleList.xml -r Reference.em -m Mask.em --SphericalMask --
angleShells 3 --angleIncrement 3. -d ./ -n 10 -b 2 --pixelSize
2.62 --particleDiameter 250
```

3.5.5 Classification

Subtomograms with differing structural features, e.g., due to a particular conformational state or different composition, can be disentangled during subsequent classification. This is usually done by constrained principle component analysis (CPCA), where a pairwise cross-correlation matrix of the subtomograms is computed and subsequently grouped by principle component analysis and k-means clustering. This allows for the removal of false positives from the dataset, as well as the enrichment of subtomograms showing distinct pronounced structural features such as the small ribosomal subunit or the membrane (Fig. 6a).

1. Generate a mask encompassing the feature of interest within your initial average (Fig. 6a), either with Chimera (shape mask), or with `initSphere` (pytom) for a spherical mask (*see* Subheading 3.4, **step 13**).
2. Compute a cross-correlation matrix of all particles by running the following command (*see* **Note 27**):

```
mpiexec --tag-output -n numberOfCPUs pytom PathToPytom/calcu-
late_correlation_matrix.py -p particleList.xml -m Mask.mrc -f
10 -b 1
```

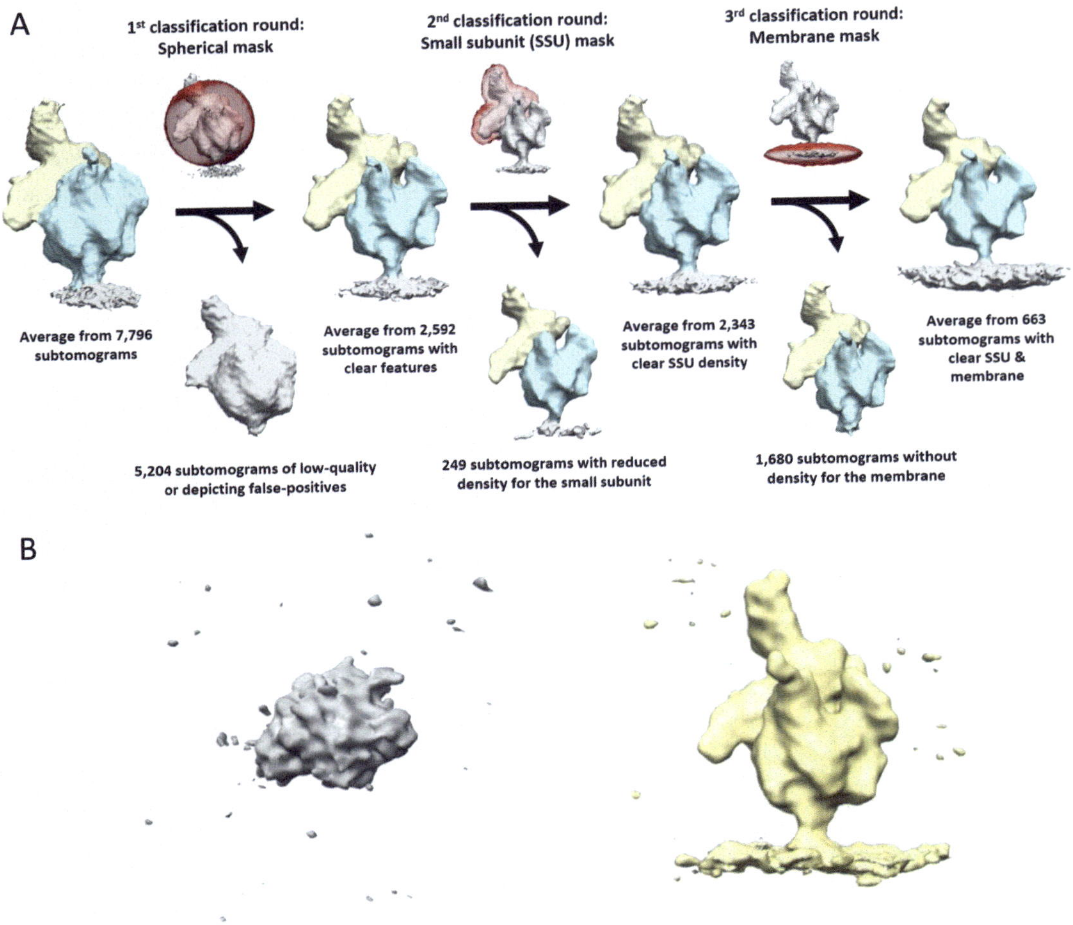

Fig. 6 Classification scheme to enrich mitoribosomes with a clear membrane density. (**a**) By performing multiple rounds of classification with different masks (red), subtomograms with a clear membrane density can be separated from subtomograms depicting noise or lacking a clear density for small subunit or membrane. (**b**) Class-averages computed from ~100 subtomograms upon the initial classification of 7796 subtomograms with a spherical mask. The left class-average (gray) represents a class of false-positives matches, e.g., ice, gold markers, or membrane densities that should be discarded. The right class-average (yellow) already shows clear mitoribosomal features, i.e., the small and large subunit as well as the membrane (both averages were filtered in Chimera with a Gaussian filter of 1.2)

3. Group the data based on the output "`correlation_matrix.csv`" using CPCA and k-means clustering (*see* **Note 28**). Here, the data are projected to five principal components and grouped 7800 subtomograms into 67 classes (Fig. 6a):

```
pytom path_to_pytom/bin/classifyCPCA.py -p particleList.xml
-o pL_classified.xml -c correlation_matrix.csv -e 5 -n 67 -a
"Average"
```

4. Open and inspect all the classes (here "`Average1-67.em`") in Chimera (Fig. 6b) and note down the class numbers that you would like to merge for your further analysis.
5. Filter the particleList to include only the classes that you have picked using the pytom function `splitByClass`:

   Load the pytom module and open the interactive shell by typing "`ipytom`." Then run the following lines to split the particlelist "`pL_classified.xml`":

```
pl=ParticleList()
pl.fromXMLFile('pL_classified.xml')
lists=pl.splitByClass()
```

   Specify the desired classes in the square brackets and write them out to a new particlelist by running the following lines:

```
ribos=lists[1] + lists[2]
ribos.toXMLFile('pickedClasses.xml')
```

   For convenience, you can also use the provided bash script `merge_pl_classes.sh` which also allows merging of classes from several particleLists and contains explanations.
6. If desired, apply further rounds of classification with different masks to separate the subtomograms according to variations in specific areas, e.g., membrane density (Fig. 6a). Alternatively, repeat the alignment with the filtered set of subtomograms.

4 Notes

1. Lysis efficiency will slightly differ depending on the tightness of the individual Glass-Teflon-Potter. Monitor the cell lysis in a light microscope and adjust the number of strokes to achieve of roughly 60%.
2. Test at least two dilutions of your sample (e.g., undiluted and 1:3). In the case where you characterize your purification protocol for the first time sample a wider range of concentrations. We found that Nanodrop measurements at 280 nm provide reproducible results with regards to mitochondria and vesicle densities and recommend the following conditions for the mitochondrial sample: 1.5 mg/ml in 20 mM Hepes pH 7.4 and 150 mM Sucrose (human) or 600 mM Sorbitol (yeast). The concentration of the mitochondrial sample is a critical parameter to achieve high-quality tomograms since it affects the ice thickness. Plunge-freezing of four grids roughly takes 30 min, so the handling time is neglectable compared to

mitochondrial isolation protocols, but mitochondria should be kept on ice.

3. Make sure to not contaminate the ethane or ethane-propane with any liquid nitrogen or water, e.g., from your breath. Try to maintain a protective atmosphere of cold nitrogen vapor in your container at all time to prevent contamination of your sample by ice crystals from the air humidity.
4. For iso-osmotic conditions, mitochondria require 150–300 mM sucrose (human) and ~600 mM sorbitol (yeast) in the isolation buffer (*see* Subheading 2.1). However, the sugar concentration should be as low as possible in the vitrified sample to provide a good contrast and to prevent beam damage in the TEM.
5. The choice of the magnification is a tradeoff between FOV and the pixel size. A large FOV enables covering large or even multiple vesicles, while the pixel size puts an upper limit to the maximum resolution. In practice, the maximum resolution is limited to approximately 50% of the Nyquist frequency, i.e., the minimal distinguishable distance is four times the pixelsize on the specimen level. For *in-organello* studies of mitochondrial translation a pixel size of ~2 Å does not limit the resolution, which is rather restricted by the low contrast arising from the sample thickness and the crowded environment of the mitochondrion.
6. It is recommended to test the beam and detector settings in a region of the grid that does not contain useful mitochondrial vesicles, or on a completely different grid to avoid unnecessary radiation damage to the sample. The exposure times for your View/Search/Focus/Trial mode should be adjusted as low as possible but high enough to yield sufficient signal in the resulting image. For your record parameter, the exposure time should be adjusted so that the accumulated dose does not exceed 80 $e^{-}/Å^2$ for 200 kV respectively 120 $e^{-}/Å^2$ for 300 kV EM for thinner samples (accumulated dose = dose per tiltangle × number of images). Saving record frames in super-resolution takes slightly longer than in simple counting, and the files are four times bigger. However, these considerations are negligible for tomography, and more critical for SPA data acquisition, where the fairly small gain in detector quantum efficiency often does not outweigh the lower throughput. Regarding the file options, it is advisable to save the files as .tif files with LZW compression as one stack, which yields compression factors of ~40. Including the tilt angle in the filename is also recommended.
7. The position of the Focus/Trial area should differ from the Exposure area by more than the beam diameter. To measure

the beam diameter, you can over-expose carbon to the beam by putting the screen down with the Record mode settings. If possible, try to have some carbon or other features in your Focus/Trial area, since discrete, high-contrast features facilitate the focusing and tracking.

8. For initial or standard data acquisition, we recommend the following settings: bidirectional tilt scheme, tilt range −60° to +60°; starting angle −20°, tilt increment of 2° or 3°. The settling time strongly depends on the stage of the microscope, but 15 s is a good starting value that can be increased if blurring is observed in the Trial image, or reduced otherwise for higher throughput. For all other parameters the provided standard settings are a good starting point. We routinely employ a dose-symmetric tilt scheme [21], which has been recently implemented in the SerialEM tilt series dialog box. It requires slightly more time per tilt series but provides a better dose distribution and is advantageous for high-resolution subtomogram averaging.
9. These are the minimum input requirements for both global and local motion, with the standard patch size of 5 × 5. For more information, e.g., on how to apply gain normalization, see the motioncor2 user manual or type "motioncor2" into your terminal.
10. `av3_sortTSbymdoc(numtomo, mdocdir, mdocprefix, rawframesuffix, framedir, projdir, dim, scale)`: `numtomo` defines the number of tomograms and corresponding mdoc files, `mdocdir` the path to your mdoc file, `mdocprefix` the prefix of the mdoc file, `rawframesuffix` the filesuffix of the unaligned frames (e.g., ".tif" or ". mrc"), `framedir` the directory containing the aligned frames, `projdir` directory of projections, `dim` the desired dimension (cut to square) scale the desired scaling factor. The function will create the number of folders defined by `numtomo`, sort the corresponding tiltseries according to the tiltangles into the folder defined in `projdir` and scale and cut the projections.
11. Choose a downscaling factor between 4 and 8 to increase the signal in the resulting volume and keep the file size reasonable for subsequent template matching. Pytom also provides an alternative tomogram reconstruction method, called INFR [22]. It requires aligned but unweighted projections, which can also be obtained using `reconstructTomogram.py` with `---weightingType 0`. Run `reconstruct_INFR.py` to perform the tomogram reconstruction with INFR. The resulting tomogram will have better contrast, which facilitates the manual and automated picking (template matching) of particles.

12. Depending on the data quality and binning, it might be necessary to filter the volume. Go to "Tools/Volume Filter" and apply a Gaussian filter with width 0.5–0.9 to your volume. It might also be necessary to select solid rendering and adjust the histogram for a good contrast.
13. Check the *xyz* coordinates in your generated particleList. They should be positive values corresponding to the dimension of the tomogram you have picked. If the tilt range is different than −60° to +60°, define the opening angle of the missing wedge respectively.
14. `reconstruct_subtomos_INFR.py`: The subtomograms will be written into the specified path in the `particleList.xml`. The option `--d` specifies the input projections, `-s` specifies the box size, `-b` the downscaling factor (be sure to use the same the downscaling factor that corresponds to the tomogram you used for picking your coordinates), and `-o` the offset of the coordinate system in case the positions were picked on cropped tomograms. The function does not have the option to apply a downscaling to the subtomograms. If downscaled subtomograms are intended, create downscaled projections and use them as an input for the subtomogram reconstruction (*see* Subheading 3.3.1, **step 4**).
15. The parameter "`Frequency`" defines the starting spatial frequency (in inverse pixels) for the lowpass filter in the first iteration of alignment, and "`BandwidthRange`" the bandwidth range that is used throughout all iterations (i.e., a high-pass filter is effectively used). Thirty iterations should usually result in a converging average.
16. Ideally, the resolution will increase and meaningful structural features will manifest themselves. However, for small particle sizes, the structure can align structures according to the missing wedge than their structures. Nevertheless, for large complexes such as the ribosome this reference-free FRM alignment typically succeeds. If the FRM alignment results in a subtomogram average with distinctive features and details, the gold standard real space alignment with the angles from the FRM alignment might improve the result even further (*see* Subheading 3.3.3).
17. If an external structure as a template is intended, apply the correct scaling and have matching density values (i.e., both positive/negative values for the electron-density). Also, make sure that handedness corresponds your reference system (left- or right-handed). To generate a template for the human mitoribosome you can use the EMDB structure EMDB-2876. Load it in Chimera ("`File/Fetch by ID`"), and save the density map as an mrc density file ("`2876.mrc`"). Determine the scaling factor to de-magnify from 1.34 Å/vox to the desired voxel

size (e.g., 20 Å/vox) and divide the box size by that factor to yield your final box size (e.g., 16). Then run the following command with the value in the square brackets to rescale it:

```
map=tom_mrcread('2876.mrc')
map=tom_rescale(map.Value,[16,16,16])
```

If the map needs to be mirrored or inverted, use the following commands (otherwise skip them):

```
map=tom_mirror(map,'x')
map=map*-1
```

Save the map by executing the following line:

```
tom_emwrite('5aj4_scaled.mrc',map)
```

18. The angular search of 7112 angles (12.85° increment) is a good standard parameter. The different angle files are located within `PathtoPytom/angles/angleLists/`.
19. The last three numbers indicate the splitting of the volume in *x*, *y*, and *z*. This should ideally correspond to the number of nodes. The division of the volume by the provided factor has to result in full integers.
20. If the results do not correspond to the features, make sure to have checked all the requirements mentioned in **Note 14**. Especially for small, elongated particles, template matching might fail. In this case, apply a higher downscaling to the tomogram.
21. `extractCandidates.py`: Option `-n` defines the number of particles,`-s` defines the radius around the peak which will be zeroed to exclude multiple picking of the same particle, `-p` defines the path to the particle list, and `--m` defines the path to write out the results in TOM-compatible motiflist format. A good template matching result will show a Gaussian distribution for the determined cross-correlation peaks ("`Value`" in `particleList.xml` (PyTom), column 1 in AV3-motiflist). However, within the crowded mitochondrial matrix the results of the template matching often show false-positive matches (Fig. 5). In order to filter the template matching results, multiply the correlation volumes prior to particle extraction with a binary mask encompassing the mitochondrion (e.g., by generating the mask with Chimera Volume Tracer). If the particle list is to be used directly for subtomogram reconstruction (*see* **step** 7, Subheading 3.4), provide an option `-t` with an argument, which defines the target directory for the reconstructed subtomograms.

22. At this step it is beneficial to exclude as many false positives as possible. However, this is not absolutely critical since a classification will also help in removing false positives (Fig. 6b).

23. `av3_filterClassLabels`: `motlin` defines the input motiflist file, `labelfile` the file containing the manual classifications from the Chooser, `class` defines the class index that will be included (e.g., 1) and `motlout` the name of the filtered output motifllist. The last three parameters - `z_height` (defines the *z* position at which, if applicable, the downscaled tomogram was cropped), `scaling` (scaling factor of the tomogram) and `rawsize` (dimension of the non-downscaled projections)—are optional, and used for the generation of a non-scaled motiflist with the coordinate system of the aligned raw projections.

24. The argument of option `-s` defines the box size, `-b` the downscaling factor of the particle coordinates compared to the projection, and `--o` the offset of the particle coordinates from the coordinate system chosen for the reconstruction, which is used in the .xml file, if any.

25. If the box is empty, make sure that the supplied coordinates in the .xml file correspond to your tomogram dimension. (0 to 3838/3710 for full-size data from a K2 detector).

26. The resulting average should show distinctive structural features if the template matching and reconstruction have worked. If this is not the case, the template matching probably resulted in a considerable number of false positives which have to be removed by repeating **steps 2–5**, checking the template matching results or repeating the template matching. If the results do not improve, manual particle selection might be the only option (*see* Subheading 3.4). Mitoribosomes are reliably detected by template matching in very thin tomograms (<150 nm) with good contrast but are hardly detected in thicker tomograms where they can still be identified by eye.

27. `calculate_correlation_matrix.py`: Option `-f` represents a low-pass filter, and `--b` a downsampling factor to be applied to the subtomograms.

28. `classifyCPCA.py`: Option `-p` defines the path to the particlelist (make sure that the path to the subtomograms within the particlelist is correct), `-o` the targetpath for the output-particlelist that will include the classlabels, `-c` filename of the correlation matrix, `-e` number of eigenvectors; `-n` the number of classes; `-a` basename of the class-averages. Five eigenvectors are usually sufficient to represent the main features of the subtomograms. On the one hand side, the number of classes should be chosen as high as possible in order to separate subtomograms depicting different conformations. On the

other hand, the number should be chosen sufficiently small, such that a class-average contains enough subtomograms to yield sufficient SNR to distinguish features. For mitoribosomes, 100 subtomograms/class should yield enough signal for the reliable assessment of class-averages (Fig. 6b).

Acknowledgement

We would like to thank Dr Stuart Howes for critical comments on the manuscript. This work was supported by funding from the Nederlandse Organisatie voor Wetenschappelijke Onderzoek (Vici 724.016.001), the European Research Council under the European Union's Horizon2020 Programme (ERC Consolidator Grant Agreement 724425—BENDER) and the Deutsche Forschungsgemeinschaft (FO 716/3-2).

References

1. Lucić V, Förster F, Baumeister W (2005) Structural studies by electron tomography: from cells to molecules. Annu Rev Biochem 74:833–865
2. Dubochet J et al (1988) Cryo-electron microscopy of vitrified specimens. Q Rev Biophys 21 (02):129
3. Ott M, Herrmann JM (2010) Co-translational membrane insertion of mitochondrially encoded proteins. Biochim Biophys Acta 1803(6):767–775
4. Asano S et al (2015) Proteasomes. A molecular census of 26S proteasomes in intact neurons. Science 347(6220):439–442
5. Förster F, Hegerl R (2007) Structure determination in situ by averaging of tomograms. Methods Cell Biol 79:741–767
6. Wan W, Briggs JAG (2016) Cryo-electron tomography and subtomogram averaging. Methods Enzymol 579:329–367
7. Nickell S et al (2005) TOM software toolbox: acquisition and analysis for electron tomography. J Struct Biol 149(3):227–234
8. Hrabe T, Chen Y, Pfeffer S, Cuellar LK, Mangold A-V, Förster F (2012) PyTom: a python-based toolbox for localization of macromolecules in cryo-electron tomograms and subtomogram analysis. J Struct Biol 178 (2):177–188
9. Daum G, Böhni PC, Schatz G (1982) Import of proteins into mitochondria. Cytochrome b2 and cytochrome c peroxidase are located in the intermembrane space of yeast mitochondria. J Biol Chem 257(21):13028–13033
10. Englmeier R, Pfeffer S, Förster F (2017) Structure of the human mitochondrial ribosome studied in situ by cryoelectron tomography. Structure 25(10):1574–1581.e2
11. Frezza C, Cipolat S, Scorrano L (2007) Organelle isolation: functional mitochondria from mouse liver, muscle and cultured fibroblasts. Nat Protoc 2(2):287–295
12. Mastronarde DN (2005) Automated electron microscope tomography using robust prediction of specimen movements. J Struct Biol 152(1):36–51
13. Zheng SQ, Palovcak E, Armache J-P, Verba KA, Cheng Y, Agard DA (2017) MotionCor2: anisotropic correction of beam-induced motion for improved cryo-electron microscopy. Nat Methods 14(4):331–332
14. Pettersen EF et al (2004) UCSF chimera - a visualization system for exploratory research and analysis. J Comput Chem 25 (13):1605–1612
15. PyTom | Python and Tomography. http://pytom.org/. Accessed 22 Oct 2018
16. Yonekura K, Braunfeld MB, Maki-Yonekura S, Agard DA (2006) Electron energy filtering significantly improves amplitude contrast of frozen-hydrated protein at 300 kV. J Struct Biol 156(3):524–536
17. Grimm R, Typke D, Bärmann M, Baumeister W (1996) Determination of the inelastic mean free path in ice by examination of tilted vesicles and automated most probable loss imaging. Ultramicroscopy 63(3–4):169–179

18. SerialEM Home Page. http://bio3d.colorado.edu/SerialEM/. Accessed 22 Oct 2018
19. Patch Tracking Example Data Set. http://bio3d.colorado.edu/imod/doc/patchTrackExample.html. Accessed 22 Oct 2018
20. Chen Y, Pfeffer S, Hrabe T, Schuller JM, Förster F (2013) Fast and accurate reference-free alignment of subtomograms. J Struct Biol 182 (3):235–245
21. Hagen WJH, Wan W, Briggs JAG (2017) Implementation of a cryo-electron tomography tilt-scheme optimized for high resolution subtomogram averaging. J Struct Biol 197 (2):191–198
22. Chen Y, Förster F (2014) Iterative reconstruction of cryo-electron tomograms using nonuniform fast Fourier transforms. J Struct Biol 185(3):309–316

Chapter 19

Mitochondrial Complexome Profiling

Heiko Giese, Jana Meisterknecht, Juliana Heidler, and Ilka Wittig

Abstract

Complexome profiling combines blue native gel electrophoresis (BNE) and quantitative mass spectrometry to define an entire protein interactome of a cell, an organelle, or a biological membrane preparation. The method allows the identification of protein assemblies with low abundance and detects dynamic processes of protein complex assembly. Applications of complexome profiling range from the determination of complex subunit compositions, assembly of single protein complexes, and supercomplexes to comprehensive differential studies between patients or disease models. This chapter describes the workflow of complexome profiling from sample preparation, mass spectrometry to data analysis with a bioinformatics tool.

Key words Complexome profiling, Blue native electrophoresis, Membrane protein complexes, Mitochondria, Mass spectrometry, Assembly

1 Introduction

Blue native electrophoresis (BNE) became a widely used method to study stoichiometry, composition, and assembly of mitochondrial protein complexes from many organisms (e.g., *Saccharomyces cerevisiae*, *Yarrowia lipolytica*, worm, fish, fly, birds, mammals, and plants) [1, 2]. In addition, BNE serves as a standard tool for diagnostics of mitochondrial disorders to characterize assembly and stability defects of the oxidative phosphorylation system (OXPHOS) and to test beneficial effects of treatments [3]. Recently, we extended BNE with high-resolution quantitative mass spectrometry and subsequent hierarchical clustering to gain a deep and comprehensive insight into the subunit composition of complexes, supercomplexes, and assembly intermediates including low abundant complexes [4–6]. The method analyses the migration of each protein from the high to the low molecular weight region of a BN-gel. Proteins with equal or similar migration pattern represent a high probability to be an interacting protein or subunit of a complex. This bottom-up approach was called complexome profiling and used in the meantime for many applications [4]:

Michal Minczuk and Joanna Rorbach (eds.), *Mitochondrial Gene Expression: Methods and Protocols*,
Methods in Molecular Biology, vol. 2192, https://doi.org/10.1007/978-1-0716-0834-0_19,

(1) Complexome profiling identified known and new assembly factors bound to distinct assembly intermediates of complex I in human cells and in the plant *Arabidopsis thaliana* [5, 7–9]. (2) A clear view on the pathological situation at molecular level was presented in mitochondria from patients with defects in complex I subunits or assembly factors [10–12]. (3) Mitochondrial complexomics provided new insights into patho-mechanisms in mitochondria of patients with Barth syndrome, a disease with affected cardiolipin remodeling [13]. (4) Adaptive processes and remodeling of OXPHOS complexes were studied under chronic hypoxia [14]. (5) Complexome profiling contributed to investigations of cytochrome c oxidase (complex IV) subunit composition and assembly in bacteria, yeast, and mammals [15–17]. (6) In addition to OXPHOS complexes, complexome profiling was frequently used to study components of mitochondrial contact site and cristae organizing system (MICOS) in yeast and human [18–21]. (7) Migration profiles of mitochondrial ribosomes contributed to better understand molecular consequences in Perrault syndrome with mutations in the gene ERAL1 and sensorineural hearing loss with defects in the gene MRPS2 [22, 23]. (8) Besides mitochondria, the method was also applied to study other cellular membranes [24].

In this chapter, we will first provide instructions for simple mitochondria preparation from tissues, organs, and cultured cells. This will be followed by a detailed description of a step-by-step procedure from BNE to sample processing for mass spectrometry and data analysis (Fig. 1a, b).

If crude preparations are executed immediately upon tissue or cell collection, soluble mitochondrial complexes from the matrix remain intact and are available for complexome analysis. Complexomes from fast and crude mitochondria preparations of human cells give usually up to 4000 protein identifications (IDs) including mitochondrial proteins and contaminations from other cellular membranes. Mitochondrial complexes are solubilized and separated by blue native electrophoresis according to established workflows [1]. Mild solubilization procedures with digitonin retain very labile complexes and higher-order assemblies of mitochondrial complexes, e.g., supercomplexes or dimeric and oligomeric ATP synthases. Dodecyl-β-D-maltoside (DDM) solubilizes single mitochondrial complexes. For the analysis of human OXPHOS complexes from cell culture, we recommend to use digitonin in general. Human complex I is more stable as part of the supercomplex and exhibits a better resolution in BNE.

Soluble complexes do not bind Coomassie dye to that extent as membrane proteins complexes with remaining lipids [15]. Therefore, we recommend for native mass estimation the use of soluble mass ladders (HMW) for soluble complexes and membrane complex ladders (bovine or chicken mitochondria) for membrane complexes [25].

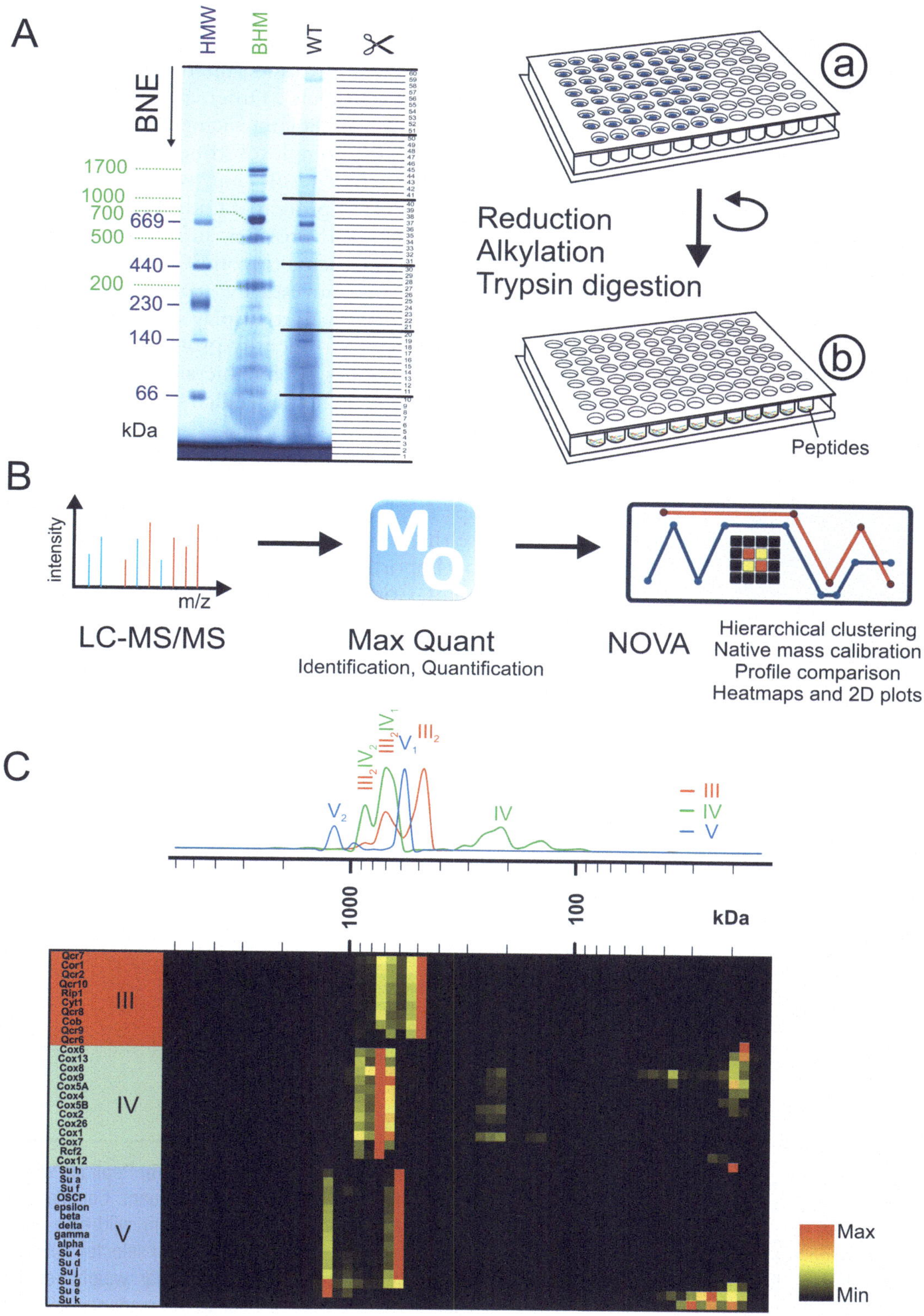

Fig. 1 Workflow of complexome profiling. (**a**) Separation of mitochondrial protein complexes by BNE. Matrix to cut a gel into even slices. Transfer of pieces to filtered microtiter plate (a). Upon thiol reduction and alkylation,

For downstream mass spectrometry analysis, we have proved to use a cutting template (created by graphics editor) together with a printed version of the gel, which greatly facilitates the process of uniformly slicing the lanes (Fig. 1a left). Other laboratories developed strategies that employ sub-millimeter slicing of BN-gels by a cryo-microtome [26]. OXPHOS complexes from yeast serve as an example to illustrate a complexome result (Fig. 1c). The comparison of profiles and visualization of protein abundance as heatmaps was used by most applications and provides an intuitive view to illustrate molecular changes in patients or conditions (Fig. 2). We developed NOVA a tool to investigate complexome data [27]. NOVA uses interactive heatmaps to display single or multiple complexome profiling data sets. To identify proteins with similar migration profiles NOVA supplies several hierarchical clustering algorithms and distance measures. For a detailed comparison, profiles can be compared as 2D plots.

Complexome data can be analyzed in different ways. One way follows hierarchical clustering of protein migration profiles. This unbiased analysis helps to identify unknown protein interactions. Another way is to use the knowledge of subunit composition and assembly factors to sort important players to visualize the molecular situation e.g., in a patient. Complexome profiles are comprehensive data sets of the entire interactome of a sample and contain many valuable information, which just lies outside of the scope of a focused investigation. To make those unused interactome information available for researchers, complete complexome data sets were uploaded to public repositories (e.g., PRIDE, ComplexomeMap) [9, 28].

2 Materials

2.1 Special Equipment and Devices

1. Motor-driven, tightly fitting 0.5–1 ml glass/Teflon Potter–Elvehjem homogenizer or Ultraturrax mini for homogenization of tissues and cells.
2. Equipment for native electrophoresis [1, 2].
3. Table top shaker (back and forth).
4. Table top orbital shaker for microtiter plates.

Fig. 1 (continued) proteins will be digested and peptides collected in microtiter plate (b). (**b**) Peptides will be dried and analyzed by nanoLC/MSMS. Proteins will be identified and quantified by MaxQuant. Complexome profiles will be generated by NOVA tool. (**c**) Selection of mitochondrial complexes from wild-type yeast mitochondria in a typical complexome profiling heatmap view. 2D plot represents profiles of selected subunits of complex III, IV, and V. Complexes III and IV show co-migration in higher molecular weight regions representing supercomplexes III_2IV_1 and III_2IV_2. Complex V or ATP synthase appears as monomer (V_1) and dimer (V_2)

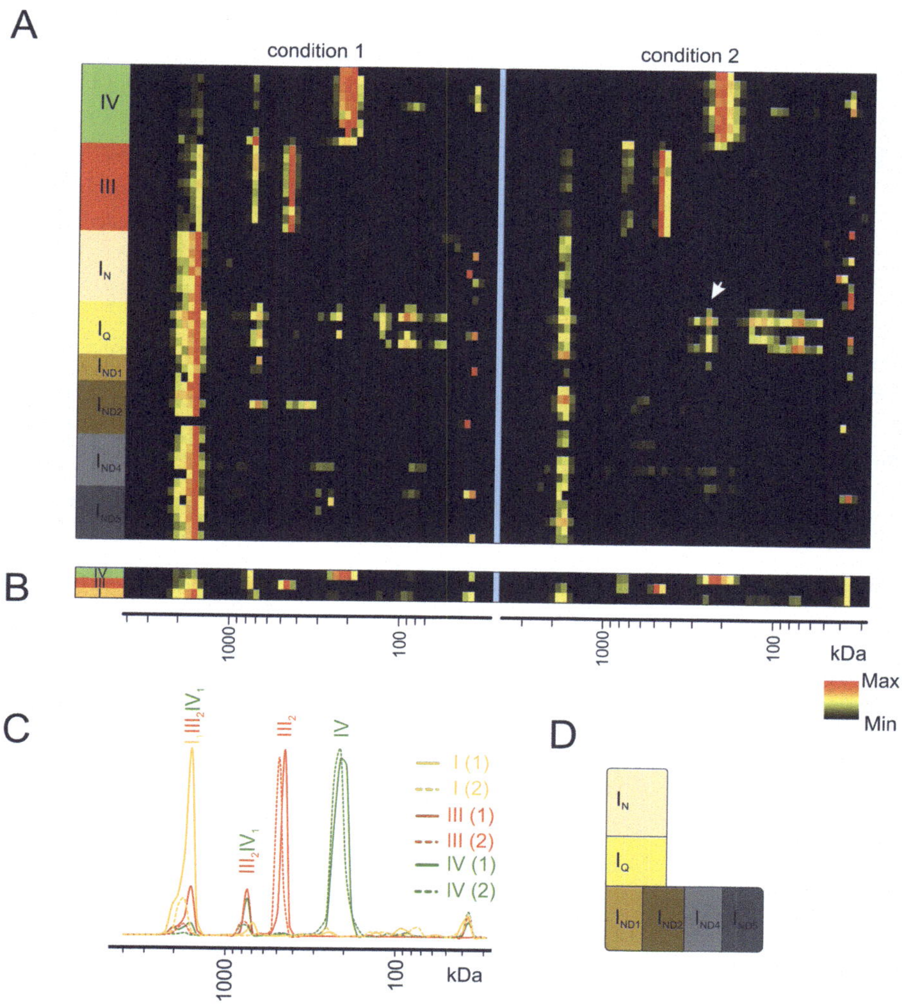

Fig. 2 Applications of complexome profiling to identify molecular consequences of disease conditions in human 143B cells. (**a**) Complex I, III, and IV as heatmap to visualize protein abundance of single subunits. Sum of all proteins from the data set of condition 2 was normalized to the control reference data set (condition 1). Heatmap represents normalization to maximum abundance between both conditions. Condition 2 exhibits a clear complex I deficiency at the molecular weight of supercomplexes $I_1III_2IV_1$ and accumulation of an assembly intermediate of subunits of the Q-module of complex I (white arrow). (**b**) Average of subunit abundance of respiratory chain complexes I, III, and IV normalized to maximum for heatmap presentation. (**c**) 2D plot to compare complex abundance. (**d**) Modules of complex I [31, 32]. Assignments: $I_1III_2IV_1$, respiratory chain supercomplexes containing one copy of complex I, one complex III dimer and one copy of complex IV; I, complex I and modules; III, dimeric complex III/cytochrome *bc*$_1$ complex; IV, complex IV/cytochrome *c* oxidase

5. Office flatbed scanner.
6. Centrifuge for microtiter plates.
7. Centrifugal vacuum concentrator (SpeedVac) with rotor for microtiter plates.

8. Equipment for nano liquid chromatography and mass spectrometry (nanoLC/MS), e.g., ultrahigh performance liquid chromatography unit Dionex Ultimate 3000 (Thermo Fisher Scientific) and Thermo Scientific™ Q Exactive Plus, connected via Nanospray Flex Ion-Source (Thermo Fisher Scientific).
9. C18 reversed-phase trap cartridge, 5 μm particle size, 100 Å (Thermo Fisher Scientific), in-house packed picofrit emitter tip (diameter 100 μm, 15 cm long, New Objectives) with 2.4 μm Reprosil C18 resin (Dr. Maisch GmbH).

2.2 Buffers and Solutions for Crude Mitochondrial Isolation and Solubilization

Buffers are prepared with ultrapure water and stored at 4 °C.

1. Phosphate-buffered saline (PBS): 137 mM NaCl, 2.7 mM KCl, 10 mM Na_2HPO_4, 1.8 mM KH_2PO_4, pH 7.4 (HCl).
2. Mitochondria isolation buffer for tissues: 250 mM sucrose, 10 mM Tris–HCl, pH 7.0, 1 mM EDTA, 5 mM 6-aminohexanoic acid, protease inhibitor cocktail.
3. Buffer for isolation of enriched mitochondria from cell culture (1/3 mitochondria isolation buffer): 83 mM sucrose, 3.3 mM Tris–HCl, pH 7, 0.3 mM EDTA, 1.7 mM 6-aminohexanoic acid, protease inhibitor cocktail.
4. Solubilization buffer: 50 mM NaCl, 50 mM imidazole/HCl, 2 mM 6-aminohexanoic acid, 1 mM EDTA, pH 7 (4 °C).
5. *n*-Dodecyl β-maltoside (DDM): 20% (w/v), dissolved in water, store aliquots at −20 °C.
6. Digitonin: 20% (w/v, Serva, used without recrystallization), dissolved in water, store aliquots at −20 °C.
7. 50% (w/v) glycerol, 0.1% Ponceau S dye.
8. 5% Coomassie dye: 5% (w/v) Coomassie blue G-250 (Serva), suspension in 500 mM 6-aminohexanoic acid.
9. High molecular weight (HMW) protein sets for gel filtration for native mass calibration.
10. Bovine heart mitochondria for native mass calibration.

2.3 Solutions for Coomassie Gel Staining

1. Fixing solution: 50% (v/v) methanol, 10% (v/v) acetic acid, 10 mM ammonium acetate, store at room temperature (*see* **Note 1**).
2. Coomassie staining solution: 0.025% (w/v) Coomassie dye in 10% (v/v) acetic acid, store at room temperature.
3. Coomassie destaining solution: 10% (v/v) acetic acid, store at room temperature.

2.4 Solutions, Reagents, and Special Material for Mass Spectrometry

Prepare all solution with LC/MS grade water. Only use LC/MS grade organic solvents.

1. 96 filter well plates (30–40 μm PP/PE, Pall Corporation) (*see* **Note 2**).
2. 96 well plates (PCRplate, PP).
3. Microtiter plate hot sealing films (*see* **Note 3**).
4. Acetonitrile (ACN).
5. Formic acid (FA).
6. Methanol.
7. 50 mM ammoniumbicarbonate (ABC) in water, store at 4 °C.
8. Coomassie destaining solution: 60% Methanol in 50 mM ABC.
9. Washing solution: 50% (v/v) ACN in 50 mM ABC.
10. 10 mM Dithiothreitol (DTT), freshly diluted in 50 mM ABC.
11. 30 mM Iodoacetamide (IAM), freshly prepared in 50 mM ABC (*see* **Note 4**).
12. Trypsin stock (sequencing grade), dilute 1 vial (20 μg) in 200 μl Trypsin resuspension buffer (50 mM acetic acid, provided with Trypsin) divide into 20 μl aliquots and store at −20 °C (*see* **Note 5**).
13. 100 mM $CaCl_2$ in water, prepare stocks and store at −20 °C (*see* **Note 5**).
14. ProteaseMAX surfactant, prepare stock containing 1% (w/v) in 50 mM ABC and store at −20 °C (*see* **Note 5**).
15. Digestion solution: 5 ng trypsin/μl in 50 mM ABC, 10% ACN, 0.01% (w/v) ProteaseMAX surfactant, 1 mM $CaCl_2$, freshly prepared.
16. Peptide isolation solution: 30% (v/v) ACN, 3% (v/v) FA in water.
17. Peptide dilution solution: 1% (v/v) ACN, 0.5% (v/v) FA in water.
18. NanoLC Eluent A: 4% (v/v) ACN, 0.1% (v/v) FA, water.
19. NanoLC Eluent B: 99% (v/v) ACN, 0.1 (v/v) % FA, water.
20. Loading solution for nLC: 4% (v/v) ACN, 0.1% (v/v) FA, water.

3 Methods

3.1 Isolation of Enriched Mitochondrial Membranes from Tissues and Cells

Carry out all procedures in a cold room at 4 °C or on ice. Isolate mitochondria immediately from cultured cells and animal organs without delay or freezing.

3.1.1 Isolation of Mitochondria from Tissues or Animal Organs

1. Weigh tissues (e.g., patient's specimens) or animal organs (e.g., liver, lung, kidney, heart, skeletal muscle, brain). Keep tissues chilled in petri dishes on ice and mince finely with sharp scissors. Collect fragments in isolation buffer to a final concentration of 1 g tissue/10 ml.
2. Transfer tissue suspension to a precooled motor-driven tightly fitting glass/Teflon Potter–Elvehjem homogenizer. Homogenize tissues at 1300 × *g* with approx. 30 strokes and place on ice.
3. Centrifuge homogenate at 500 × *g* for 3 min at 4 °C to gain a crude nuclear pellet. Transfer the supernatant into a new tube (*see* **Note 6**).
4. Centrifuge at 10,000 × *g* for 10 min at 4 °C to gain an enriched mitochondria pellet. Discard the supernatant.
5. Resuspend mitochondria enriched fraction in isolation buffer and determine protein concentration.
6. Prepare aliquots of 200 μg mitochondrial proteins. Centrifuge at 10,000 × *g* for 10 min. Discard supernatant.
7. Snap-freeze mitochondria enriched pellet in liquid nitrogen. Store aliquots at −80 °C.
8. Aliquots are ready for solubilization of mitochondrial complexes and separation by blue native electrophoresis.

3.1.2 Isolation of Enriched Mitochondrial Fraction from Cell Culture

1. Determine mass of empty tubes using an accuracy balance.
2. Collecting of cells:
   (a) Adherent cells: Wash cells of a cell culture dish (flask or petri dish) twice with PBS and scrape cells in 1 ml PBS using a cell lifter or scraper. Transfer cells to a pre-weight tube.
   (b) Suspension cells: Transfer cells to a 15 ml tube. Centrifuge cells at 500 × *g* for 5 min and wash twice with PBS. Resuspend cells in 1 ml PBS and transfer to a pre-weight tube.
3. Centrifuge cells at 500 × *g* for 5 min at 4 °C and discard supernatant.
4. Determine mass of tubes. Calculate the wet weight of the cell pellets.
5. Optional: Shock-freeze cell pellets in liquid nitrogen and store at −80 °C (*see* **Note 7**).
6. Resuspend cell pellets in diluted isolation buffer for cell culture to a final concentration of 100 mg/ml and incubate on ice for 5 min.

7. Transfer the cell suspension to a pre-cooled motor-driven tightly fitting glass/Teflon Potter–Elvehjem homogenizer and homogenize with 40 strokes at 1300 rpm (*see* **Note 8**).
8. Centrifuge the cell homogenate at 500 × *g* for 5 min at 4 °C to get a crude nuclear pellet.
9. Prepare aliquots of the supernatant corresponding to 10 mg wet weight. Centrifuge at 10,000 × *g* for 10 min at 4 °C to obtain a mitochondria enriched pellet. Discard the supernatant.
10. Snap-freeze aliqouts in liquid nitrogen and store at −80 °C.

3.2 Solubilization of Mitochondrial Membranes for Blue Native Electrophoresis

Perform all steps on ice or in a cold room. Use chilled centrifuge rotors.

1. Resuspend enriched mitochondria pellets in 20 μl solubilization buffer.
2. Solubilization (*see* **Note 9**):
   (a) For analysis of single mitochondrial complexes add 2.5 μl 20% DDM (2.5 g/g detergent/protein) to 200 μg mitochondrial pellets from tissues.
   (b) For analysis of single and higher protein complex assemblies add 6 μl 20% Digitonin to 200 μg mitochondria from tissues or 5 μl 20% Digitonin to 10 mg enriched mitochondria from cells.
3. Centrifuge samples at 20,000 × *g* for 20 min at 4 °C. Transfer supernatant into a new tube.
4. Optional: If at least two conditions (control vs. patient, wild type vs. mutant) are compared, determine protein concentration and prepare tubes for equal protein loading. Adjust volume to equal levels with solubilization buffer (*see* **Note 10**).
5. Add 2.5 μl 50% glycerol, 0.1% Ponceau S dye, and 3 μl volume of 5% Coomassie solution.
6. Load suspension to BNE gels (*see* **Note 11**).
7. Load molecular mass ladders for soluble and membrane proteins (Fig. 1, left).
8. Run blue native electrophoresis [1, 2].

3.3 Coomassie Staining

Perform all steps using a tabletop shaker (back and forth).

1. Transfer BN-gels immediately after electrophoresis to fixing solution and incubate for 30 min.
2. Discard fixing solution and stain in Coomassie solution for 30 min.
3. Replace Coomassie solution by destaining solution for several hours until background is clear.

4. Wash BN-gel intensively at least three times with water for 10 min (*see* **Note 12**).
5. Use an office scanner or gel documentation system to obtain a digital copy of your gel.
6. Create a gel picture with a cutting matrix using graphics editors (Fig. 1a, left). For Midi-gels (14 × 14 cm or larger) use 48–60 slices. For Mini-gels (10 × 10 cm) 32 slices.

3.4 Protein Digestion for nanoLC/MS

If not otherwise stated carry out all assays at room temperature. Use a tabletop orbital shaker for incubations.

1. Add 150 μl 50 mM ABC to a filtered microtiter plate (Fig. 1a, right, plate a).
2. Place native gel on top of a glass tray.
3. Cut each native gel lane in equal fractions according to cutting matrix using a scalpel or razor blade (Fig. 1, left). Immediately mince each slice and transfer gel cubes to microtiter wells (Fig. 1a, right, *see* **Note 13**).
4. Optional: The plate is now ready for long time storage at −20 °C.
5. Place filtered microtiter plate “a” (Fig. 1a, right) with gel cubes on top of a second microtiter (waste) plate or fitting box to collect and discard flow through. Centrifuge at 1500 × *g* for 3 min to remove liquid.
6. Destain gel cubes by adding 150 μl 60% Methanol, 50 mM ABC to filtered microtiter plate and incubate for about 60 min under gentle shaking.
7. Place filtered microtiter plate on top of a waste plate and remove liquid by centrifugation for 3 min at 1500 × *g*.
8. Repeat destaining another two times if needed.
9. Wash gel pieces with 50% ACN, 50 mM ABC. Remove the solution by centrifugation for 3 min at 1500 × *g*.
10. Add 120 μl 10 mM DTT in 50 mM ABC and incubate for 60 min at 56 °C. Remove solution by centrifugation for 3 min at 1500 × *g*.
11. Add 120 μl 30 mM IAM in 50 mM ABC and incubate for 45 min at room temperature in the dark. Remove the solution by centrifugation for 3 min at 1500 × *g* (*see* **Note 4**).
12. Wash two times with 150 μl 60% Methanol, 50 mM ABC for 15 min on a shaker in the dark. Remove the solution by centrifugation for 3 min at 1500 × *g* (*see* **Note 4**).
13. Allow the gel pieces to dry for 30–45 min in the workbench, without agitations.

14. Prepare digestion solution and add 20 μl to each well (*see* **Note 14**).
15. Incubate 5 min at 4 °C to allow reswelling of gel pieces.
16. Add 80 μl 50 mM ABC to cover all gel pieces (*see* **Note 15**).
17. Transfer microtiter plate to a tempered cabinet for at least 12 h at 37 °C, without agitation.
18. Place a new microtiter plate "b" (Fig. 1a, right, plate b) below the filter plate, fix both together with tape and centrifuge to collect peptides for at least 5 min at 1500 × *g* (*see* **Note 16**).
19. Add 30 μl 30% ACN, 3% FA to filtered microtiter plate and incubate for 20 min to release remaining peptides.
20. Collect peptides by centrifugation into microtiter plate "b" (Fig. 1a, right, plate b).
21. Evaporate the peptide solutions in a SpeedVac to dryness.
22. Optional: Purify peptides on stage tips (*see* **Note 17**).
23. Reconstitute peptides in 15 μl 1% ACN, 0.5% FA.
24. Seal the microtiter plate with hot sealing foil (*see* **Note 3**).
25. Allow peptides to resolve completely for at least 1 h under gentle agitation. Shortly spin down.
26. The samples are now ready for analysis by nanoLC/MS.
27. The microtiter plates can be stored at −20 °C for at least 4 weeks.

3.5 nanoLC/MS

We recommend using a pre-column setup to concentrate and purify peptide prior analytical column separation.

1. Place microtiter plate into autosampler.
2. Adjust nanoLC/MS method for complexome profiling (Table 1).
3. Start with a blank sample.
4. Measure from low to high molecular weight gel lane region.
5. End with a blank sample.
6. Measure next lane from low to high molecular weight region.
7. End with a blank sample.
8. Copy raw files to an analysis computer.

3.6 Raw Data Analysis

We recommend using MaxQuant [29].

1. Load raw files into MaxQuant.
2. Create experimental design file. Each slice corresponds to one experiment with one fraction.
3. Analyze projects with more than one lane as a batch. This creates a single protein data file for all lanes.

Table 1
nanoLC/MS conditions

Parameters	**Conditions**		
nLC			
Pre-column	C18 PepMap100, 5 μm, 100 Å		
Analytical column	In-house packed picofrit emitter tip. Diameter 100 μm, 30 cm, 2.4 μm C18		
Gradient	Time (min)	Eluent A (%)	Eluent B (%)
	0	99	1
	5	99	1
	35	1	99
	40	1	99
	42	99	1
Flow rate	300 nl/min		
Injection volume	5 μl		
MS			
Resolution	70,000		
AGC Target	3 × E6		
Maximum injection time	160 ms		
Scan range	300–2000 *m/z*		
Spectrum data type	Profile		
MSMS			
Resolution	17,500		
AGC target	1 × E5		
Maximum injection time	150 ms		
TopN	10		
Isolation window	2.0 *m/z*		
Spectrum data type	Centroid		
Dynamic exclusion	30 s		

nLC nano liquid chromatography, *MS* mass spectrometry, *MSMS* tandem mass spectrometry, *AGC* automatic gain control

4. Keep default settings for group-specific parameters.
5. Keep default settings for global parameters with following exceptions:
   Sequences: Load species reference proteome database.
   Lable-free quantification: enable –iBAQ-, disable –Log fit- (*see* **Note 18**).

6. Start processing.
7. Use file –proteingroup.txt- for further analysis.
8. Keep raw data files and –txt- folder for uploading to your and public repositories.

3.7 Complexome Profiling Data Analysis

We recommend using NOVA, a software to analyze complexome profiling data. Please find system requirements, download and tutorials at www.bioinformatik.uni-frankfurt.de/tools/nova. Here, we describe analysis of a single BN-lane and how to compare multiple BN-lanes.

3.8 Analysis of Single BN-Lane

1. Start NOVA.
2. Open the MaxQuant protein output file (proteingroups.txt).
3. Select the portion of the data from the MaxQuant output file to investigate (e.g., IBAQ values) by adjusting the options in the—layout—submenu. Check the preview window to see if your data settings are correct: Protein identifications should be listed in the first column (ID) followed by the IBAQ values of each slice in the subsequent columns. Use the options provided in the submenu—modification—to sort the IBAQ columns so that the first column represents the highest and the last column the lowest molecular weight slice. → OK.
4. For hierarchical clustering of proteins with comparable migration behavior, select—clustering—from the—Methods—menu. Use default/recommend settings or select preferential normalization and clustering function → Execute.
5. Create a mass scale: Double click on the area above the heatmap to setup the mass scale. Fill in the unit (e.g., kDa) and set—interpolation: exponential. Add data points to the scale for slices according to native molecular mass ladders or use internal native mass of known protein complexes (Table 2). → Save.
6. Explore your data sets with the provided visualization tools (e.g., profile viewer, tree viewer, and edit group tags according to complexes of interest).
7. Select the—project—menu to save project to a NOVA project file (npf).
8. Export data for further analysis or publication using the options in the—Export—menu.

3.9 Comparison of Multiple BN-Lanes from a Batch

1. Start with opening the reference data set of a multiple data set (e.g., control or wild type) by following the **steps 1–5** from Subheading 3.8. To align multiple data sets, it is necessary that comparable protein identifications have an identical ID column

Table 2
Native mass ladders[a]

Native complexes, supercomplexes, and proteins	Native mass ladders[a] (kDa) HMW	BHM	Internal mass calibration[b] (kDa) Human mitochondria	Mouse mitochondria
$I_1III_2IV_1$ (Supercomplex S1)		1700	1665	1676
I_1III_2 (Supercomplex S0)		1500	1454	1463
I (Complex I)		1000	970	980
V (ATP synthase)		597	619	593
III_2 (dimeric Complex III)		482	484	483
IV (Complex IV)		205	211	213
II (Complex II)		123	123	123
Thyroglobulin	669			
Ferritin	476			
Catalase	239			
Lactate dehydrogenase	146			
BSA	66			

BSA bovine serum albumin, *HMW* high molecular mass standard
[a]Native protein mass of HMW, native masses of bovine heart mitochondria (BHM) according to Wittig et al. [25]
[b]Native masses are calculated from mature masses of known subunit composition and stoichiometry of mitochondrial complexes

and comparable slices have the same column name. Replace slice column names with numbers using the options provided in the—modification—submenu (*see* **step 3** from Subheading 3.8).

2. Add other data sets for comparison: Select comparison from the methods menu. Click the add-button and follow the instructions in **step 3** from Subheading 3.8 to add an additional data set. Remember to rename the slice column names so that they match to those of the reference data set. Repeat until all data sets are added. We recommend to normalize the intensities of the added data sets to the intensities of the reference data set by enabling this option. → OK.
3. Continue with **step 6–8** from Subheading 3.8.

4 Notes

1. Use carbonyl-free methanol to prevent random alkylation of proteins which interferes with mass spectrometric analysis.
2. Filtered microtiter plates allow incubation and washing steps. Liquids can be removed and peptides can be collected by centrifugation.
3. We recommend heat sealing. Self-adhesive films could contaminate needles during peptide loading and may lead to autosampler malfunction.
4. Keep iodoacetamide solution light protected.
5. Stocks can be stored at least 4 weeks at −20 °C.
6. To prevent significant loss of material do not perform this step for tiny tissue samples.
7. Omit this step if you are interested in soluble mitochondrial complexes.
8. Check cell disintegration using trypan blue staining and light microscopy. Continue homogenization if more than 50% of cells are still intact.
9. Digitonin is mild and preserves labile protein assemblies. DDM or Triton X-100 solubilize more stable protein–protein interactions.
10. 20–100 μg protein/lane are sufficient for a complexome. A volume of up to 30 μl is suitable.
11. Solubilized complexes are stable on ice for several hours.
12. BN-gel can be stored in water up to 1 week.
13. This procedure is very time consuming. Keep the gel wet during procedure. Avoid contaminations with human keratins using gloves and working in a laminar flow bench.
14. ProteaseMAX is degraded over the course of digestion.
15. Gel pieces should completely be overlaid. Do not exceed maximum volume of microtiter plate.
16. Don't discard this solution because it contains your peptides.
17. Using stage tip purification minimizes the risk to clog analytical column on nanoLC. Protocols are available in [30].
18. We recommend to use intensity-based absolute quantification (IBAQ) as they correlate to absolute protein abundance. We do not recommend label-free quantification (LFQ) values as slices do not represent comparable sample fractions.

Acknowledgments

The work was supported by the Bundesministerium für Bildung und Forschung (BMBF 01GM1906D; mitoNET—Deutsches Netzwerk für mitochondriale Erkrankungen) and by the Deutsche Forschungsgemeinschaft, Sonderforschungsbereich 815 (Projects Z1 (Redox-Proteomics)).

References

1. Wittig I, Braun HP, Schägger H (2006) Blue native PAGE. Nat Protoc 1:418–428
2. Heidler J, Strecker V, Csintalan F, Bleier L, Wittig I (2013) Quantification of protein complexes by blue native electrophoresis. Methods Mol Biol 1033:363–379
3. Repp BM, Mastantuono E, Alston CL, Schiff M, Haack TB, Rötig A, Ardissone A, Lombès A, Catarino CB, Diodato D, Schottmann G, Poulton J, Burlina A, Jonckheere A, Munnich A, Rolinski B, Ghezzi D, Rokicki D, Wellesley D, Martinelli D, Wenhong D, Lamantea E, Ostergaard E, Pronicka E, Pierre G, Smeets HJM, Wittig I, Scurr I, de Coo IFM, Moroni I, Smet J, Mayr JA, Dai L, de Meirleir L, Schuelke M, Zeviani M, Morscher RJ, McFarland R, Seneca S, Klopstock T, Meitinger T, Wieland T, Strom TM, Herberg U, Ahting U, Sperl W, Nassogne MC, Ling H, Fang F, Freisinger P, Van Coster R, Strecker V, Taylor RW, Häberle J, Vockley J, Prokisch H, Wortmann S (2018) Clinical, biochemical and genetic spectrum of 70 patients with ACAD9 deficiency: is riboflavin supplementation effective? Orphanet J Rare Dis 13:120
4. Wessels HJ, Vogel RO, van den Heuvel L, Smeitink JA, Rodenburg RJ, Nijtmans LG, Farhoud MH (2009) LC-MS/MS as an alternative for SDS-PAGE in blue native analysis of protein complexes. Proteomics 9:4221–4228
5. Heide H, Bleier L, Steger M, Ackermann J, Dröse S, Schwamb B, Zörnig M, Reichert AS, Koch I, Wittig I, Brandt U (2012) Complexome profiling identifies TMEM126B as a component of the mitochondrial complex I assembly complex. Cell Metab 16:538–549
6. Wessels HJ, Vogel RO, Lightowlers RN, Spelbrink JN, Rodenburg RJ, van den Heuvel LP, van Gool AJ, Gloerich J, Smeitink JA, Nijtmans LG (2013) Analysis of 953 human proteins from a mitochondrial HEK293 fraction by complexome profiling. PLoS One 8:e68340
7. Guerrero-Castillo S, Baertling F, Kownatzki D, Wessels HJ, Arnold S, Brandt U, Nijtmans L (2017) The assembly pathway of mitochondrial respiratory chain complex I. Cell Metab 25:128–139
8. Ligas J, Pineau E, Bock R, Huynen MA, Meyer EH (2019) The assembly pathway of complex I in *Arabidopsis thaliana*. Plant J 97(3):447–459
9. Senkler J, Senkler M, Eubel H, Hildebrandt T, Lengwenus C, Schertl P, Schwarzländer M, Wagner S, Wittig I, Braun HP (2017) The mitochondrial complexome of *Arabidopsis thaliana*. Plant J 89:1079–1092
10. Alston CL, Compton AG, Formosa LE, Strecker V, Oláhová M, Haack TB, Smet J, Stouffs K, Diakumis P, Ciara E, Cassiman D, Romain N, Yarham JW, He L, De Paepe B, Vanlander AV, Seneca S, Feichtinger RG, Płoski R, Rokicki D, Pronicka E, Haller RG, Van Hove JL, Bahlo M, Mayr JA, Van Coster R, Prokisch H, Wittig I, Ryan MT, Thorburn DR, Taylor RW (2016) Biallelic mutations in TMEM126B cause severe complex I deficiency with a variable clinical phenotype. Am J Hum Genet 99:217–227
11. Alston CL, Heidler J, Dibley MG, Kremer LS, Taylor LS, Fratter C, French CE, Glasgow RIC, Feichtinger RG, Delon I, Pagnamenta AT, Dolling H, Lemonde H, Aiton N, Bjørnstad A, Henneke L, Gärtner J, Thiele H, Tauchmannova K, Quaghebeur G, Houstek J, Sperl W, Raymond FL, Prokisch H, Mayr JA, McFarland R, Poulton J, Ryan MT, Wittig I, Henneke M, Taylor RW (2018) Bi-allelic mutations in NDUFA6 establish its role in early-onset isolated mitochondrial complex I deficiency. Am J Hum Genet 103:592–601
12. Sánchez-Caballero L, Ruzzenente B, Bianchi L, Assouline Z, Barcia G, Metodiev MD, Rio M, Funalot B, van den Brand MA, Guerrero-Castillo S, Molenaar JP, Koolen D, Brandt U, Rodenburg RJ, Nijtmans LG, Rötig A (2016) Mutations in complex I assembly factor TMEM126B result in muscle weakness and isolated complex I deficiency. Am J Hum Genet 99:208–216
13. Chatzispyrou IA, Guerrero-Castillo S, Held NM, Ruiter JPN, Denis SW, IJlst L, Wanders RJ, van Weeghel M, Ferdinandusse S, Vaz FM, Brandt U, Houtkooper RH (2018) Barth

syndrome cells display widespread remodeling of mitochondrial complexes without affecting metabolic flux distribution. Biochim Biophys Acta Mol basis Dis 1864:3650–3658

14. Fuhrmann DC, Wittig I, Dröse S, Schmid T, Dehne N, Brüne B (2018) Degradation of the mitochondrial complex I assembly factor TMEM126B under chronic hypoxia. Cell Mol Life Sci 75:3051–3067
15. Schimo S, Wittig I, Pos KM, Ludwig B (2017) Cytochrome c oxidase biogenesis and metallochaperone interactions: steps in the assembly pathway of a bacterial complex. PLoS One 12: e0170037
16. Strecker V, Kadeer Z, Heidler J, Cruciat CM, Angerer H, Giese H, Pfeiffer K, Stuart RA, Wittig I (2016) Supercomplex-associated Cox26 protein binds to cytochrome c oxidase. Biochim Biophys Acta 1863:1643–1652
17. Vidoni S, Harbour ME, Guerrero-Castillo S, Signes A, Ding S, Fearnley IM, Taylor RW, Tiranti V, Arnold S, Fernandez-Vizarra E, Zeviani M (2017) MR-1S interacts with PET100 and PET117 in module-based assembly of human cytochrome c oxidase. Cell Rep 18:1727–1738
18. Eydt K, Davies KM, Behrendt C, Wittig I, Reichert AS (2017) Cristae architecture is determined by an interplay of the MICOS complex and the F1FO ATP synthase via Mic27 and Mic10. Microb Cell 4:259–272
19. Weber TA, Koob S, Heide H, Wittig I, Head B, van der Bliek A, Brandt U, Mittelbronn M, Reichert AS (2013) APOOL is a cardiolipin-binding constituent of the Mitofilin/MINOS protein complex determining cristae morphology in mammalian mitochondria. PLoS One 8: e63683
20. Anand R, Strecker V, Urbach J, Wittig I, Reichert AS (2016) Mic13 is essential for formation of crista junctions in mammalian cells. PLoS One 11:e0160258
21. Huynen MA, Mühlmeister M, Gotthardt K, Guerrero-Castillo S, Brandt U (2016) Evolution and structural organization of the mitochondrial contact site (MICOS) complex and the mitochondrial intermembrane space bridging (MIB) complex. Biochim Biophys Acta 1863:91–101
22. Chatzispyrou IA, Alders M, Guerrero-Castillo-S, Zapata Perez R, Haagmans MA, Mouchiroud L, Koster J, Ofman R, Baas F, Waterham HR, Spelbrink JN, Auwerx J, Mannens MM, Houtkooper RH, Plomp AS (2017) A homozygous missense mutation in ERAL1, encoding a mitochondrial rRNA chaperone, causes Perrault syndrome. Hum Mol Genet 26:2541–2550
23. Gardeitchik T, Mohamed M, Ruzzenente B, Karall D, Guerrero-Castillo S, Dalloyaux D, van den Brand M, van Kraaij S, van Asbeck E, Assouline Z, Rio M, de Lonlay P, Scholl-Buergi S, Wolthuis DFGJ, Hoischen A, Rodenburg RJ, Sperl W, Urban Z, Brandt U, Mayr JA, Wong S, de Brouwer APM, Nijtmans L, Munnich A, Rötig A, Wevers RA, Metodiev MD, Morava E (2018) Bi-allelic mutations in the mitochondrial ribosomal protein MRPS2 cause sensorineural hearing loss, hypoglycemia, and multiple OXPHOS complex deficiencies. Am J Hum Genet 102:685–695
24. Prior KK, Wittig I, Leisegang MS, Groenendyk J, Weissmann N, Michalak M, Jansen-Dürr P, Shah AM, Brandes RP (2016) The endoplasmic reticulum chaperone calnexin is a NADPH oxidase NOX4 interacting protein. J Biol Chem 291:7045–7059
25. Wittig I, Beckhaus T, Wumaier Z, Karas M, Schägger H (2010) Mass estimation of native proteins by blue native electrophoresis: principles and practical hints. Mol Cell Proteomics 9:2149–2161
26. Müller CS, Bildl W, Haupt A, Ellenrieder L, Becker T, Hunte C, Fakler B, Schulte U (2016) Cryo-slicing blue native-mass spectrometry (csBN-MS), a novel technology for high resolution complexome profiling. Mol Cell Proteomics 15:669–681
27. Giese H, Ackermann J, Heide H, Bleier L, Dröse S, Wittig I, Brandt U, Koch I (2015) NOVA: a software to analyze complexome profiling data. Bioinformatics 31:440–441
28. Vizcaíno JA, Csordas A, del-Toro N, Dianes JA, Griss J, Lavidas I, Mayer G, Perez-Riverol Y, Reisinger F, Ternent T, Xu QW, Wang R, Hermjakob H (2016) 2016 update of the PRIDE database and its related tools. Nucleic Acids Res 44:D447–D456
29. Cox J, Mann M (2008) MaxQuant enables high peptide identification rates, individualized p.p.b.-range mass accuracies and proteome-wide protein quantification. Nat Biotechnol 26:1367–1372
30. Rappsilber J, Mann M, Ishihama Y (2007) Protocol for micro-purification, enrichment, pre-fractionation and storage of peptides for proteomics using StageTips. Nat Protoc 2:1896–1906
31. Wirth C, Brandt U, Hunte C, Zickermann V (2016) Structure and function of mitochondrial complex I. Biochim Biophys Acta 1857:902–914
32. Formosa LE, Dibley MG, Stroud DA, Ryan MT (2018) Building a complex: assembly of mitochondrial respiratory chain complex I. Semin Cell Dev Biol 76:154–162

Chapter 20

Blue-Native Electrophoresis to Study the OXPHOS Complexes

Erika Fernandez-Vizarra and Massimo Zeviani

Abstract

Blue-native polyacrylamide gel electrophoresis (BN-PAGE) is a technique optimized for the analysis of the five components of the mitochondrial oxidative phosphorylation (OXPHOS) system. BN-PAGE is based on the preservation of the interactions between the individual subunits within the integral complexes. To achieve this, the complexes are extracted from the mitochondrial inner membrane using mild detergents and separated by electrophoresis in the absence of denaturing agents. The electrophoretic procedures can then be combined with a variety of downstream detection techniques. Since its development in the 1990s, BN-PAGE has been applied in the study of mitochondria from all kinds of organisms and extensive amounts of data have been produced using this technique, being key for the understanding of many aspects of OXPHOS physiopathology.

Key words Blue-native gel electrophoresis, Oxidative phosphorylation system, Mitochondrial complexes I, II, III, IV, and V, First-dimension BN-PAGE, Second-dimension BN-PAGE, In gel activity assays

1 Introduction

*B*lue-*n*ative *p*oly*a*crylamide *g*el *e*lectrophoresis (BN-PAGE), a technique developed in the early 1990s by Schägger and Von Jagow [1], has nowadays become a reference method for the quantitative and qualitative analyses of the mitochondrial oxidative phosphorylation system (OXPHOS) complexes. It is based on extraction of the OXPHOS multi-protein complexes from the mitochondrial membranes using mild neutral detergents and electrophoretic separation in native conditions, using a combination of buffers that maintain the interactions between the components of the individual complexes [2–4]. This technique can be applied to mitochondria isolated from any source [5] (examples displayed in Fig. 1). In addition, with the specific optimization for its use in clinically relevant human samples, such as primary cultured fibroblasts derived from skin biopsies and amniocytes [6, 7], peripheral

Michal Minczuk and Joanna Rorbach (eds.), *Mitochondrial Gene Expression: Methods and Protocols*, Methods in Molecular Biology, vol. 2192, https://doi.org/10.1007/978-1-0716-0834-0_20,

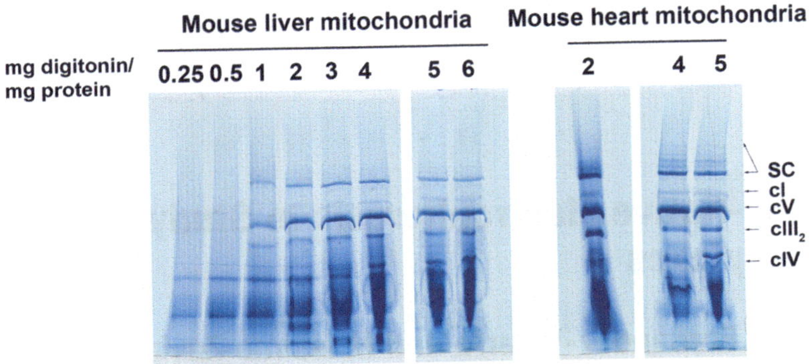

Fig. 1 1D BN-PAGE on isolated mitochondria solubilized with digitonin. Mitochondria from C57BL/6J mice were isolated from liver and heart according to the protocol described in Subheading 3.1. The effect of changing digitonin/protein ratios from 0.25 to 6 mg of digitonin/mg of mitochondrial protein was tested. The recommended ratio is 4 mg/mg, but a range between 2 and 6 mg/mg did not significantly alter the OXPHOS complex and supercomplex band pattern. Samples were electrophoresed on a 3–13% manually casted native gel and the bands were detected by Coomassie staining. *SC* supercomplexes (associations of complexes I, III and IV), *cI* complex I, *cV* complex V, *cIII*$_2$ complex III dimer, *cIV* complex IV

blood leukocytes (Fig. 2b), or small amounts of skeletal muscle biopsies [7] (Fig. 3). BN-PAGE has become a routine analysis method in mitochondrial disease diagnosis and research [8].

To quantify the amounts of the active fully assembled enzymes, BN-PAGE is usually combined either with Coomassie staining (Fig. 1), Western blot (WB), and immunodetection of the individual OXPHOS complexes using antibodies against specific structural subunits (Figs. 2 and 3) or with *in gel activity* (IGA) experiments, based on the histochemical assays for complexes I, II, IV, and V [9] (Fig. 4). Another way to identify the migration of the different OXPHOS components in a BN-PAGE is to cut the electrophoresis lane in slices and determine their peptide content by mass spectrometry to create a “complexomic profile” as detailed in Chapter 19 by Wittig et al.

Additionally, there is the possibility to separate each individual subunit from their corresponding complex using a second dimension (2D) denaturing SDS-PAGE, run after a first dimension (1D) BN-PAGE (Fig. 3). This kind of experiment provides qualitative information about the assembly state of the OXPHOS complexes, enabling the detection of specific subunits in assembly intermediates in addition to the fully assembled complex [1, 3, 8]. After 2D BN-PAGE, proteins can be visualized with WB and immunodetection techniques, but also, although with much less

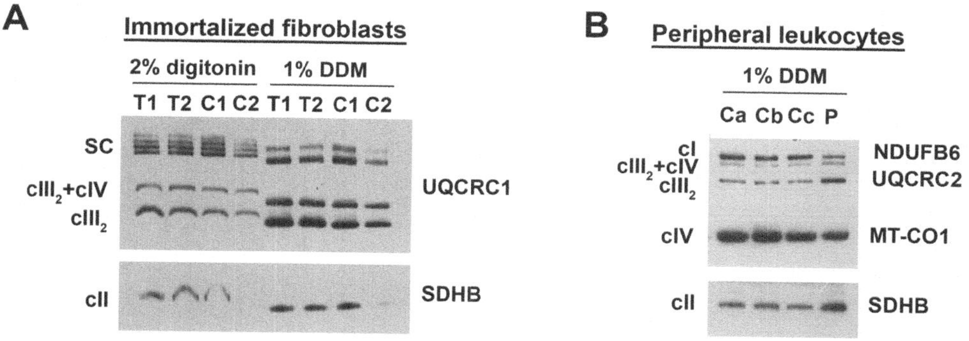

Fig. 2 1D BN-PAGE and immunodetection of permeabilized (digitonized) cells, solubilized with digitonin and DDM. (**a**) 5 × 10^6 immortalized fibroblast cells were processed as described in Subheading 3.5, finally solubilized using either 2% digitonin or 1% DDM (final concentrations). Samples were electrophoresed on a commercial precast 3–12% gel and transferred to a PVDF membrane. Complex III and complex II were immunodetected using anti-UQCRC1 and anti-SDHB (Table 5), respectively. T1, T2: Immortalized fibroblast cell lines carrying pathological mutations in TTC19 [24, 25]; C1 and C2: Wild-type control immortalized fibroblast cell lines. (**b**) Leukocyte pellets from 5 ml of peripheral blood were treated as described in Subheading 3.5 and membranes solubilized using a final concentration of 1% DDM. Samples were electrophoresed on a 5–13% manually casted gel and blotted on a PVDF membrane. Immunodetection of complexes I, II, III, and IV was performed with specific antibodies against NDUFB6, SDHB, UQCRC2, and MT-CO1 (Table 5). Ca, Cb, and Cc: leukocyte samples collected from three healthy volunteers; P: leukocyte sample from a mitochondrial disease patient showing combined complex I + complex IV deficiency. *SC* supercomplexes (associations of complexes I, III and IV), *cI* complex I, *cV* complex V, *cIII*$_2$ + *cIV* supercomplex band due to the association of complex III and complex IV, *cIII*$_2$ complex III dimer, *cIV* complex IV, *cII* complex II

sensitivity and specificity, by Coomassie and silver staining. Other detection possibilities include labeling the OXPHOS subunits with fluorescent dyes as well as through metabolic incorporation of radioactive L-[^{35}S]-Methionine [7, 4, 10–12].

Mainly two detergents are used for the extractions: digitonin and n-dodecyl β-D-maltoside (DDM), although some laboratories also make use of Triton X-100 [13, 14]. Digitonin extraction has the advantage of keeping the interactions between complexes I, III, and IV in the so-called supercomplexes or respirasomes [15, 16], whereas DDM and Triton X-100 disrupt these higher-order interactions, separating the individual complexes. Therefore, depending on the desired analysis one must choose the type of detergent to use.

We will now describe in detail the methods used for our research focused on rodent and human cells and tissues. However, the method can be adapted to any source of mitochondria (e.g., insects, plants, or yeast) and just a few examples of this can be found in refs. 17–20.

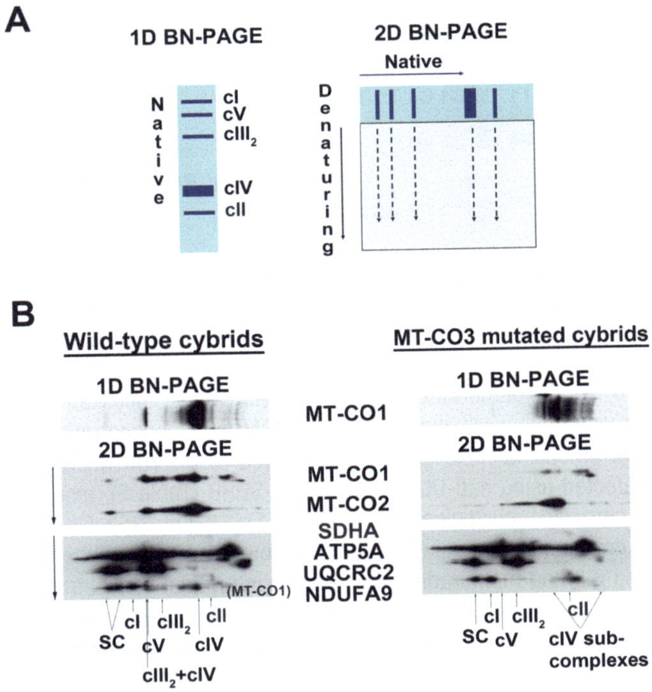

Fig. 3 Denaturing 2D BN-PAGE. (**a**) Schematic representation of the denaturing 2D BN-PAGE principle. OXPHOS complexes are separated by BN-PAGE in the 1D native gel. The 2D denaturing SDS-PAGE is run on a perpendicular orientation to separate each complex individual subunits according to their molecular mass. (**b**) BN-PAGE samples from 5×10^6 cytoplasmic hybrid (cybrid) cells, carrying either wild-type mitochondrial DNA or a homoplasmic *MT-CO3* mutation [26, 27], were prepared as described in Subheading 3.5, with a final solubilization using a final concentration of 1% DDM. Samples were run on a commercial precast 3–12% gel. The 1D BN-PAGE was blotted and immunodetected with anti-MT-CO1. The 2D BN-PAGE commercial gels were blotted and immunodetected with MT-CO1, MT-CO2 and the complex I (NDUFA9), complex II (SDHA), complex III (UQCRC2), and complex V (ATP5A) antibodies contained in the "Total OXPHOS Blue Native WB Antibody Cocktail" (Abcam, ab110412). *SC* supercomplexes (associations of complexes I, III and IV), *cI* complex I, *cV* complex V, $cIII_2 + cIV$ supercomplex band due to the association of complex III and complex IV, $cIII_2$ complex III dimer, *cIV* complex IV, *cII* complex II. (MT-CO1) indicates the presence of residual MT-CO1 signal in the blot corresponding to the wild-type cybrids

2 Materials

2.1 Isolation of Mitochondria from Different Sources

1. Glass-teflon Elvehjem–Potters of various volumes.
2. Rotating motor head.
3. Refrigerated centrifuge for 50- and 15-ml conical Falcon-type tubes.

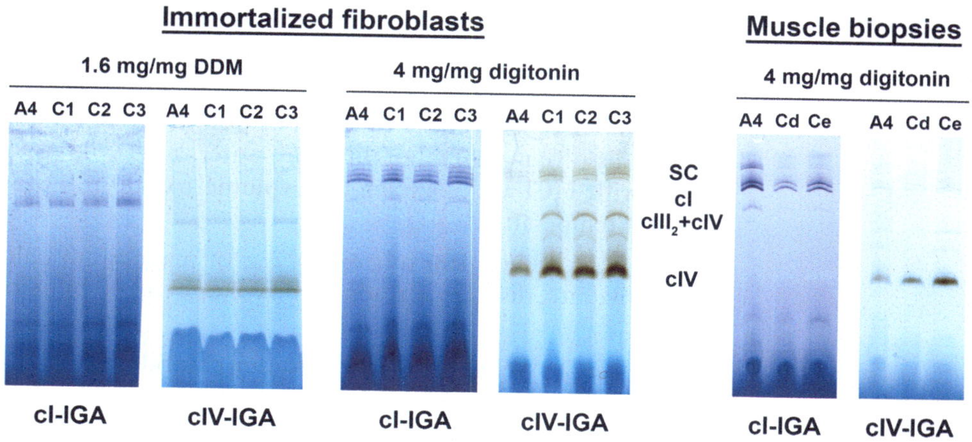

Fig. 4 In gel activity (IGA) assays performed on immortalized fibroblasts and a skeletal muscle biopsy taken from a mitochondrial complex IV deficiency patient (A4) carrying a pathological mutation in *NDUFA4*/*COXA4* [28, 29]. Two samples of 5×10^6 immortalized fibroblasts each, from A4 and three control lines were prepared as described in Subheading 3.5 with a slight modification: after **step 8**, a sample was taken to determine the protein concentration using a detergent-compatible protein assay (*see* **Note 14**). The final amount of detergent was then adjusted to achieve a ratio of 1.6 mg of DDM/mg or protein on one batch of samples, and 4 mg digitonin/mg of protein on the other batch. 25 mg of skeletal muscle biopsy material from patient A4 and two controls (Cd and Ce) were prepared as described in Subheading 3.2 and solubilized using 4 mg digitonin/mg protein. Samples were electrophoresed on precast 3–12% gels. In gel activity assays (IGA) for complex I and complex IV were performed. The cI-IGA reactions were left for 3–6 h and the cIV-IGA were left overnight at room temperature. *SC* supercomplexes (associations of complexes I, III and IV), *cI* complex I, $cIII_2 + cIV$ supercomplex band due to the association of complex III and complex IV, *cIV* complex IV

4. Refrigerated microfuge for 1.5-ml Eppendorf-type tubes.
5. Homogenization Medium A: 0.32 M Sucrose, 10 mM Tris–HCl pH 7.4, 1 mM EDTA. For 1 l, weigh 109.5 g of sucrose, dissolve in 800 ml of ultrapure water, add 2 ml of 0.5 M disodium EDTA stock solution and 20 ml of 0.5 M Tris–HCl, pH 7.4. Check and adjust, if necessary, the pH to 7.4 and complete the volume up to 1 l. Autoclave at low pressure or sterilize by filtration. Store at 4 °C.
6. Hypertonic Buffer IB 10×: 0.35 M Tris–HCl pH 7.8, 0.25 M NaCl, 50 mM $MgCl_2$. To prepare 100 ml, add 70 ml of 0.5 M Tris–HCl pH 7.8, 5 ml of 5 M NaCl and 5 ml of 1 M $MgCl_2$. Complete to 100 ml with ultrapure water and sterilize by filtration. Store at 4 °C.
7. Isotonic Buffer IB 1×: 35 mM Tris–HCl pH 7.8, 25 mM NaCl, 5 mM $MgCl_2$. Dilute 1:10 Hypertonic Medium IB 10×. For 100 ml, add 10 ml of IB 10× and 90 ml of ultrapure water. Sterilize by filtration. Store at 4 °C.
8. Hypotonic Buffer IB 0.1×: 3.5 mM Tris–HCl pH 7.8, 2.5 mM NaCl, 0.5 mM $MgCl_2$. Dilute 1:10 Isotonic Medium IB 1×. For 100 ml, add 10 ml of IB 1× and 90 ml of ultrapure water. Sterilize by filtration. Store at 4 °C.

9. 0.5 M EDTA: Weigh 93.1 g of disodium EDTA, dissolve in 400 ml of ultrapure water, adjust the pH to 8.0, and complete the volume up to 500 ml. Store at room temperature.
10. 0.5 M Tris–HCl pH 7.4 or 7.8: For 500 ml, weigh 30.3 g of Tris, dissolve in 400 ml of ultrapure water, adjust pH to 7.4 or 7.8 with HCl and complete the volume to 500 ml. Store at room temperature.
11. 1 M $MgCl_2$: For 100 ml, weigh 2 g of magnesium chloride hexahydrate, dissolve and adjust the volume to 100 ml. Store at 4 °C.
12. 5 M NaCl: Weigh 29.3 g of sodium chloride, dissolve, and adjust the volume to 100 ml.
13. Protein quantification reagents (for example: Bio-Rad DC™ Protein Assay or Pierce™ BCA Protein Assay kits).

2.2 Mitochondrial Enrichment from Cultured Cells and Peripheral Leukocytes by Digitonin Treatment

1. Phosphate Buffer Saline (PBS) pH 7.4 for tissue culture.
2. Digitonin Solution 1: 8 mg/ml of 50% purity or 4 mg/ml of high purity. For 25 ml, dissolve 0.2 g of 50% purity or 0.1 g of high-purity digitonin in 25 ml (final volume) of PBS. Keep solution at −20 °C. Discard solutions older than 3 months.

2.3 Mitochondrial Membrane Solubilization

1. Solubilization buffer: 1.5 M Aminocaproic Acid, 50 mM Bis-Tris/HCl pH 7.0. For 50 ml dissolve 9.84 g of 6-aminocaproic acid and 0.52 g of Bis-Tris in 35 ml of ultrapure water, adjust the pH to 7.0 with HCl and complete the volume up to 50 ml. Store at 4 °C.
2. Digitonin Solution 2: 10% digitonin. For 1 ml, weigh either 200 mg of 50% purity or 100 mg of high purity digitonin. Dissolve in ultrapure water. Store at −20 °C (*see* **Note 1**). Avoid repeated freeze-thawing cycles. Discard solutions older than 3 months.
3. DDM Solution: 10% n-dodecyl β-D-maltoside. For 1 ml, weigh 100 mg of DDM. Dissolve in ultrapure water. Store at −20 °C.
4. Blue-Native Sample Buffer: 0.75 M Aminocaproic Acid, 50 mM Bis-Tris–HCl pH 7.0, 0.5 mM EDTA, 5% SERVA Blue G (Coomassie Brilliant Blue G-250). For 50 ml, dissolve 4.92 g of 6-aminocaproic acid and 0.52 g of Bis-Tris in 40 ml ultrapure water, adjust pH to 7.0 with HCl, add 2.5 g of SERVA Blue G, dissolve and complete volume up to 50 ml. Store at 4 °C.

2.4 First-Dimension Native Electrophoresis

1. Mini-gel electrophoresis equipment.
2. Equipment for manually casted gels (see below) or commercial precast gels (*see* **Notes 2** and **3**).

3. Power supply.
4. Peristaltic pump, rubber tubbing, and either a plastic yellow tip or a 20 G needle to fit between the two gel casting glass plates.
5. Gradient maker.
6. Magnetic stirrer plate.
7. AB Mix: Acrylamide:Bisacrylamide 49% (48:1.5). Dissolve 48 g Acrylamide and 1.5 g Bisacrylamide in 100 ml of ultrapure water. Protect from light and keep at 4 °C.
8. 1D Gel Buffer 3×: 1.5 M Aminocaproic Acid, 150 mM Bis-Tris pH 7.0. For 500 ml, dissolve 98.4 g of 6-aminocaproic acid and 15.7 g of Bis-Tris in 400 ml of ultrapure water, adjust pH to 7.0 with HCl and complete volume up to 500 ml. Store at 4 °C.
9. Glycerol.
10. *N,N,N′,N′*-Tetramethylethylenediamine (TEMED).
11. 10% Ammonium Persulfate (APS). For 1 ml, weigh 100 mg of ammonium persulfate, dissolve in 1 ml (final volume) of ultrapure water. Prepare fresh for optimal results, or use solutions kept at 4 °C for a maximum of 2 weeks.
12. Cathode Buffer A: 50 mM Tricine, 15 mM Bis-Tris/HCl pH 7.0, 0.02% SERVA Blue G. For 500 ml, dissolve 4.48 g of Tricine and 1.57 g of Bis-Tris in 400 ml of ultrapure water, adjust the pH to 7.0 with HCl, add 5 ml of 2% SERVA Blue G and complete the volume to 500 ml. Store at 4 °C.
13. Cathode Buffer B: 50 mM Tricine, 15 mM Bis-Tris/HCl pH 7.0, 0.002% Serva Blue G. For 500 ml, dissolve 4.48 g of Tricine and 1.57 g of bis-Tris in 400 ml of ultrapure water, adjust the pH to 7.0 with HCl, add 0.5 ml of 2% SERVA Blue G and complete the volume to 500 ml. Store at 4 °C.
14. Anode Buffer: 50 mM Bis-Tris/HCl pH 7.0. For 2 l dissolve 20.92 g of Bis-Tris in 1.5 l of ultrapure water, adjust the pH to 7.0 with HCl and complete the volume to 2 l. Store at 4 °C.
15. 2% SERVA Blue G stock solution. Dissolve 2 g of SERVA Blue G (Coomassie Brilliant Blue G 250) in 100 ml of ultrapure water. Store at room temperature.

2.5 Second-Dimension Native Electrophoresis

1. Mini-gel electrophoresis equipment.
2. Precast gels if that is the preferred option (*see* **Note 4**).
3. Power supply.
4. Strip Dissociating Solution: 1% 2-Mercaptoethanol, 1% SDS. For 10 ml, add 0.1 ml of 2-Mercaptoethanol, 0.5 ml of a 20% SDS stock solution, and 9.4 ml of ultrapure water. Keep at room temperature.

5. 20% SDS stock solution. For 100 ml, weigh 20 g of Sodium Dodecyl Sulfate (SDS) and dissolve in 100 ml (final volume) of ultrapure water. Keep at room temperature.
6. AB Mix: Acrylamide:Bisacrylamide 49% (48:1.5).
7. 2D Gel Buffer 3×: 3 M Tris–HCl pH 8.45, 0.3% SDS. For 500 ml, weigh 181.7 g of Tris and dissolve in 400 ml of ultrapure water, adjust the pH to 8.45 with HCl, add 7.5 ml of 20% SDS. Complete volume up to 500 ml. Store at room temperature.
8. Glycerol.
9. TEMED.
10. 10% APS.
11. 2D Cathode Buffer: 0.1 M Tris, 0.1 M Tricine, 0.1% SDS, pH 8.25. For 1 l, weigh 12.11 g of Tris, 17.92 g of tricine and add 5 ml of 20% SDS. It is not necessary to adjust the pH. Prepare fresh before electrophoresis.
12. 2D Anode Buffer: 0.2 M Tris–HCl pH 8.9. For 1 l, weigh 24.23 g of Tris, dissolve in 400 ml of ultrapure water, adjust the pH to 8.9 with HCl, complete volume up to 1 l. Prepare fresh before electrophoresis.

2.6 Coomassie Blue Staining and Destaining

1. Staining and Fixing Solution: 0.2% Coomassie Blue R250, 50% Methanol, 7% Acetic Acid.

   For 1 l, weigh 2 g of Coomassie Blue R250 and dissolve in 500 ml of methanol and 70 ml Acetic Acid. Complete volume up to 1 l with ultrapure water. Filter to eliminate Coomassie Blue precipitates and keep at room temperature.
2. Destaining Solution: 20% Methanol, 7% Acetic Acid.

   For 2 l, mix 400 ml of methanol and 140 ml of acetic acid. Complete the volume up to 2 l with ultrapure water.

2.7 Western Blotting and Immunodetection

1. PVDF transfer membranes.
2. Whatman™ 3MM chromatography paper.
3. Methanol ≥99.8%, HPLC grade.
4. Wet electrophoretic transfer system.
5. Power supply.
6. 20× stock solution of 1D Bicarbonate Transfer Buffer: 0.2 M $NaHCO_3$, 60 mM Na_2CO_3. For 1 l, weigh 16.80 g of $NaHCO_3$ and 6.36 g of Na_2CO_3 (anhydrous). Keep at room temperature.
7. 1D Bicarbonate Transfer Buffer: 10 mM $NaHCO_3$, 3 mM Na_2CO_3.

   For 1 l, add 50 ml of 20× stock solution and 950 ml of ultrapure water. Prepare before transfer, keep at 4 °C until used.

8. 20× stock solution of 2D Transfer Buffer: 0.25 M Tris, 1.92 M Glycine.

   For 1 l, weigh 30.3 g of Tris and 144 g of Glycine, dissolve in 800 ml of ultrapure water, complete volume up to 1 l. Store at room temperature.

9. 2D Transfer Buffer: 12.5 mM Tris, 96 mM Glycine, 20% Methanol, 0.025% SDS.

   For 1 l, add 50 ml of 20× stock solution of 2D Transfer Buffer, 200 ml of Methanol, 1.25 ml of 20% SDS, complete volume up to 1 l with ultrapure water.

10. Blocking agents such as: nonfat powdered milk and/or bovine serum albumin (BSA) heat-shock fraction, free of IgGs.

11. PBS-T: 1× PBS, 0.1% Tween-20. For 2 l, add 200 ml of 10× PBS, 1.8 ml of ultrapure water and 2 ml of Tween-20.

12. 10× PBS: Dissolve 80 g NaCl, 2 g KCl, 26.8 g $Na_2H-PO_4 \cdot 7H_2O$ and 2.4 g KH_2PO_4 in 800 ml ultrapure water, adjust to pH 7.4 with HCl and complete volume up to 1 l. Sterilize by autoclaving. Store at room temperature.

13. Primary antibodies against the desired target proteins.

14. Horse radish peroxidase (HRP)-conjugated secondary antibodies.

15. ECL™ Western blotting detection reagents.

2.8 In Gel Activity (IGA) Assays

1. Complex I IGA solution: 5 mM Tris–HCl pH 7.4, 0.14 mg/ml NADH, 1 mg/ml Nitro Blue Tetrazolium (NBT). For 10 ml, add 10 mg of NBT, 100 μl of a 14 mg/ml NADH (disodium salt, grade I) stock solution, 100 μl of 0.5 M Tris–HCl pH 7.4, complete the volume up to 10 ml with ultrapure water and dissolve well. Prepare fresh before the assay and protect from light.

2. Complex II IGA solution: 5 mM Tris–HCl, pH 7.4, 0.2 mM Phenazine Methosulfate (PMS), 20 mM Succinate and 1 mg/ml NBT.

   For 10 ml, add 10 mg NBT, 200 μl of a 1 M Succinate stock solution, 8 μl of a 0.25 M PMS stock solution, 100 μl of 0.5 M Tris–HCl pH 7.4, complete the volume up to 10 ml with ultrapure water and dissolve well. Prepare fresh before the assay and protect from light.

3. 1 M Succinate stock solution.

   For 10 ml, weigh 2.7 g of Sodium Succinate dibasic hexahydrate dissolve in 10 ml of ultrapure water (final volume). Make 1 ml aliquots and store them at −20 °C.

4. 0.25 M PMS stock solution.

   For 1 ml, weigh 76.6 mg of Phenazine Methosulfate, dissolve in 1 ml (final volume) of DMSO. Protect from light and store at −20 °C.

5. Complex IV IGA solution: 50 mM Potassium Phosphate buffer pH 7.4, 1 mg/ml 3,3′-Diaminobenzidine tetrahydrochloride hydrate (DAB), 24 U/ml Catalase, 1 mg/ml Cytochrome c, 75 mg/ml Sucrose.

   For 10 ml, weigh 10 mg of DAB, 10 mg of Cytochrome c and 750 mg of Sucrose, add 2 ml of 0.25 M Potassium Phosphate buffer pH 7.4, 10 μl of a ≈24,000 U/ml Catalase (from bovine liver) stock solution and complete the volume up to 10 ml with ultrapure water. Prepare fresh before the assay and protect from light.

6. Complex V: 35 mM Tris–HCl pH 7.8, 270 mM Glycine, 14 mM $MgSO_4$, 0.2% $Pb(NO_3)_2$, and 8 mM ATP.

   For 10 ml, weigh 203 mg of Glycine and 20 mg of $Pb(NO_3)_2$, add 700 μl of 0.5 M Tris–HCl pH 7.8, 140 μl of a 1 M $MgSO_4$ stock solution and 400 μl of a 0.2 M ATP stock solution, complete the volume up to 10 ml with ultrapure water. Prepare fresh before the assay and protect from light.

7. 1 M $MgSO_4$ stock solution.

   For 50 ml, weigh 12.32 g of $MgSO_4 \cdot 7H_2O$, dissolve in 40 ml of ultrapure water and complete the volume up to 50 ml. Store at room temperature.

8. 0.2 M ATP stock solution.

   For 10 ml weigh, 1.10 g of Adenosine 5′-Triphosphate disodium salt hydrate, grade I, dissolve in 10 ml of ultrapure water (final volume). Make 1 ml aliquots and store them at −20 °C.

3 Methods

3.1 Isolation of Mitochondria from Fresh Mouse or Rat Tissues

Any method based on tissue homogenization and differential centrifugation can be used as the source of mitochondria for BN-PAGE analysis. The method described below includes some washing steps that yield a cleaner mitochondrial preparation without employing long and laborious purification steps [12, 21].

1. Remove the organ of interest and place it in a pre-weighed 50-ml beaker with ice-cold Homogenization Medium A.
2. Weigh the beaker with the Medium A and the sample, to know the amount of tissue that has been extracted.
3. Cut the tissue into small pieces with a pair of scissors.

4. Sift the tissues and wash them with more Homogenization Medium A in order to remove blood, hair, and connective tissue. Put them back in the beaker and repeat until the tissue is well cleaned.
5. Add fresh Homogenization Medium A to the glass body of the potter, in a proportion of 5 ml/g of tissue.
6. Transfer the pieces of tissue to the potter.
7. Homogenize with four to ten up-and-down strokes in the Elvehjem–Potter with the motor-driven Teflon pestle at 600 rpm. The number of strokes will depend on the tissue: five strokes for soft tissues like liver, kidney, or brain; ten strokes for skeletal or cardiac muscle.
8. Transfer the homogenized tissue to the 50- or 15-ml sterile Falcon-type conical tubes.
9. Centrifuge at 1000 × *g* in either a fixed or swinging bucket rotor for 5 min at 4 °C in order to pellet unbroken tissue, cells, and nuclei.
10. Collect the supernatant containing the mitochondria and transfer it to a clean conical tube.
11. Centrifuge at 9000 × *g* in a fixed rotor for 10 min at 4 °C in order to sediment a crude mitochondrial pellet.
12. Eliminate the supernatant.
13. Carefully resuspend the crude mitochondrial pellet with 5 ml of Homogenization Medium A, using a glass Pasteur pipette.
14. Transfer the mitochondrial suspension to four Eppendorf tubes, previously placed on ice (approximately 1.3 ml of suspension in each tube).
15. Centrifuge the Eppendorf tubes for 2 min at 17,000 × *g* in a microfuge at 4 °C.
16. Using a sterile Pasteur pipette, remove the supernatant trying to draw out all the liquid and part of the light-colored fluffy layer on the top of the pellet, without disturbing the darker part where mitochondria are.
17. To wash the mitochondria, fill up two of the four tubes with Homogenization Medium A and resuspend. Transfer the mitochondrial suspension of one tube to one of the tubes without liquid and resuspend.
18. Centrifuge the two resulting tubes as in **step 15**.
19. Repeat the same procedure once again until one tube, containing all the material, is left.
20. Resuspend the final pellet in 1 ml of Homogenization Buffer A. Take an aliquot for protein quantification.

21. Centrifuge at 17,000 × *g* at 4 °C for 2 min.
22. The resulting mitochondrial pellet (*see* **Note 5**) can now be used for solubilization (Subheading 3.4).

3.2 Mitochondria-Enriched Fractions from Small Amounts of Frozen Tissues

1. Place 25–50 mg of frozen biopsy or necropsy tissue on a Petri dish on ice.
2. Cut the tissue into small pieces in cold Homogenization Medium A. Carefully remove the buffer.
3. Homogenize in 10 volumes of fresh Homogenization Medium A in a motor-driven Elvehjem Teflon–Glass potter at 600 rpm with five to ten strokes. This will depend on the tissue: five strokes for soft tissues like liver, kidney or brain, ten strokes for skeletal or cardiac muscle.
4. Transfer the homogenate to an Eppendorf-type tube.
5. Centrifuge at 800 × *g* during 5 min at 4 °C, to remove nuclei and cell debris.
6. Transfer supernatant to a fresh tube.
7. Centrifuge at 9000 × *g* during 10 min at 4 °C, to obtain an enriched mitochondrial fraction.
8. Remove supernatant. Resuspend pellet in Medium A.
9. Take an aliquot to measure protein concentration.
10. Centrifuge at 9000 × *g* in microfuge during 10 min at 4 °C.
11. The resulting pellet is now ready for solubilization (Subheading 3.4).

3.3 Isolation of Mitochondria from Cultured Cells

1. Harvest exponentially growing cells by trypsinization. Use the cells contained in ten 150-mm plates that are about 80–90% confluent, giving a cell count in the order of 15×10^7 cells.
2. Transfer the cells to 50-ml conical Falcon-type tubes.
3. Wash twice with cold PBS by centrifuging at 600 × *g* in the clinical centrifuge for 5 min at 4 °C. In the last wash, transfer the cells to a 15-ml Falcon-type conical tube and centrifuge as before.
4. Place the tube containing the cells on ice. Measure the volume occupied by the packed cells, which is typically 1–2 ml.
5. Resuspend the cells in one-half volume of packed cells of Hypotonic Buffer IB 0.1×.
6. Pipette the cell suspension into the glass body of a 5-ml potter.
7. Wash the tube where the cells were collected with IB 0.1× using another half volume of the originally packed cells. Pipette this into the potter and thoroughly mix the cells with the buffer.

8. Perform ten strokes in the Elvehjem–Potter homogenizer with the motor-driven Teflon pestle at 1000 rpm.
9. Quickly add 1/10 of the initial volume of packed cells of Hypertonic Buffer IB 10×, to make the medium isotonic and prevent excessive breakage of mitochondria.
10. Transfer the homogenized cells to a 15-ml conical centrifuge tube. The homogenizer can be washed twice with 500 μl of Isotonic Buffer IB 1× to collect as much of the homogenate as possible.
11. Centrifuge at 1200 × *g* for 3 min at 4 °C, in a fixed or swinging rotor to sediment nuclei and unbroken cells (P1 pellet).
12. Draw out the mitochondria-containing supernatant and transfer it to a clean conical tube placed on ice.
13. To increase the yield of mitochondria: resuspend the resulting P1 pellet in one-half of its volume of Hypotonic Buffer IB 0.1× and repeat **steps 6–11**.
14. Collect the supernatant from this second round of homogenization and centrifugation and add it to the tube containing the first supernatant.
15. Centrifuge at 1200 × *g* for 3 min at 4 °C, to eliminate possible nuclear contaminants.
16. Pipette the supernatant in four Eppendorf tubes previously placed on ice.
17. Centrifuge at 17,000 × *g* in the microfuge for 2 min at 4 °C, to sediment the mitochondrial fraction.
18. Remove the supernatants.
19. Wash the mitochondrial pellets with Homogenization Medium A, transferring from four to two tubes, continuing until all the material is in one tube (as in **steps 15–19** in Subheading 3.1).
20. Resuspend the final pellet in 1 ml of Medium A and take an aliquot to measure protein concentration.
21. Centrifuge at 17,000 × *g* during 2 min at 4 °C. Eliminate supernatant, the pellet (*see* **Note 5**) is now ready for solubilization (Subheading 3.4).

3.4 Membrane Solubilization from Mitochondrial Pellets

1. Resuspend the pellet in the appropriate amount of Solubilization Buffer (1.5 M Aminocaproic acid, 50 mM Bis-Tris/HCl pH 7.0) to obtain a concentration of 10 mg of mitochondrial protein/ml (*see* **Note 6**).
2. Solubilize the mitochondrial membranes by adding either 1.6 mg DDM/mg protein, that is 16 μl of DDM solution (10% DDM) per mg of protein, to separate the individual

complexes or 4 mg Digitonin/mg protein, that is 40 μl of Digitonin Solution 2 (10% digitonin) per mg of protein, to maintain the supercomplexes.

3. Incubate on ice for 5 min.
4. Centrifuge at 20,000 × *g* in microfuge at 4 °C during 30 min.
5. Pass the supernatant to a clean tube (*see* **Note 7**) and add 1/2 volume of Blue-Native Sample Buffer as of volume of detergent added (8 μl/mg of mitochondrial protein for DDM solubilized samples and 20 μl/mg of mitochondrial protein for digitonin-solubilized samples).
6. Load the equivalent to 50–100 μg of protein per sample (*see* **Note 8**) on a gradient native gel (Subheading 3.6).

3.5 Sample Preparation from Cultured Cells and Peripheral Blood Leukocytes

For these kinds of samples, mitochondrial-enriched fractions are usually obtained by digitonin treatment of the cellular pellet (*see* **Note 9**).

Adherent cells are harvested by trypsinization and counted using a manual hemocytometer or automated cell counter (*see* **Note 10**).

Leukocytes were obtained from 5 ml of peripheral blood collected in EDTA Blood Collection tubes and were separated by hypotonic lysis of red cells and centrifugation as described in [22]. The resulting leukocyte pellet was treated in the same way as a 2 × 10^6 primary fibroblast pellet.

The cell pellets washed with cold PBS twice are ready for sample preparation:

1. For 2 × 10^6 primary culture cells or 5 × 10^6 immortalized cells, resuspend the cell pellet in 200 μl cold PBS.
2. Add 200 μl (1 volume) of cold Digitonin Solution 1 (4 mg/ml in PBS).
3. Incubate on ice during 10 min.
4. Add 1 ml of cold PBS.
5. Centrifuge at 10,000 × *g* for 5 min at 4 °C.
6. Remove supernatant. Wash pellet using 1 ml of cold PBS.
7. Centrifuge at 10,000 × *g* for 5 min at 4 °C.
8. Remove supernatant. The digitonized pellet is now ready for the final solubilization (*see* **Note 11**).
9. Resuspend the pellet in 100 μl of Solubilization Buffer (*see* **Note 12**).
10. Solubilize the membranes by adding either 10 μl of DDM Solution (10% DDM) or 20 μl of Digitonin Solution 2 (10% digitonin) (*see* **Notes 13** and **14**).
11. Incubate on ice for 5 min.

12. Centrifuge at 20,000 × *g* at 4 °C during 30 min.
13. Pass the supernatant to a clean tube (*see* **Note 7**) and add 10 μl of Blue-Native Sample Buffer.
14. Directly load 25 μl of sample (*see* **Note 8**) on a gradient native gel (Subheading 3.6).

3.6 First-Dimension Native Electrophoresis (See Note 15)

1. Assemble the glass plate sandwich with 1.5 mm spacers onto the casting stand.
2. Take the pump, magnetic stirrer plate, gradient maker, and assembled casting stand to a cold room (*see* **Note 16**).
3. Prepare two gel solutions with the polyacrylamide concentrations corresponding to the two extremes of the gradient according to Table 1:
   (a) 5–13% gradient for DDM prepared samples (individual complex separation).
   (b) 3–13% gradient for digitonin-prepared samples (supercomplex separation).
4. Place the tube containing the 5% or 3% mix and the 13% mix on ice.
5. Make sure the pump is turned off and that the valve between the two chambers is closed before pouring the two mixes. The valve between the front mixing chamber and the pump (if present) can be open at all times.
6. Add the APS 10% and TEMED immediately before transferring the gel mixes to the gradient maker.
7. Pour the 5% or 3% solution in the reservoir (back) chamber and the 13% solution in the mixing chamber with a magnetic stirrer inside. Start the stirring on the stirrer plate, at a middle speed enough to allow thorough mixing without creating a vortex.

Table 1
Composition of the gel mixes necessary to cast either a 3–13% or a 5–13% linear gradient BN-PAGE in an 8 × 10 cm and 1.5-mm-thick mini-gel

Native gels	3% (6 ml)	5% (6 ml)	13% (4 ml)
AB Mix	0.36 ml	0.61 ml	1.04 ml
1D Gel Buffer 3×	2 ml	2 ml	1.33 ml
Ultrapure Water	3.6 ml	3.35 ml	0.8 ml
Glycerol	–	–	0.72 ml
10% APS	40 μl	40 μl	14 μl
TEMED	4 μl	4 μl	3 μl

8. Start the pump and once the first drop of gel has gone out, introduce the needle or tip (at the end of the tubing) at the top and between the glass plate sandwich. Keep the valve between the two chambers closed until the bottom of the gel sandwich is covered with 13% gel mix. The flow should be continuous without generating turbulence (around 1 ml/min).
9. Open the in-between valve and allow the 5%/3% gel mix to pass into the mixing right chamber. Keep pouring the gel until it reaches a height of 1.5 cm under the small glass plate top edge.
10. Very gently, pour a layer of 1 ml of water to ensure that the gel polymerizes straight.
11. Immediately fill both chambers of the gradient maker with water and pump it through the system to avoid polymerization of residual acrylamide and clogging of the tubes.
12. Leave the gel to polymerize completely in the cold room (*see* **Notes 17** and **18**).
13. Thoroughly remove the water or buffer on top of the gel and prepare a 4% Sample Gel to be casted on top of the gradient (Table 2).
14. Pour the Sample Gel and introduce the 10- or 15-well comb, making sure no air bubbles are formed.
15. Once the Sample Gel is completely polymerized uncast the gel and remove the comb. Place the gel in the electrophoresis cell. Wash the wells with Cathode Buffer A to remove traces of non-polymerized acrylamide and salts. Fill the wells with Cathode Buffer A.
16. Fill the inner compartment (cathode) with Cathode Buffer A until half of its capacity in a way that the wells filled with blue buffer are still visible.
17. Fill the outer bottom compartment (anode) with Anode Buffer.
18. Load the samples into the wells.

Table 2
Composition of the gel mix necessary to cast the 4% native sample gel

Sample gel	4% (3 ml)
AB Mix	0.25 ml
1D Gel Buffer 3×	1 ml
Ultrapure Water	1.75 ml
10% APS	25 μl
TEMED	3 μl

19. Once all the samples are loaded. Carefully fill up the inner cathode compartment with Cathode Buffer A and attach the lid to start the electrophoresis.
20. Run the gel at 90 V for 30 min and then at 12 mA, limiting the voltage to 300 V, until the front reaches the end of the gel (*see* **Note 19**). When the front is about half way, Cathode Buffer A can be substituted by Cathode Buffer B in order to see the complex bands better (recommended for most applications).
21. The running of the gels takes about 4 h in total.
22. Depending on the desired analysis, the gel can either be fixed and stained with Coomassie (Subheading 3.8), electroblotted into a PVDF membrane (Subheading 3.9.1), or used for in gel activity (IGA) assays (Subheading 3.10) as well as to perform native (*see* **Note 20**) or denaturing 2D electrophoresis as described below in Subheading 3.7 (*see* **Note 21**).

3.7 Second-Dimension Denaturing Electrophoresis

For the denaturing 2D BN-PAGE, each of the lanes previously run through a native gel are excised and electrophoresed on one Tricine-SDS-PAGE gel [23], on a 90° orientation (Fig. 3).

1. Carefully and cleanly excise the 1D BN-PAGE lane/s containing the sample to be analyzed with a razor blade or scalpel (*see* **Note 22**). Place on the large glass gel plate, when manually casting the 2D gel/s. Place on a glass or plastic surface, if precast gels will be used for the denaturing electrophoresis.
2. Cover the gel strip/s with Dissociation Solution under a fume hood.
3. Incubate for 1–2 h at room temperature, covering the strips to avoid excessive evaporation.
4. Remove thoroughly the excess of Dissociation Solution using filter paper, being careful that the strip does not stick to the paper. This is essential for proper polymerization of the manually casted 2D gel.

For Manually Casted Gels

5. Place the short plate on top of the large glass and the two *1 mm* spacers on both sides to assemble the sandwich with the strip in it. The use of thinner spacers, prevents the strip from slipping to the bottom during the pouring of the gel. Place the sandwich on the casting stand.
6. Two denaturing gels are poured: First a 16.5% polyacrylamide gel, up to about 2 cm from the 1D strip, then a 10% polyacrylamide gel on top of the 16.5% one, up to 0.5 cm of the 1D strip (Table 3).
7. Let polymerize each of the two denaturing gels adding a thin layer of water that will be removed before adding the next gel.

Table 3
Composition of the gel mixes necessary to cast the 16.5% and 10% second dimension denaturing SDS-PAGE

Denaturing gels	16.5% (5 ml)	10% (2 ml)
AB Mix	1.66 ml	0.4 ml
2D Gel Buffer 3×	1.66 ml	0.66 ml
Water	1.13 ml	0.73 ml
Glycerol	0.55 ml	0.21 ml
APS 10%	20 μl	7.5 μl
TEMED	7 μl	2.5 μl

The quantities are for one 8 × 10 cm and 1.0-mm-thick mini-gel

Table 4
Composition of the gel mix necessary to cast the 10% native strip-sample gel

Native gel	10% (2 ml)
AB Mix	0.4 ml
1D Gel Buffer 3×	0.66 ml
Water	0.73 ml
Glycerol	0.21 ml
APS 10%	7.5 μl
TEMED	2.5 μl

8. Finally, a native 10% polyacrylamide gel (Table 4) is poured around the 1D BN-PAGE strip (*see* **Notes 23** and **24**).
9. Once the last gel is completely polymerized. Transfer the gel sandwich/es to the electrophoresis tank.
10. Fill the inner compartment with 2D Cathode Buffer and the outer compartment with 2D Anode Buffer.
11. Run the electrophoresis at 8–10 mA/gel during 20–30 min, then raise to 15 mA until the front arrives to the end of the gel. An alternative is to run at 4–5 mA/gel overnight.

For Precast Commercial Gels

1. Remove the 2D well comb from the precast gel. The buffer remaining on the well does not need to be removed.
2. Introduce the treated 1D BN-PAGE strip containing the lane to be analyzed in the 2D well. Take care that no air bubbles remain between the strip and the gel.

3. Once the 1D BN-PAGE lane is properly fitted in the 2D well, remove the protective sticker from the bottom of the precast gel and assemble the gel/s into the electrophoresis system.
4. Fill both the cathode and anode compartments with the appropriate SDS Running Buffer.
5. Load molecular mass standards in the small extra well as in a normal SDS-PAGE.
6. The manufacturer recommends running the gels at a constant voltage of 200 V for 35 min, but running them at lower voltages (100–150 V) for longer times will result in a better separation.

For Both Manual and Precast Gels

1. Depending on the desired analysis, the gel/s can either be fixed and stained with Coomassie (Subheading 3.8) or electroblotted into a PVDF membrane, *see* **step 2** in Subheading 3.9.

3.8 Coomassie Blue Gel Staining and Unstaining

1. Release the gel from the glass or plastic plates. Cut out the top part of the gel/s (the Sample Gels for the manual cast gels or the wells for the precast gels).
2. Place the gel in a tray of an appropriate size.
3. Cover the gel with Staining and Fixing Solution. Incubate for 1 h at room temperature on an orbital or rocking shaker. Make sure the gel is not stuck to the bottom of the tray to ensure homogenous staining.
4. Replace the Staining Solution with Destaining Solution, quickly rinsing the gel once with the same solution.
5. Incubate for 4 h in Destaining solution at room temperature and/or overnight at 4 °C until the OXPHOS complex bands are clearly seen. Change the solution 3–4 times during the destaining process.

3.9 Western Blotting and Immunodetection (See Note 25)

3.9.1 Western Blotting of Native 1D BN-PAGE

1. Activate the cut PVDF membrane (7.5 × 10 cm) by soaking it in methanol for 2 s and washing it for 5 min with ultrapure water.
2. Soak the activated membrane and the gel in 1D Transfer Buffer (bicarbonate) for 5 min.
3. Assemble the transfer sandwich with the briefly soaked sponge, two pieces of 8.5 × 11 cm Whatman paper, activated PVDF membrane, gel, two pieces of paper and sponge.
4. Fill up the transfer tank and perform electroblotting in the cold room or with external cooling at a constant current of 300 mA (which will give a voltage of approximately 60 V) for 1 h.

5. Disassemble the transfer sandwich, discard the gel and papers and rinse the membrane with 1× PBS for 1 min.
6. Proceed to immunodetection (*see* **Note 26**).

3.9.2 Western Blotting of Denaturing 2D BN-PAGE

Transfer of 2D BN-PAGE gels is performed in the same way as a regular SDS-PAGE Western blot. Follow the same steps as in Subheading 3.9.1 but use 2D Transfer Buffer (Tris-Glycine, Methanol, and SDS). Perform electroblotting at a constant voltage of 100 V for 1 h or at 20 V overnight.

3.9.3 Immunodetection of the OXPHOS Complexes in 1D and 2D BN-PAGE

For this procedure a standard Western blot protocol is used. The conditions routinely used for our applications are as follow:

1. Block the blot with 5% milk in PBS-T during 1 h at room temperature.
2. Perform three washes of 10 min each with PBS-T.
3. Incubate with the appropriately diluted primary antibody in 3% BSA overnight at 4 °C.
4. Perform three washes of 10 min each with PBS-T.
5. Incubate with the appropriately diluted HRP-conjugated secondary antibody for 1 h at room temperature.
6. Perform five washes of 10 min each with PBS-T.
7. Proceed to chemiluminescent detection following the instructions of the ECL reagent manufacturer (*see* **Note 27**).

3.10 In Gel Activity (IGA) Assays

1. Release the 1D BN-PAGE gel from the glass or plastic plates. Cut out the top part of the gel/s (wells).
2. Place the gel in a tray of appropriate size.
3. Rinse quickly with ultrapure water.
4. Cover each mini-gel with 10 ml of the IGA solution to detect the complex of interest.
5. Incubate on an orbital or rocking shaker at room temperature.
6. Complex I and complex II are the fastest to react and produce a visible signal, taking from around 10 min in samples from isolated mitochondria to around 2 h in samples from digitonin-treated cell pellets.
7. Complex IV and complex V are the slowest to react, taking several hours to produce a signal in samples from isolated mitochondria to overnight incubations in samples from digitonin-treated cells.
8. Once the signal has reached the desired intensity, remove the IGA solution and wash the gel with ultrapure water. Take a photograph or scan the gel at this point.

4 Notes

1. 10% digitonin solutions tend to precipitate, especially after freeze and thaw cycles. If this happens, Digitonin can be re-solubilized by heating this solution at 90 °C for 5 min. Make sure the solution has cooled down before adding it to the sample.
2. A convenient alternative to the manually casted gels is the use of commercial precast native 3–12% and 4–16% gradient gels available from Invitrogen.
3. Invitrogen also offers a commercial running buffer for native gels that can substitute the Anode Buffer and, together with a Coomassie Blue-containing additive, both Cathode Buffer A and B.
4. Denaturing precast SDS-PAGE gels with a 2D well and commercial buffers are also available from Invitrogen and can be used for 2D BN-PAGE.
5. Mitochondrial pellets can be kept at −80 °C before proceeding to solubilization.
6. If the yield of your mitochondrial preparation is very low in a way that resuspending it at a protein concentration of 10 mg/ml will result in an extremely low volume, samples can be resuspended at a concentration of 5 mg/ml. Maintain the proportion of detergent to protein.
7. When collecting the soluble material from membrane solubilization, after the 20,000 × *g* centrifugation, take care not to aspirate any of the pellet or it will interfere with the electrophoresis run.
8. Samples can be loaded onto the gel directly after solubilization and addition of Blue-Native Sample Buffer but they can also be stored at −80 °C before the electrophoresis. The samples can be frozen and thawed at least three times without noticeable effects in the quality.
9. Digitonin binds to cholesterol, opening pores in the cell membrane to allow the enrichment in membranous organelles as opposed to soluble cytoplasmic components. This method is much more suitable for slow-growing primary cells or when the starting material is scarce (like for example leukocytes from a blood sample). It can only be used if the OXPHOS complexes are going to be analyzed by Western blot and immunodetection or in gel activity assays, as it does not yield enough complexes to be visualized directly by Coomassie staining.

10. For primary fibroblasts the starting amount is two 100 mm dishes about 90% confluent ($\approx 2 \times 10^6$ cells) or one 100 mm dish of immortalized or tumor cells ($\approx 5 \times 10^6$ cells).
11. Digitonin-treated cell pellet samples can be kept at −80 °C before proceeding to solubilization.
12. Cell pellets after Digitonin treatment with Digitonin Solution 1 can be difficult to resuspend as a significant amount of insoluble material is formed during the process. This depends on the cell type but it is a common occurrence. Try to resuspend as thoroughly as possible, but if some insoluble material remains it will not interfere with your preparation as it will be removed in the last centrifugation step.
13. Either use 10 μl of DDM Solution (10% DDM) to obtain a final concentration of 1% for studying the individual OXPHOS complexes or use 20 μl of Digitonin Solution 2 (10% digitonin) to obtain a final concentration of 2%, if the purpose is to analyze supercomplexes.
14. Protein amounts can be measured after Digitonin treatment of the cell pellets (*see* **step 8** of Subheading 3.5) using a detergent-compatible protein quantification assay. In this case, the amount of detergent for the final solubilization can be adjusted to the amount of protein in the same way as for isolated mitochondrial fractions.
15. The 1D BN-PAGE is a linear gradient gel poured from the top, in a way that the dense solution is poured first.
16. Prior to pouring the gel, make sure there are no leakages in the system, including the gradient maker valves, the rubber tubing and the gel casting sandwich, by passing water through the whole setting. Make sure the gel sandwich is completely dry before pouring the gel.
17. It is recommendable to let the gel polymerize in the cold room but it can also be taken to room temperature to speed up the polymerization process.
18. 1D BN-PAGE gradient gels can be poured the evening before the electrophoresis. After the gel is completely polymerized, just replace the layer of water with 1× 1D Gel Buffer and cover with plastic film to avoid excessive evaporation. Keep at 4 °C until used.
19. For precast gels, the manufacturer recommends running the gels at a constant voltage of 150 V.
20. An interesting variation of the 2D BN-PAGE is to run the 1D BN-PAGE of samples solubilized with digitonin and another native 2D BN-PAGE in the presence of DDM to release the individual complexes from the supercomplexes. The native 2D

BN-PAGE is prepared in the same way as the 1D native gel (*see* Subheading 3.6) and 0.02% DDM is added to the 1D Cathode Buffer [4].

21. After a 1D native gel is run, it can be kept at 4 °C overnight before proceeding to 2D BN-PAGE. Disassemble the gel sandwich from the electrophoresis cell and without taking it out of the glass (or plastic) plates, wrap it in plastic film to avoid drying. To ensure proper hydration, it can be stored in a plastic box with a couple drops of 1× 1D Gel Buffer.
22. The lanes of a 1D gel must be cut straight and in clean way to avoid the formation of bubbles that will interfere with protein electrophoretic mobility. Wetting the scalpel or razor blade used to cut the gel helps with this task.
23. Slightly tip the casting stand while pouring the 2D Sample Gel to avoid the formation of bubbles between the 1D strip and the gel. Slowly and gradually take it back to a straight position to finish.
24. When manually casting the 2D BN-PAGE gels, a comb with a single small well can be introduced in the 2D Sample Gel to allow the loading of a molecular mass standard ladder.
25. The procedures for protein blotting onto membranes after 1D and 2D BN-PAGE and detection using antibodies are essentially the same as those used for regular SDS-PAGE. Standard methods and protocols for these procedures can be obtained from multiple sources. In this chapter, we describe only specific details optimized for our applications.
26. Some primary antibodies give a faint signal or no signal at all in 1D BN-PAGE Western blot. Every antibody that works in SDS-PAGE must also work in 2D BN-PAGE. Table 5 provides a list of the antibodies commonly used to detect each one of the human and mouse OXPHOS complexes in 1D BN-PAGE and Western blotting.
27. In some cases, as in the examples shown in Figs. 2a and 3b, a proportion of supercomplex species can remain after solubilization with medium-low concentrations of DDM.

Acknowledgements

We are grateful to Dr. José L. Capablo (Neurology Department, Miguel Servet University Hospital, Zaragoza, Spain) and Robert D.S. Pitceathly (MRC Centre for Neuromuscular Diseases, UCL Institute of Neurology and National Hospital for Neurology and Neurosurgery, London, UK) for providing pathological human samples. Our research was funded by Core Grant from the MRC (Grant MC_UU_00015/5), ERC Advanced Grant FP7-322424

Table 5
Antibodies for detection of OXPHOS complexes in Western blots of 1D BN-PAGE

Complex	Target subunit	Clonality	Supplier	Catalog number	Dilution
I	NDUFB6 NDUFB8 NDUFS3	Mouse monoclonal Mouse monoclonal Mouse monoclonal	Abcam Abcam Abcam	ab110244 ab110242 ab110246	1:1000 1:1000 1:1000
II	SDHB	Mouse monoclonal	Abcam	ab14714	1:1000
III	UQCRC1 UQCRC2 UQCRFS1	Mouse monoclonal Mouse monoclonal Mouse monoclonal	Abcam Abcam Abcam	ab110252 ab14745 ab14746	1:1000 1:1000 1:1000
IV	MT-CO1	Mouse monoclonal	Abcam	ab14705	1:1000
V	ATP5A	Mouse monoclonal	Abcam	ab110273	1:1000

and NRJ-Institut de France Grant to M.Z.; and by a "Miguel Servet" Grant (CP09/00156) from the Instituto de Salud Carlos III (Ministerio de Economía y Competitividad), "Marie Curie" European Reintegration Grant (PERG04-GA-2008-239372) and Association Française contre les Myopathies Trampoline Grant (AFM 14921) and Research Grant (AFM 16086) to E.F.-V.

References

1. Schagger H, von Jagow G (1991) Blue native electrophoresis for isolation of membrane protein complexes in enzymatically active form. Anal Biochem 199(2):223–231
2. Schagger H (1995) Native electrophoresis for isolation of mitochondrial oxidative phosphorylation protein complexes. Methods Enzymol 260:190–202
3. Schagger H (1996) Electrophoretic techniques for isolation and quantification of oxidative phosphorylation complexes from human tissues. Methods Enzymol 264:555–566
4. Wittig I, Braun HP, Schagger H (2006) Blue native PAGE. Nat Protoc 1(1):418–428
5. Eubel H, Braun HP, Millar AH (2005) Blue-native PAGE in plants: a tool in analysis of protein-protein interactions. Plant Methods 1 (1):11. https://doi.org/10.1186/1746-4811-1-11
6. Klement P, Nijtmans LG, Van den Bogert C, Houstek J (1995) Analysis of oxidative phosphorylation complexes in cultured human fibroblasts and amniocytes by blue-native-electrophoresis using mitoplasts isolated with the help of digitonin. Anal Biochem 231 (1):218–224. https://doi.org/10.1006/abio.1995.1523
7. Nijtmans LG, Henderson NS, Holt IJ (2002) Blue native electrophoresis to study mitochondrial and other protein complexes. Methods 26 (4):327–334
8. Calvaruso MA, Smeitink J, Nijtmans L (2008) Electrophoresis techniques to investigate defects in oxidative phosphorylation. Methods 46(4):281–287
9. Zerbetto E, Vergani L, Dabbeni-Sala F (1997) Quantification of muscle mitochondrial oxidative phosphorylation enzymes via histochemical staining of blue native polyacrylamide gels. Electrophoresis 18(11):2059–2064. https://doi.org/10.1002/elps.1150181131
10. Fernandez-Silva P, Acin-Perez R, Fernandez-Vizarra E, Perez-Martos A, Enriquez JA (2007) In vivo and in organello analyses of mitochondrial translation. Methods Cell Biol 80:571–588
11. McKenzie M, Lazarou M, Ryan MT (2009) Chapter 18. Analysis of respiratory chain complex assembly with radiolabeled nuclear- and mitochondrial-encoded subunits. Methods Enzymol 456:321–339. S0076-6879(08) 04418-2
12. Fernández-Vizarra E, Ferrín G, Pérez-Martos A, Fernández-Silva P, Zeviani M,

Enríquez JA (2010) Isolation of mitochondria for biogenetical studies: an update. Mitochondrion 10(3):253–262

13. McKenzie M, Lazarou M, Thorburn DR, Ryan MT (2006) Mitochondrial respiratory chain supercomplexes are destabilized in Barth Syndrome patients. J Mol Biol 361(3):462–469
14. McKenzie M, Lazarou M, Thorburn DR, Ryan MT (2007) Analysis of mitochondrial subunit assembly into respiratory chain complexes using blue native polyacrylamide gel electrophoresis. Anal Biochem 364(2):128–137
15. Schagger H (2002) Respiratory chain supercomplexes of mitochondria and bacteria. Biochim Biophys Acta 1555(1–3):154–159
16. Acin-Perez R, Fernandez-Silva P, Peleato ML, Perez-Martos A, Enriquez JA (2008) Respiratory active mitochondrial supercomplexes. Mol Cell 32(4):529–539
17. Bratic A, Wredenberg A, Gronke S, Stewart JB, Mourier A, Ruzzenente B, Kukat C, Wibom R, Habermann B, Partridge L, Larsson NG (2011) The bicoid stability factor controls polyadenylation and expression of specific mitochondrial mRNAs in Drosophila melanogaster. PLoS Genet 7(10):e1002324. https://doi.org/10.1371/journal.pgen.1002324
18. Eubel H, Jansch L, Braun HP (2003) New insights into the respiratory chain of plant mitochondria. Supercomplexes and a unique composition of complex II. Plant Physiol 133(1):274–286
19. Cruciat CM, Hell K, Folsch H, Neupert W, Stuart RA (1999) Bcs1p, an AAA-family member, is a chaperone for the assembly of the cytochrome bc(1) complex. EMBO J 18(19):5226–5233
20. Nijtmans LG, Artal Sanz M, Bucko M, Farhoud MH, Feenstra M, Hakkaart GA, Zeviani M, Grivell LA (2001) Shy1p occurs in a high molecular weight complex and is required for efficient assembly of cytochrome c oxidase in yeast. FEBS Lett 498(1):46–51
21. Fernandez-Vizarra E, Fernandez-Silva P, Enriquez JA (2006) Isolation of mitochondria from mammalian tissues and cultured cells. In: Celis JE (ed) Cell biology: a laboratory handbook, vol 3. Elsevier-Academic, Amsterdam, pp 69–77
22. Ma YY, Zhang XL, Wu TF, Liu YP, Wang Q, Zhang Y, Song JQ, Wang YJ, Yang YL (2011) Analysis of the mitochondrial complex I–V enzyme activities of peripheral leukocytes in oxidative phosphorylation disorders. J Child Neurol 26(8):974–979. 0883073811399905
23. Schagger H (2006) Tricine-SDS-PAGE. Nat Protoc 1(1):16–22
24. Ghezzi D, Arzuffi P, Zordan M, Da Re C, Lamperti C, Benna C, D'Adamo P, Diodato D, Costa R, Mariotti C, Uziel G, Smiderle C, Zeviani M (2011) Mutations in TTC19 cause mitochondrial complex III deficiency and neurological impairment in humans and flies. Nat Genet 43(3):259–263. ng.761
25. Bottani E, Cerutti R, Harbour ME, Ravaglia S, Dogan SA, Giordano C, Fearnley IM, D'Amati G, Viscomi C, Fernandez-Vizarra E, Zeviani M (2017) TTC19 plays a husbandry role on UQCRFS1 turnover in the biogenesis of mitochondrial respiratory complex III. Mol Cell 67(1):96–105.e104. https://doi.org/10.1016/j.molcel.2017.06.001
26. Tiranti V, Corona P, Greco M, Taanman JW, Carrara F, Lamantea E, Nijtmans L, Uziel G, Zeviani M (2000) A novel frameshift mutation of the mtDNA COIII gene leads to impaired assembly of cytochrome c oxidase in a patient affected by Leigh-like syndrome. Hum Mol Genet 9(18):2733–2742
27. Vidoni S, Harbour ME, Guerrero-Castillo S, Signes A, Ding S, Fearnley IM, Taylor RW, Tiranti V, Arnold S, Fernandez-Vizarra E, Zeviani M (2017) MR-1S interacts with PET100 and PET117 in module-based assembly of human cytochrome c oxidase. Cell Rep 18(7):1727–1738. https://doi.org/10.1016/j.celrep.2017.01.044
28. Pitceathly RD, Rahman S, Wedatilake Y, Polke JM, Cirak S, Foley AR, Sailer A, Hurles ME, Stalker J, Hargreaves I, Woodward CE, Sweeney MG, Muntoni F, Houlden H, Consortium UK, Taanman JW, Hanna MG (2013) NDUFA4 mutations underlie dysfunction of a cytochrome c oxidase subunit linked to human neurological disease. Cell Rep 3(6):1795–1805. https://doi.org/10.1016/j.celrep.2013.05.005
29. Pitceathly RDS, Taanman JW (2018) NDUFA4 (renamed COXFA4) is a cytochrome-c oxidase subunit. Trends Endocrinol Metab 29(7):452–454. https://doi.org/10.1016/j.tem.2018.03.009

Chapter 21

Identification of Putative Mitochondrial Protease Substrates

Eduard Hofsetz, Pitter F. Huesgen, and Aleksandra Trifunovic

Abstract

Mitochondrial proteases constitute a fundamental part of the organellar protein quality control system to ensure the timely removal of damaged or obsolete proteins. The analysis of proteases is often limited to the identification of bona fide substrates that are degraded in the presence and become more abundant in the absence of the respective protease. However, proteases in numerous organisms from bacteria to humans can process specific substrates to release shortened proteins with potentially altered activities. Here, we describe an adaptation of the substrate-trapping approach, as well as the N-terminal profiling protocol Terminal Amine Isotope Labeling of Substrates (TAILS) for the identification of bona fide substrates and mitochondrial proteins that undergo complete or partial proteolysis.

Key words Mitochondria, Proteases, Substrates, Proteolysis, N Termini profiling, TAILS, Substrate-trapping, Immunoprecipitations

1 Introduction

Protein homeostasis inside mitochondria highly relies on chaperones and proteases to maintain proper folding and to remove damaged proteins that might otherwise form organelle- and cell-toxic aggregates. Beside quality control, mitochondrial proteases (mitoproteases) also modulate and regulate many essential mitochondrial functions, such as trafficking, processing and activation of mitochondrial proteins, mitochondrial dynamics, mitophagy, and apoptosis. Therefore, impaired mitoprotease function is associated with various pathological conditions, including: cancer, metabolic syndromes, and neurodegenerative disorders, with at least 12 human hereditary diseases that are caused by mutations in genes encoding mitoproteases and pseudo-mitoproteases [1]. Mammalian mitochondria harbor more than 20 different proteases that are involved in protein import, processing, and degradation of over 1500 proteins within the mitochondrial proteome [1, 2].

Michal Minczuk and Joanna Rorbach (eds.), *Mitochondrial Gene Expression: Methods and Protocols*, Methods in Molecular Biology, vol. 2192, https://doi.org/10.1007/978-1-0716-0834-0_21,

Protein quality control within mitochondria is mainly attributed to four ATP-dependent proteases (m-AAA-, i-AAA-, LONP1-, and ClpXP protease) [3–6]. These proteases form large barrel-shaped homo- or hetero-oligomeric complexes that recognize, unfold, and subsequently translocate the substrates into the catalytic core to perform partial or complete proteolysis. While inner mitochondrial membrane proteases (m-AAA and i-AAA) participate in protein surveillance as well as proteolytic processing under certain conditions [7, 8], until recently, mitochondrial matrix proteases (LONP1 and ClpXP) were generally viewed as quality control proteases that completely degrade proteins that differ widely in stability and length [9, 10]. However, we recently demonstrated that CLPP is essential for the controlled proteolysis of ERAL1 needed for the maturation of mitoribosomes [9]. In bacteria, ClpXP also regulates controlled proteolysis and in specific cases can perform specific processing, as shown for *Caulobacter crescentus* DnaX subunits that exist as two distinct forms, a full-length τ form and a shorter γ form generated through partial processing by ClpXP [11]. Furthermore, a new study reported that LONP1 protease, beside taking care of misfolded and aggregated proteins, is very important for the processing of import peptides of a subset of mitochondrial matrix proteins [12]. Therefore, it became clear that we just started unraveling the importance and the extent of the involvement of mitochondrial matrix proteases in controlled, partial or full proteolysis.

AAA^+ protease substrates can be identified by various approaches. Generally, bona fide substrate levels increase in absence of the protease while their transcript levels remain unaltered. A combined "omics" approach of proteomic and RNA-seq analysis of any protease proficient/deficient system can generate valuable substrate candidates, however, further validation is inevitable. Co-immunoprecipitations with the protease of interest is a common method to identify interacting proteins. However, protease-substrate interactions are short-lived by nature and can last only a few seconds in vitro [13]. To overcome this limitation, substrates are "trapped" within the protease by mutating either the Walker B motif in the ATPase domain or a catalytical residue within the protease chamber [9, 14]. These mutations prolong the interaction and greatly increase the chances to co-purify substrates during immunoprecipitations. Since the mutation of catalytical residues is not limited to AAA^+ proteases we will describe how substrates of mitochondrial proteases can be identified with catalytically inactive proteases in the first part of the protocol.

Most proteins in the mitochondrial matrix are imported via a positively charged N-terminal mitochondrial targeting signal (MTS) that is cleaved off by the mitochondrial processing peptidase (MPP) complex [15, 16]. Some proteins undergo further processing by additional proteases before the mature protein is released

[17]. The N-terminus of mature proteins is classified as the expected N terminus that can be predicted with high precision by bioinformatic tools such as Mitoprot or MitoFates. All other N termini further within the proteins are thus considered unexpected. While cytosolic proteins with unexpected N termini can be the result of alternative translation initiation sites, this process can be largely excluded for mitochondrial proteins with an N-terminal MTS.

Recently, the analysis of substrate processing by proteases was recognized as a further post-translational modification to regulate protein function [18, 19]. Several methods for selective enrichment and analysis of protein N- and C termini have been developed (Niedermaier and Huesgen, Biochim Biophys Acta, 2018, in press). Among these, N termini enrichment by negative selection using the Terminal Amine Isotope Labeling of Substrates (TAILS) has become one of the most widely used approaches. Detailed TAILS protocols are already available and we strongly encourage the reader to refer to them for fundamental aspects of this method [20–22]. Therefore, in the second part of this protocol we will describe the application of TAILS for the characterization of mitochondrial proteases and their proteolytic footprints, as well as to identify new substrates and cleavage sites.

Both substrate-trapping and N termini enrichment protocols can be used to study mitochondrial proteases and their substrates in a cell culture-based model or in vivo. To provide the reader with a suitable starting protocol, we use mouse embryonic fibroblasts (MEFs) and heart tissue as examples for the respective protocols (*see* Fig. 1).

2 Materials

2.1 Equipment

1. Benchtop centrifuge.
2. Homogenizing potter or dounce equipment.
3. Refrigerator at −80 and −20 °C.
4. Magnetic Rack for 1.5 mL reaction tubes.
5. Gel electrophoresis equipment.
6. Cell Culture equipment.
7. Temperature controlled incubation shaker.
8. Mass spectrometry system.

2.2 Reagents and Consumables

1. Chemically resistant 1.5, 15, and 50 mL tubes and pipette tips.
2. Double-distilled water.
3. Magnetic beads (e.g., Anti-FLAG® M2 Magnetic Beads; Sigma).

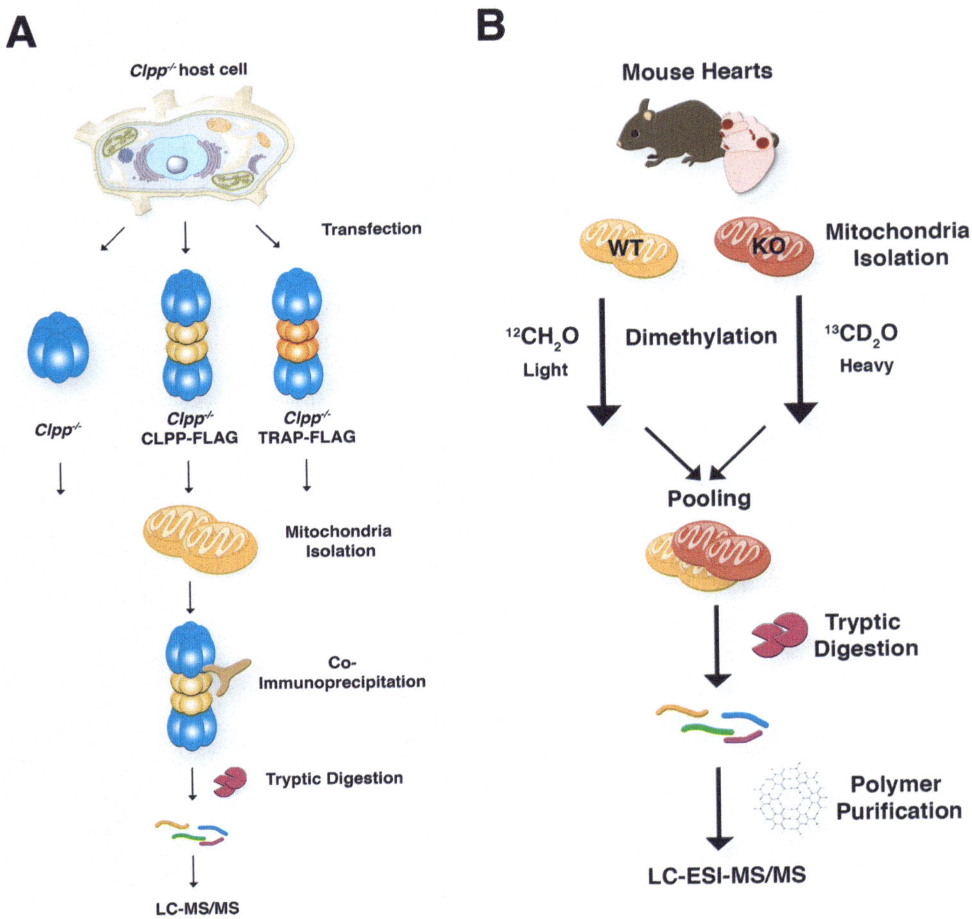

Fig. 1 Mitochondrial protease characterization via substrate-trapping and N-terminal profiling. (**a**) Protocol outline for the three-armed analysis of ClpXP substrates in MEFs. KO cells are transfected with one of the three constructs, and mitochondria are isolated from each condition. Mitochondria are further lysed and CLPP-interacting proteins are co-immunoprecipitated using anti-FLAG magnetic beads. Elutions undergo tryptic digestion and mass spectrometry analysis. (**b**) Protocol outline for N-terminal profiling of mitochondrial proteins. Heart mitochondria are isolated from protease proficient (WT) and deficient (KO) mice and N termini are differentially labeled with light and heavy formaldehyde, respectively. Samples are pooled and digested with trypsin. Tryptic N termini are removed via polymer-purification and dimethylated peptides are prepared for mass spectrometry analysis

4. Phosphate Buffered Saline (PBS).
5. Mannitol.
6. Sucrose.
7. TES.
8. Tween-20.
9. KCl.
10. EDTA.

11. 6 M GuaHCl solution.
12. Bicinchoninic acid (BCA) or equivalent protein assay.
13. Liquid Nitrogen.
14. Methanol (MeOH).
15. Chloroform ($CHCl_3$).
16. 1 M 4-(2-hydroxyethyl)-1-piperazineethanesulfonic acid (HEPES) pH 7.5.
17. 1 M Dithiothreitol (DTT).
18. 0.5 M Iodoacetamide (IAA).
19. 250 mM Chloroacetamide (CAA).
20. 2 M Formaldehyde (CH_2O; $^{13}CD_2O$; $^{12}CD_2O$).
21. Deuterium oxide (D_2O).
22. 1 M Sodium cyanoborohydride ($NaBH_3CN$; $NaBD_3CN$) in 5 M NaOH.
23. 100% Formic acid (FA).
24. 1 M Tris–HCl pH 6.8.
25. 5 M NaOH.
26. Trypsin.
27. Lys-C protease.
28. HPG-ALD II polymer solution.
29. 7 kDa MW cut-off dialysis membrane.
30. pH test strips.
31. 10 kDa MW cut-off dialysis membrane.
32. C18 double layered stage tips.
33. Acetonitrile (ACN).
34. Solutions for silver staining of polyacrylamide gel.

2.3 Buffers

1. Mitochondria Isolation Buffers of choice as described in [23] e.g.,:

   Mitochondria Isolation Buffers for mouse embryonic fibroblasts (MEFs):

   MIB1 (20 mM HEPES, 220 mM Mannitol, 70 mM Sucrose, 1 mM EDTA 0.2% BSA, pH 7.6).

   MIB2 (20 mM HEPES, 220 mM Mannitol, 70 mM Sucrose, 1 mM EDTA, pH 7.6).

   Mitochondria Isolation Buffers for heart tissue:

   MIB3 (100 mM sucrose, 50 mM KCl, 20 mM TES, 1 mM EDTA, 0.2% BSA, pH 7.2).

   MIB4 (100 mM sucrose, 50 mM KCl, 20 mM TES, 1 mM EDTA, pH 7.2).

2. IP Lysis Buffer (e.g., Pierce™ IP Lysis Buffer; Thermo).
3. IP Washing buffer (IP Lysis buffer + 0.08% Tween-20).
4. IP Elution Buffer (e.g., 0.1 M Glycine pH 2.5).

3 Methods

Substrate-Trapping of Mitochondrial Proteases: *Substrate identification via "trapping" is a straightforward approach, however, certain considerations must be met carefully to obtain optimal results. If possible, the protocol should be performed in protease-deficient (KO) cell systems (see* **Note 1***). Transfections can be performed with any established protocol that suits the desired cell culture and that can be scaled up to acquire sufficient material (see* **Note 2***).*

3.1 Generation of Necessary Expression Constructs

To discriminate between interacting proteins, such as adaptor proteins, and protease substrates, a three-armed analysis must be performed. The analysis includes:

A: Negative control (KO background cells)

B: Active protease expression (in KO background cells)—WT

C: Inactive protease expression (in KO background cells)—TRAP

Proteins that are enriched in C over A and B represent putative substrate candidates, whereas proteins that are enriched in B and C over A include interacting proteins that aren't necessarily substrates (*see* **Note 3**).

If the catalytical residues of protease of interests are not described, a sequence comparison with bacterial homologues can be of help with the generation of inactive constructs. Here, we will use ClpXP as a protocol example (*see* Fig. 1a) that was additionally fused to a C-terminal 2×FLAG tag [9].

3.2 Transfection and Mitochondrial Isolations

Transfections can be performed with any setup available if sufficient amounts of mitochondria can be obtained afterward. Mitochondrial isolation protocols depend on the cell type and we provide a short protocol for mitochondrial isolation from MEFs. If in vivo approaches are preferred, we describe a short protocol for mitochondrial isolation from mouse heart tissue in Subheading 3.7. More stringent purification protocols via sucrose or Percoll gradients can be considered to reduce non-mitochondrial contaminations within the samples but will greatly increase the required material and procedure time and is thus not recommended here.

Example for mitochondrial isolation from MEFs:

1. Detach cells from plates (total area should be at least 350 cm^2).
2. Centrifuge at 800 × *g* for 5 min at 4 °C.
3. Remove supernatant and wash cells with ice-cold PBS.

4. Repeat centrifugation from **step 2**.
5. Resuspend cell pellet in 5 mL MIB1 and incubate for 30 min on ice.
6. Homogenize the cells using a Teflon tissue grinder at 1000 rpm until the solution is homogeneous (*see* **Note 4**).
7. Centrifuge at 800 × *g* for 5 min at 4 °C.
8. Collect supernatant (repeat homogenization if necessary and combine supernatants).
9. Centrifuge at 12,000 × *g* for 15 min at 4 °C to pellet mitochondria.
10. Remove supernatant and resuspend pellet in 1 mL MIB2.
11. Aliquot into 1.5 mL reaction tubes.
12. Centrifuge at 12,000 × *g* for 15 min at 4 °C.
13. Resuspend pellet in desired volume of MIB2 and store at −80 °C.

3.3 Co-immunoprecipitation of the Protease and Associated Substrates/Interactors

1. Lyse mitochondria in 1 mL IP Lysis buffer on ice for 45 min (Keep 5% input).
2. Centrifuge at 20,000 × *g* for 45 min.
3. Measure protein concentration and adjust for equal protein amounts/volume.
4. Add equilibrated anti-FLAG magnetic beads to the samples.

   Equilibration: (shortly before use)

   (a) Place tubes on a magnetic rack and remove storage buffer.

   (b) Wash three times with PBS.

   (c) Resuspend in IP Lysis buffer.
5. Incubate 2 h on a rotating wheel or overnight at 4 °C.
6. Place tubes on a magnetic rack and collect the unbound fraction (UB).
7. Wash beads in 1 mL IP Washing buffer.
8. Place tubes on a magnetic rack and collect the supernatant (W_1).
9. Repeat the washing step three times and discard supernatants.
10. Elute proteins in 100 μL IP Elution Buffer and collect the supernatant (E_1).
11. Repeat elution and collect E_2.
12. Add ~10 μL 1 M Tris–HCl pH 7.5.
13. Check neutral pH with strips.
14. Freeze samples in liquid nitrogen and store at −80 °C.

3.4 SDS-PAGE and Western Blot

1. Use 5% of input, UB, W_1, E_1, and E_2 for SDS-PAGE analysis.
2. Ensure that no FLAG-tagged protein is present in UB and W_1 fraction (Adjust beads volume or washing buffer conditions if necessary).
3. Combine E_1 and E_2 if necessary for mass spectrometry.

3.5 In Solution Digestion

1. Determine protein concentration if possible.
2. Add DTT to a final concentration of 5 mM to the sample's mix and incubate at RT for 1 h.
3. Add CAA to a final concentration of 40 mM, mix, and incubate in the dark for 30 min.
4. Add Lys-C protease at an enzyme: substrate ratio of $\geq$1:75 and incubate at 25 °C for 4 h.
5. Add Trypsin at an enzyme: substrate ratio of $\geq$1:75 and incubate at 25 °C overnight.
6. Add formic acid to a final concentration of 1%.
7. Continue with stage-tip protocol according to the instructions of your proteomics facility or as described later (*see* protocol in Subheading 3.11).
8. Perform mass spectrometry analysis.

3.6 Considerations and Interpretation of the Results

Proteomic analysis of any biological sample can result in the identification of hundreds to thousands of peptides, leaving the inexperienced scientist with the task of "looking for the needle in a meadow." Careful interpretation is therefore mandatory to identify putative protease substrates. In this protocol, we described a three-armed approach with the expression of either WT-, TRAP- or no protease.

To address correct enrichments, WT and TRAP samples should be normalized toward the bait protein of the IP (e.g., protease-FLAG). This is of special importance if the expression of either construct is detrimental for the cell and results in different expression levels.

Once normalized, the negative control must be subtracted from both samples. This step can be performed manually, to avoid losing potential candidates. However, substrate candidates that are abundant in the negative control should be validated more carefully.

Combining the trapping approach with other methods, such as mitochondrial proteome quantification or N termini profiling can be helpful in the generation of a putative protease substrates list.

N-Terminal Profiling of the Mitochondrial Proteome: *To identify the N-terminal cleavage signature of a mitochondrial protease, proficient and deficient cells for the protease of interest are necessary.*

These can be knockout cells (or tissues), as well as gene knockdowns, if they are sufficiently effective. The TAILS protocol allows for duplex or triplex labeling, thus hyperactive conditions (such as constitutive protease expressions) can be added to the experimental setup. For simplicity, we will only describe the protocol for proficient (WT) and deficient (KO) duplex labeling (see *Fig. 1b*). *We recommend using at least five biological replicates for each condition to ensure sufficient statistical power.*

3.7 Mitochondrial Isolation

Mitochondrial protease and substrate abundance can be very low when whole cell lysates are used to perform the experiments. We thus strongly advise using crude mitochondrial isolations of the desired background. Protocols for mitochondrial isolation from diverse tissues and cell cultures are available and we recommend following them. If no protocol is available for the desired cell/tissue, a detailed starting protocol can be found here [23]. All samples should be processed in parallel if possible.

Example for mitochondria isolation from mouse heart tissue:

1. Harvest the mouse heart and remove containing blood.
2. Homogenize the tissue in 5 mL MIB3 using a Teflon tissue grinder at 1000 rpm until the solution is homogeneous (*see* **Note 4**).
3. Transfer the solution into a 50 mL tube and fill up to 20 mL with MIB3.
4. Centrifuge for 5 min at 8500 × *g* (4 °C).
5. Discard supernatant with floating fat (*see* **Note 5**).
6. Resuspend the pellet in 30 mL MIB3 by vigorous shaking.
7. Centrifuge for 5 min at 800 × *g* (4 °C).
8. Transfer the supernatant into a new 50 mL tube and store on ice.
9. Repetition of **steps 5–7** can increase mitochondrial recovery.
10. Combine supernatants from **step 8**.
11. Centrifuge for 5 min at 8500 × *g* (4 °C) to pellet mitochondria.
12. Resuspend the mitochondrial pellet in 50–200 μL MIB4 (*see* **Note 6**).

3.8 Protein Purification

1. Resuspend the mitochondrial pellets in 6 M GuaHCl solution. In case of nucleic acid contamination, shear the samples with a 22 G needle syringe or via sonication.
2. Measure protein concentration with a BCA assay and adjust samples to equal concentrations and volume. Total protein amount of mitochondrial samples should exceed >1 mg (samples can be shock-frozen in liquid nitrogen and stored at −80 °C at this point).

3. Precipitate proteins with MeOH/$CHCl_3$ in chemically stable tubes.
4. Add 4× starting volume MeOH (−20 °C) and mix.
5. Add 2× starting volume $CHCl_3$ (−20 °C) and mix.
6. Add 3× starting volume water (4 °C) and mix.
7. Centrifuge for 5 min at >10,000 × *g* (4 °C).
8. Remove the upper and lower phases, leaving the protein pellet from the interphase.
9. Add 3× starting volume MeOH (−20 °C) and mix.
10. Wash pellet 2–3× with 1 mL MeOH (−20 °C) by vortexing to remove any $CHCl_3$.
11. Air dry pellets carefully in a fume hood until a light shimmer of liquid remains.
12. Dissolve pellets in 1 mL 2 M GuaHCl, 100 mM HEPES.
13. Determine protein concentration with BCA assay (*see* **Note 7**).

3.9 TAILS N Termini Enrichment

1. Confirm a sample pH of 7–8 with pH strips, adjust with 1 M HCl or 1 M NaOH if necessary.
2. Add DTT to 10 mM final concentration and incubate at 37 °C for 30 min.
3. Cool samples to room temperature.
4. Add IAA to 30 mM final concentration and incubate for 30 min at RT in the dark.
5. Quench alkylation by adding DTT to a final concentration of 25 mM and incubate for 15 min at RT.
6. Add formaldehyde and cyanoborohydride to 20 mM final concentration.
   WT: light formaldehyde ($^{12}CH_2O$).
   KO: heavy formaldehyde ($^{13}CD_2O$) (*see* **Note 8**).
7. Adjust pH to 6–7 with formic acid (e.g., to 0.2% final) if necessary.
8. Incubate overnight at 37 °C.
9. Add additional 20 mM formaldehyde and cyanoborohydride (now both 40 mM).
10. Incubate 2 h at 37 °C for complete labeling.
11. Quench labeling by adding Tris–HCl pH 6.8 to 100 mM final concentration.
12. Adjust pH to 6–7 with formic acid if necessary.
13. Save approximately 5 μg for quality control (A).
14. Combine equal protein amounts of each one WT and KO sample (*see* **Note 9**).

15. Precipitate proteins with MeOH/$CHCl_3$ in chemically stable tubes.
16. Resuspend pellet in 60 μL 50 mM NaOH.
17. Add 480 μL H_2O and HEPES pH 7.5 to 100 mM final concentration.
18. Confirm a sample pH of 7.5–8 with pH strips, adjust the pH if necessary.
19. Measure protein concentration with BCA (optional but recommended).
20. Add trypsin at a ratio of 1:100 to the protein and gently invert the sample.
21. Incubate overnight at 37 °C.
22. Dialyze the HPG-ALD II polymer solution with a 7 kDa MW cut-off membrane overnight against water.
23. Add trypsin at a ratio of 1:200 to the protein and gently invert the sample.
24. Incubate for 2 h at 37 °C.
25. Save 10% (60 μL) after digestion as "preTAILS" sample control (B).
26. Adjust all preTAILS to e.g., 1 μg/μL.
27. Add HPG-ALD II polymer to the protein samples at a ratio of 5:1 (w/w).
28. Add cyanoborohydride to 20 mM final concentration.
29. Adjust pH to 6–7 with formic acid (e.g., to 0.05% final) if necessary.
30. Incubate overnight at 37 °C.
31. Save a small aliquot of ~2 μg peptides for quality control gel (C).
32. Quench the reaction by adding Tris–HCl pH 6.8 to 100 mM final concentration.
33. Incubate at 37 °C for 30 min.

3.10 Unbound Peptide (TAILS) Recovery

1. Wash 10 kDa MW cut-off 0.5 mL spin filter devices with 400 μL 100 mM NaOH.
2. Centrifuge at 10,000 × *g* for 10 min.
3. Add 400 μL H_2O.
4. Centrifuge at 10,000 × *g* for 10 min.
5. Equilibrate with 400 μL 100 mM Tris–HCl pH 6.8.
6. Centrifuge at 10,000 × *g* for 10 min.
7. Load ≤400 μL TAILS.
8. Centrifuge at 10,000 × *g* for 15 min.

9. Retain Flow-through in new tubes and repeat for volumes ≥400 μL.
10. Wash spin filters with 400 μL 100 mM Tris–HCl pH 6.8.
11. Centrifuge at 10,000 × *g* for 15 min.
12. Combine Flow-through fractions =>**TAILS** (D).

3.11 Desalt 10 μg PreTAILS and 10% (120 μL) TAILS with C18 Double Layer Stage Tips

1. Activate: 20 μL 50% ACN; 0.1% FA.
2. Wash: 40 μL 2% ACN; 0.1% FA.
3. Load sample (up to 250 μL).
4. Wash: 2× sample volume 2% ACN; 0.1% FA.
5. Empty and dry the stage tip.
6. Elute in 20 μL 50% ACN; 0.1% FA.
7. Dry for ~10 min in a speed vac.
8. Resuspend peptides in 10 μL 2% ACN; 0.1% FA.
9. Use ≥2.5 μL for LC-ESI-MS/MS analysis.

3.12 Optional: SDS-PAGE and Silver Staining

1. Prepare 12% polyacrylamide gels.
2. Load ~2 μg pre-digest (A), post-digest (preTAILS) (B), polymer-bound (C) and TAILS (D) samples in LDS buffer.
3. Run electrophoresis at constant 100 V.
4. Wash and fix the gel overnight in 40% MeOH 10% acetic acid.
5. Wash the gel in water to remove acetic acid.
6. Continue with silver staining protocol as described in [24] (*see* Fig. 2).

3.13 MS Measurement and Bioinformatic Analysis of N Termini

1. Analyze both preTAILS and TAILS samples by LC-ESI-MS/MS. Settings will depend on the instrument configuration that is available and should be discussed with an experienced operator. We usually analyze an estimated amount of 1 μg desalted peptides with the instrument settings commonly used for standard quantitative shotgun proteomics as a starting point.
2. Settings for matching spectra to peptide sequences again depend on the instrument and software used. We typically use MaxQuant version >1.6 [25] due to its ease of use and well-recognized capabilities in MS1 quantification. Typical settings are:
   (a) For preTAILS (*see* **Note 10**): Cleavage specificity of the enzyme used for proteome digestion with up to two or three missed cleavages, fixed labeling with the chosen dimethyl isotopes (*see* **Note 8**) at Lys residues, variable oxidation (+16), PSM and protein-level false discovery rate of 0.01.

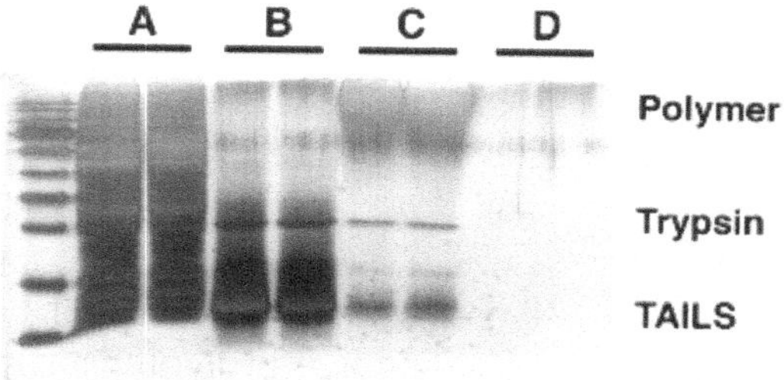

Fig. 2 Silver stained polyacrylamide gel of two heart mitochondrial samples during TAILS. (A) Dimethyl-labeled proteins. (B) Trypsin-digested proteins ("preTAILS"). (C) Free peptides and polymer-bound peptides. (D) TAILS after polymer purification. Polymer-peptides, trypsin and free peptides in the gel are indicated

(b) For TAILS: Cleavage specificity of the enzyme used during protein digestion with semi-specific specificity settings for the enzyme used for proteome digestion with variable N-terminus (*see* **Note 9**)

3. Match identified N-terminal peptides to their position in the precursor protein. This positional annotation is essential to distinguish when expected start sites form neo-N-termini generated by proteolytic processing and to predict their functional consequences. For the MaxQuant search results, this information can be found in the "peptides" output file. Such positional annotation can also be obtained using the TopFINDer functionality in the TopFIND database [26].
4. Determine significantly altered N termini, either with stringent fold change cut-offs and (preferred) appropriate statistical tests. We recommend filtering the data to retain only N termini quantified in >50% of the sample pairs, then apply a LIMMA moderated t-test [27, 28] at $p < 0.05$ and twofold change in abundance as cut-off (log2(wt/ko) >1 or <−1).

3.14 Biological Interpretation of N Terminome Data

As mentioned in the Trapping protocol, careful interpretation is crucial toward understanding the results of large datasets. In most cases, it is important to investigate the N termini on the single peptide level, not aggregated, and averaged on the protein level, even when the number of N termini can reach dozens for highly abundant proteins. N termini are usually first distinguished between "expected" termini, i.e., known and predicted N termini resulting from protein synthesis and known maturation steps such as MTS, and "unexpected" protein neo-N termini generated by proteolytic activity.

Typically, the predicted mature N terminus after the MTS is among the most abundant N-terminal peptides (expected N terminus). While expected N termini do not directly reveal cleavage sites of a protease of interest, an increased amount of expected N termini in the protease-deficient sample may point toward protease-substrate interactions. Accumulating N termini may reveal substrates that are normally degraded by the protease of interest or reflect accumulation of unprocessed precursor proteins. Comparison with quantitative proteome data derived from analysis of pre-TAILS samples or parallel label-free or SILAC based quantitative mitochondrial proteome analysis can help to distinguish between these two scenarios: Expected N termini of degradation substrates are likely to reflect overall protein amounts, whereas expected N termini of processed substrates accumulate while the overall protein amount may not change. However, it is important to consider also alternative explanations such as changes in transcription and translation.

Unexpected N termini include all N termini that match to positions within the protein sequence that are not annotated maturation sites. For mitochondrial proteins, we consider all termini starting at positions >2 amino acids after the predicted MTS as unexpected. Unexpected termini found in larger abundance in the wild type may point to cleavage sites executed by the protease of interest, whereas unexpected N termini found in higher abundance in the knockout mutant may result from compensating proteolytic activities of other proteases. N termini that deviate from the total abundance of the protein abundance are more likely to be direct substrate candidates. As mentioned earlier, many protease-generated neo-N termini scattered across the protein sequence may be observed for highly abundant proteins such as SDHA or ATP5A1 where even short-lived degradation intermediates of constitutive turnover may be abundant enough to be detected. The different N termini frequently show divergent behavior, particularly when the constitutive turnover of the protein is affected by the protease of interest (resulting in N termini with lower abundance in the mutant) and/or maintained by compensating activities (revealed by additional N termini increased in the mutant).

We recommend validating each of these candidates by other means such as Western blotting. However, the shorter the remaining peptide becomes, the more difficult it is to detect it with common available antibodies.

A third possibility to analyze the TAILS dataset is to compare the cleavage windows, i.e., the aligned cleavage sites derived from the identified sequences. These aligned sequences can reveal distinct cleavage site motifs, for example unexpected N termini that are significantly decreased in the protease-deficient sample may reveal the specificity of the protease of interest, while N termini that increase in abundance can point to activated compensating proteases. This analysis is particularly helpful to discriminate potential direct and indirect effects if the cleavage site preference of the protease of interest is known.

In general, it is important to consider that many observed effects can also be generated indirectly by altered proteolytic potential in the protease web. Although the described protocols identify strong protease substrate candidates, they lack proof of a direct protease-substrate relationship. We thus recommend employing in vitro degradation assays with reconstituted proteases and recombinant substrates as the gold standard to verify protease specificity and substrates. Recommended protocols and conditions strongly depend on the mode of action of the protease of interest and are therefore beyond the scope of this protocol.

4 Notes

1. When multimeric complexes are analyzed, the expression of catalytically inactive proteases should be performed in a KO background to guarantee the absence of any proteolytic activity by the respective protease (complex). If KO cells are not viable, a sufficiently high expression level can outcompete the endogenous active protein.
2. We recommend transfecting enough cells to obtain ~1 mg of isolated mitochondria. For cell cultures notoriously difficult to transfect, such as mouse embryonic fibroblasts (MEFs) or neural cell cultures, electroporation was a valid approach in our hands.
3. While many adaptor proteins are known for bacterial proteases, only few have been proposed for mitochondrial proteases. Any known interacting protein, such as associated ATPases can be used as quality controls.
4. Mitochondrial isolation protocols from rigid tissues such as striated muscles or hearts can include the use of proteases such as trypsin, collagenase, or subtilisin in the initial homogenizing step. If possible, proteases should be avoided at any step during mitochondrial isolations, especially if intermembrane space or outer membrane proteins are investigated as this proteolytic digest will generate new N termini before labeling that cannot easily be distinguished from endogenous N termini.
5. The removal of floating fat is especially important for tissues with high fat content such as liver or adipose tissues.
6. The mitochondrial pellet should appear yellow-brownish. If surrounding fat or blood around the mitochondria is still visible, resuspend the pellet in 1 mL MIB1, transfer into a 2 mL reaction tube and continue from **section 3.7 step 6**.
7. Typically, protein concentration of tissue mitochondria drops by 40–50% after MeOH/$CHCl_3$ precipitation.

8. For comparison of two conditions (duplex labeling), dimethylation with light ($^{12}CH_2O$) and heavy ($^{13}CD_2O$) formaldehyde isotopes and sodium cyanoborohydride are recommended, resulting in mass shifts of +28.0313 and +34.0631, respectively, for each modified amine.
9. Use equal protein amounts for each channel in WT-KO pairs. Biological replicates do not need to have equal protein amounts, although this would be preferred to obtain similar identification rates. Suitable pairs should be combined for maximal protein amount after pairing.
10. Analysis of preTAILS samples also provides a control for dimethyl labeling efficiency. Either chose no label for the control channel, or search with variable dimethyl modification of Lys residues with the chosen isotopes (*see* **Note 8**).

References

1. Quirós P, Langer T, López-Otín C (2015) New roles for mitochondrial proteases in health, ageing and disease. Nat Rev Mol Cell Biol 16:345–359. https://doi.org/10.1038/nrm3984
2. Smith A, Robinson A (2015) MitoMiner v3.1, an update on the mitochondrial proteomics database. Nucleic Acids Res 44:D1258–D1261. https://doi.org/10.1093/nar/gkv1001
3. Baker T, Sauer R (2012) ClpXP, an ATP-powered unfolding and protein-degradation machine. Biochim Biophys Acta Mol Cell Res 1823:15–28. https://doi.org/10.1016/j.bbamcr.2011.06.007
4. Gur E, Sauer R (2008) Recognition of misfolded proteins by Lon, a AAA+ protease. Genes Dev 22:2267–2277. https://doi.org/10.1101/gad.1670908
5. Koppen M, Metodiev M, Casari G, Rugarli E, Langer T (2006) Variable and tissue-specific subunit composition of mitochondrial m-AAA protease complexes linked to hereditary spastic paraplegia. Mol Cell Biol 27:758–767. https://doi.org/10.1128/mcb.01470-06
6. Graef M, Seewald G, Langer T (2007) Substrate recognition by AAA+ ATPases: distinct substrate binding modes in ATP-dependent protease Yme1 of the mitochondrial intermembrane space. Mol Cell Biol 27:2476–2485. https://doi.org/10.1128/mcb.01721-06
7. Anand R, Wai T, Baker M, Kladt N, Schauss A, Rugarli E, Langer T (2014) Thei-AAA protease YME1L and OMA1 cleave OPA1 to balance mitochondrial fusion and fission. J Cell Biol 204:919–929. https://doi.org/10.1083/jcb.201308006
8. Nolden M, Ehses S, Koppen M, Bernacchia A, Rugarli E, Langer T (2005) The m-AAA protease defective in hereditary spastic paraplegia controls ribosome assembly in mitochondria. Cell 123:277–289. https://doi.org/10.1016/j.cell.2005.08.003
9. Szczepanowska K, Maiti P, Kukat A, Hofsetz E, Nolte H, Senft K, Becker C, Ruzzenente B, Hornig-Do H, Wibom R, Wiesner R, Krüger M, Trifunovic A (2016) CLPP coordinates mitoribosomal assembly through the regulation of ERAL1 levels. EMBO J 35:2566–2583. https://doi.org/10.15252/embj.201694253
10. Matsushima Y, Goto Y, Kaguni L (2010) Mitochondrial Lon protease regulates mitochondrial DNA copy number and transcription by selective degradation of mitochondrial transcription factor A (TFAM). Proc Natl Acad Sci U S A 107:18410–18415. https://doi.org/10.1073/pnas.1008924107
11. Vass R, Chien P (2013) Critical clamp loader processing by an essential AAA+ protease in Caulobacter crescentus. Proc Natl Acad Sci U S A 110:18138–18143. https://doi.org/10.1073/pnas.1311302110
12. Zurita Rendón O, Shoubridge E (2018) LONP1 is required for maturation of a subset of mitochondrial proteins, and its loss elicits an integrated stress response. Mol Cell Biol. https://doi.org/10.1128/mcb.00412-17
13. Sen M, Maillard R, Nyquist K, Rodriguez-Aliaga P, Pressé S, Martin A, Bustamante C (2013) The ClpXP protease unfolds substrates using a constant rate of pulling but different gears. Cell 155:636–646. https://doi.org/10.1016/j.cell.2013.09.022

14. Lowth B, Kirstein-Miles J, Saiyed T, Brötz-Oesterhelt H, Morimoto R, Truscott K, Dougan D (2012) Substrate recognition and processing by a Walker B mutant of the human mitochondrial AAA+ protein CLPX. J Struct Biol 179:193–201. https://doi.org/10.1016/j.jsb.2012.06.001
15. Endo T, Mitsui S, Roise D (1995) Mitochondrial presequences can induce aggregation of unfolded proteins. FEBS Lett 359:93–96. https://doi.org/10.1016/0014-5793(95)00015-2
16. Hawlitschek G, Schneider H, Schmidt B, Tropschug M, Hartl F, Neupert W (1988) Mitochondrial protein import: identification of processing peptidase and of PEP, a processing enhancing protein. Cell 53:795–806. https://doi.org/10.1016/0092-8674(88)90096-7
17. Vögtle F, Prinz C, Kellermann J, Lottspeich F, Pfanner N, Meisinger C (2011) Mitochondrial protein turnover: role of the precursor intermediate peptidase Oct1 in protein stabilization. Mol Biol Cell 22:2135–2143. https://doi.org/10.1091/mbc.e11-02-0169
18. Rinschen M, Hoppe A, Grahammer F, Kann M, Völker L, Schurek E, Binz J, Höhne M, Demir F, Malisic M, Huber T, Kurschat C, Kizhakkedathu J, Schermer B, Huesgen P, Benzing T (2017) N-Degradomic analysis reveals a proteolytic network processing the podocyte cytoskeleton. J Am Soc Nephrol 28:2867–2878. https://doi.org/10.1681/asn.2016101119
19. Calvo S, Julien O, Clauser K, Shen H, Kamer K, Wells J, Mootha V (2017) Comparative analysis of mitochondrial N-termini from mouse, human, and yeast. Mol Cell Proteomics 16:512–523. https://doi.org/10.1074/mcp.m116.063818
20. Demir F, Niedermaier S, Kizhakkedathu JN, Huesgen PF (2017) Profiling of protein N-termini and their modifications in complex samples. Methods Mol Biol 1574:35–50
21. Lange P, Huesgen P, Nguyen K, Overall C (2014) Annotating N termini for the Human Proteome Project: N termini and N-α-acetylation status differentiate stable cleaved protein species from degradation remnants in the human erythrocyte proteome. J Proteome Res 13:2028–2044. https://doi.org/10.1021/pr401191w
22. Kleifeld O, Doucet A, Prudova A, auf dem Keller U, Gioia M, Kizhakkedathu J, Overall C (2011) Identifying and quantifying proteolytic events and the natural N terminome by terminal amine isotopic labeling of substrates. Nat Protoc 6:1578–1611. https://doi.org/10.1038/nprot.2011.382
23. Frezza C, Cipolat S, Scorrano L (2007) Organelle isolation: functional mitochondria from mouse liver, muscle and cultured filroblasts. Nat Protoc 2:287–295. https://doi.org/10.1038/nprot.2006.478
24. Kumar G (2018) Principle and method of silver staining of proteins separated by sodium dodecyl sulfate-polyacrylamide gel electrophoresis. Methods Mol Biol 1853:231–236
25. Tyanova S, Temu T, Cox J (2016) The MaxQuant computational platform for mass spectrometry-based shotgun proteomics. Nat Protoc 11:2301–2319. https://doi.org/10.1038/nprot.2016.136
26. Fortelny N, Yang S, Pavlidis P, Lange P, Overall C (2014) Proteome TopFIND 3.0 with TopFINDer and PathFINDer: database and analysis tools for the association of protein termini to pre- and post-translational events. Nucleic Acids Res 43:D290–D297. https://doi.org/10.1093/nar/gku1012
27. Gomez-Auli A, Hillebrand L, Biniossek M, Peters C, Reinheckel T, Schilling O (2016) Impact of cathepsin B on the interstitial fluid proteome of murine breast cancers. Biochimie 122:88–98. https://doi.org/10.1016/j.biochi.2015.10.009
28. Ritchie M, Diyagama D, Neilson J, van Laar R, Dobrovic A, Holloway A, Smyth G (2006) Journal search results - Cite This For Me. BMC Bioinformatics 7:261. https://doi.org/10.1186/1471-2105-7-261

Index

A

B

C

D

E

F

G

H

I

Michal Minczuk and Joanna Rorbach (eds.), *Mitochondrial Gene Expression: Methods and Protocols*, Methods in Molecular Biology, vol. 2192, https://doi.org/10.1007/978-1-0716-0834-0,

K

L

M

N

O

P

The manufacturer's authorised representative in the EU is Springer Nature Customer Service Centre GmbH, Europaplatz 3, 69115 Heidelberg, Germany. If you have any concerns regarding our products, please contact ProductSafety@springernature.com

Printed and bound by CPI Group (UK) Ltd, Croydon, CR0 4YY
23/09/2026
02221546-0019